THE ROLE *of* BETA RECEPTOR AGONIST THERAPY *in* ASTHMA MORTALITY

THE ROLE *of* BETA RECEPTOR AGONIST THERAPY *in* ASTHMA MORTALITY

Edited by
Richard Beasley
Neil E. Pearce

CRC Press
Boca Raton Ann Arbor London Tokyo

Library of Congress Cataloging-in-Publication Data

The Role of beta receptor agonist therapy in asthma mortality /
edited by Richard Beasley, Neil E. Pearce.
p. cm.
Includes bibliographical references and index.
ISBN 0-8493-6761-1 (acid-free paper)
1. Asthma--Chemotherapy--Complications. 2. Adrenergic beta agonists--Side effects. 3. Asthma--Mortality. 4. Asthma--mortality. I. Beasley, Richard. II. Pearce, Neil.
[DNLM: 1. Adrenergic Beta Receptor Agonists--pharmacology. 2. Adrenergic Beta Receptor Agonists--therapeutic use. 3. Asthma--drug therapy. WF 553 R7442 1993]
RC591.R65 1993
616.2′38061--dc20
DNLM/DLC
for Library of Congress 92-48346
CIP

Direct all inquiries to CRC Press, Inc., 2000 Corporate Blvd., N.W., Boca Raton, Florida 33431.

International Standard Book Number 0-8493-6761-1

Library of Congress Card Number 92-48346

Printed in the United States of America 1 2 3 4 5 6 7 8 9 0

Printed on acid-free paper

FOREWORD

I feel honoured to have been invited to introduce this excellent monograph which surveys and analyzes the nature, actions, and unwanted actions of one of the most widely used class of drugs in respiratory medicine — the beta agonists.

Until recently there were few reasons to question their basic safety; after all their actions are only part of the wider actions of adrenaline. Further, following the introduction of corticosteroids and cromoglycate, the emphasis on reversible airflow obstruction as the essence of asthma was overtaken by the concept of bronchial inflammation. Indeed, deaths from asthma are frequently attributed to inadequate use of corticosteroids, and protocols of therapy have been based on this assumption.

The introduction of the new, powerful, $beta_2$ agonist, fenoterol, together with the relatively high (though still low) death rate from asthma in New Zealand, led to revival of suspicion that these drugs might be responsible. The problems of investigating such a suspicion were formidable: a disorder with no agreed operational definition, high prevalence, and a wide range of severity; a drug with few side effects other than the suspicion of a very low incidence of death; the usual treatment regimen included self-administration; there was often poor documentation of the events preceding the death. Further, confirmation of these suspicions would have implications not only for the treatment of this common disorder, but for the drug regulatory authorities and the pharmaceutical industry itself.

This monograph examines rigorously the many facets of this problem, including the pharmacology of beta agonists, their clinical usage, epidemiological aspects of asthma and its treatment, and epidemiological methodology. While an immediate contribution will be to the clinical management of asthma, on which it is likely to have a profound effect, its ultimate influence will be far wider. By addressing a situation that has many parallels in medicine, it has contributed to their better understanding and their solution.

As Popper has made clear, nothing in science is capable of proof, only disproof. Beasley, Pearce, and colleagues have marshalled the evidence to incriminate fenoterol in the increased death rate from asthma in New Zealand in the 1970s, as well as reviewing evidence linking another beta agonist (isoprenaline forte) to the epidemics of the 1960s, and raising more general questions about the efficacy and safety of this class of drug. The burden now lies with those who would disprove this hypothesis. Unless or until this happens, no longer will clinicians be able to prescribe these drugs as if their only effect is their undoubted symptomatic benefit.

The editors and contributors, in tackling a specific problem, have illuminated a much wider area of medicine from which the full benefits are yet to be derived. They have earned our congratulations and our thanks.

J. B. Howell
Emeritus Professor of Medicine

PREFACE

Asthma is one of the few treatable diseases in which there has been a widespread increase in reported morbidity and mortality over recent decades. These adverse trends have occurred despite major increases in our knowledge and understanding of the pathophysiology of the disease, improved diagnostic awareness, and the availability of more potent and specific forms of therapy. In this context, it is important to consider whether some aspects of our current management may be adversely affecting the natural history of the disease.

In this book, the possible role of beta-agonist therapy in asthma mortality is critically reviewed. An attempt has been made to produce a comprehensive overview of existing knowledge, bringing together relevant information that has been published in many different journals, covering a wide range of disciplines. This multidisciplinary approach spans the fields of epidemiology, pharmacology, clinical medicine, and public health. It includes an historical perspective and sections on experimental and epidemiological methods for examining the possible relationship between beta-agonist therapy and asthma mortality. The authors of the chapters in this book are internationally recognized experts in their fields, and have all made major contributions to our understanding of these issues.

Although this has been a controversial area, it is pleasing that the controversy has led to further research, the results of which have improved our understanding of beta-agonist therapy, and the way in which it should be used in the management of asthma. However, as highlighted in this book, there are still many unanswered questions that will need to be resolved through further research.

It is always difficult to decide when it is the right time to prepare such a book. However, we felt that it was important that existing scientific evidence is reviewed at this stage, in this rapidly expanding field. Unfortunately, a review of the possible role of the many nonpharmacological factors that may have contributed to the increase in prevalence, morbidity, and mortality from asthma was beyond the scope of this book. Likewise, recommendations for the therapeutic use of beta-agonist drug treatment are not addressed in this book, but they are well covered in many other texts on asthma.

We hope that this book will be of interest to clinicians, pharmacologists, epidemiologists, and all those interested in addressing the problems of increasing asthma morbidity and mortality.

Richard Beasley, M.D.

Neil Pearce, Ph.D.

THE EDITORS

Richard Beasley, M.D., is Professor of Medicine at the Wellington School of Medicine, University of Otago Medical School and Consultant Physician at Wellington Hospital, Wellington, New Zealand.

Dr. Beasley graduated in 1979 from the University of Otago Medical School with an MBChB degree and became a fellow of the Royal Australasian College of Physicians in 1985. He then took up a New Zealand Medical Research Council-Wellcome Trust Research Fellowship at the University of Southampton, United Kingdom, before returning to the Wellington School of Medicine in 1987 and was appointed to the Chair of Medicine in 1993. He was awarded his M.D. degree from the University of Southampton in 1990, and returned to that institution as a Medical Research Council (U.K.) Visiting Senior Scientist in 1992.

Dr. Beasley is a member of the American Thoracic Society, British Thoracic Society, European Respiratory Society, Thoracic Society of Australia and New Zealand, and the Collegium Internationale Allergologicum. He is President of the Australian Chapter of the International Association of Asthmology and has served on a number of advisory committees including the Expert Panel of the FDA Pulmonary-Allergy Drugs Advisory Committee.

Dr. Beasley is author of more than one hundred papers in the medical literature. His current major research interests in the field of asthma are related to epidemiology, pharmacology, and management.

Neil Pearce, Ph.D., is a Senior Research Fellow in the Department of Medicine in the Wellington School of Medicine. Dr. Pearce obtained his training at the Wellington School of Medicine, completing his Ph.D. degree in epidemiology in 1985. From 1985 to 1987 he carried out epidemiological research in the Department of Epidemiology, University of North Carolina at Chapel Hill, funded by an Overseas Research Fellowship of the Health Research Council of New Zealand.

Since 1987 he has primarily carried out teaching and research in epidemiology at the Wellington School of Medicine, but during 1992 to 1993 he is based at the International Agency for Research on Cancer in Lyon, France, was recipient of a Visiting Scientist Award. He is currently engaged in full-time epidemiological research in the Wellington School of Medicine with funding from the Health Research Council of New Zealand; his asthma epidemiology research is conducted as a member of the Wellington Asthma Research Group (directed by Drs. Beasley, Burgess, Crane, and Pearce), which is funded by a Programme Grant from the Health Research Council of New Zealand.

Dr. Pearce is a member of the Australasian Epidemiology Association, the International Epidemiology Association, the International Society for Pharmacoepidemiology, the Society for Epidemiologic Research, and the Thoracic Society of Australia and New Zealand. Dr. Pearce has co-authored a textbook of occupational epidemiology, and more than one hundred papers. His current major research interests include asthma epidemiology, occupational and environmental epidemiology, cancer epidemiology, and epidemiological methods.

CONTRIBUTORS

Peter Barnes, M.A., D.M., D.Sc., F.R.C.P.
Professor
Department of Thoracic Medicine
National Heart and Lung Institute
London, England

Richard Beasley, M.B.Ch.B., F.R.A.C.P., M.D.
Professor
Department of Medicine
Wellington School of Medicine
Wellington, New Zealand

Carl D. Burgess, M.B.Ch.B., M.D., M.R.C.P., F.R.A.C.P.
Senior Lecturer
Department of Medicine
Wellington School of Medicine
Wellington, New Zealand

K. Fan Chung, M.D., F.R.C.P.
Senior Lecturer
Department of Thoracic Medicine
National Heart and Lung Institute
London, England

Julian Crane, M.B., B.S., M.R.C.P., F.R.A.C.P.
Senior Lecturer
Department of Medicine
Wellington School of Medicine
Wellington, New Zealand

J. Mark Elwood, M.D., D.Sc., F.R.C.P.(C)
Director
Hugh Adam Cancer Epidemiology Unit
and
Professor
Department of Preventive and Social Medicine
Otago Medical School
Dunedin, New Zealand

Christine A. Haffner, M.A., M.R.C.P.
Research Fellow
Department of Medicine
Queen Elizabeth Hospital
Birmingham, England

Rodney T. Jackson, M.B., Ch.B., M.Med.Sc., Ph.D.
Senior Lecturer
Department of Community Health
Auckland Medical School
University of Auckland
Auckland, New Zealand

Martin Kendall, M.D., F.R.C.P.
Senior Lecturer
Department of Medicine
Queen Elizabeth Hospital
Birmingham, England

Tamar Lasky, Ph.D.
Research Assistant
Department of Epidemiology and Preventive Medicine
University of Maryland School of Medicine
Baltimore, Maryland, USA

Stella R. O'Donnell, D.Sc., Ph.D., B.Sc., M.P.S., M.R. Pharm.S.
Professor
Department of Physiology and Pharmacology
The University of Queensland
Brisbane, Australia

Neil Pearce, B.Sc., Dip.Sci., Dip.ORS, Ph.D.
Senior Research Fellow
Department of Medicine
Wellington School of Medicine
Wellington, New Zealand

Robin G. Shanks, D.Sc., M.D., F.R.C.P., F.R.C.P., Ed., F.R.C.P., I., M.R.I.A.
Professor
Department of Therapeutics and Pharmacology
The Queen's University of Belfast
Belfast, Northern Ireland

Paul D. Stolley, M.D., M.P.H.
Professor
Department of Epidemiology and Preventive Medicine
School of Medicine
University of Maryland
Baltimore, Maryland, USA

Anne E. Tattersfield, M.B.B.S., M.R.C.P., M.D., F.R.C.P.
Professor
Division of Respiratory Medicine
City Hospital
Nottingham, England

Colin S. Wong, M.B.Ch.B., F.R.A.C.P., M.D.
Consultant Physician
Department of Respiratory Medicine
City Hospital
Nottingham, England

TABLE OF CONTENTS

Section 1
Historical Overview

Chapter 1

THE DEVELOPMENT OF BETA RECEPTOR AGONIST DRUGS

Stella R. O'Donnell

TABLE OF CONTENTS

0-8493-6761-1/93/$0.00 + $.50

I. INTRODUCTION

Sympathomimetic bronchodilators have been important drugs in the treatment of asthma for most of the 20th century. This chapter traces the developments that led to the logical synthesis of many thousands of chemical compounds in the search for the ideal $beta_2$ receptor agonist bronchodilator. Only a few compounds met the clinical and other requirements for a commercially viable product, and drugs introduced over 20 years ago are still the main clinically useful drugs in the group. The beta receptor agonist drugs were designed by medicinal chemists working closely with drug development pharmacologists. In this way chemical and physical properties necessary to improve the bronchodilator selectivity of prototype compounds could be pinpointed. The drugs that have resulted from the successful modification of the chemical structure of isoprenaline provide an excellent example of the success of rational methods of drug discovery.

This chapter also stresses how adrenaline and isoprenaline were used in asthma before the adrenoceptor concept was proposed and how the selective properties of drugs, such as salbutamol and terbutaline, were known before publication of the ''beta receptor subtypes'' hypothesis. Thus, the beta receptor agonist drugs have not only been invaluable in the treatment of asthma but their availability has also played an important role in substantiating receptor theories that have been central to the thinking of classical pharmacologists for nearly a century.

II. THE FIRST BETA RECEPTOR AGONIST DRUGS

A. ADRENALINE IS DISCOVERED

The potent pressor effects of an intravenous injection of sheep adrenal extracts were reported in 1895,[1] and an impure form of the active principal was isolated in 1897 and named epinephrine. An alternative preparation was marketed in Germany under the name ''Suprarenin''. The active principle was soon purified[2] and marketed by Parke-Davis as ''Adrenaline''. Outside the United States adrenaline was adopted as the approved name for this substance, whereas the United States retained the name epinephrine. Elucidation of the chemical structure of adrenaline (Figure 1) soon followed and the isomers were separated. The history of the isolation and identification of adrenaline has been reviewed.[3]

Physiologists took an interest in adrenaline in the early 1900s believing it to be the neurotransmitter chemical released from sympathetic nerves.[4] However, although the closely related amine, noradrenaline, was synthesized soon after adrenaline, it was not until 1946 that Von Euler[5] demonstrated that noradrenaline, and not adrenaline, was the neurotransmitter chemical released by sympathetic nerves.

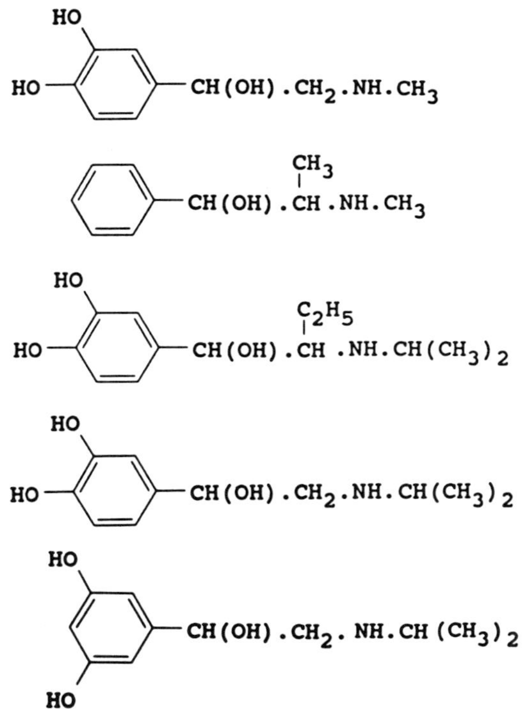

Adrenaline

Ephedrine

Isoetharine

Isoprenaline

Orciprenaline

FIGURE 1. Chemical structures of some of the first beta receptor agonist bronchodilator drugs.

B. ADRENALINE IS USED FOR ASTHMA

A report on the use of "adrenal substance" in asthma appeared in 1900,[6] and once pure adrenaline was available it was given subcutaneously to asthmatics.[7] Later, adrenaline was applied directly to the bronchial mucosa as an inhaled solution and the concentration in the inhalation solution was subsequently increased to improve its effectiveness, although this caused side effects, such as palpitations and tremor.[8] Inhaled adrenaline was still being used in the 1950s, and the correct use of the available nebulizers or atomizers, the importance of avoiding overdosage, and the need to start therapy only under medical guidance were stressed to patients. Patients were also cautioned not to panic if they had pink mucus because this was due to the oxidation products of adrenaline.[8]

When adrenaline was first synthesized in the early 1900s, one of the hypotheses used to explain asthma invoked vasodilatation. Because the vasoconstrictor effects of adrenaline were being studied at that time, it seemed logical that adrenaline should be effective in asthma. The marked effectiveness of adrenaline was used to support this "vascular" theory of asthma.[9] An alternative hypothesis that asthma occurred because of bronchospasm subsequently received support when adrenaline was shown to relax isolated airway preparations. By the 1950s adrenaline was well recognized as one of the most powerful bronchodilators available to physicians for treating asthma, and it was used in many forms including an intramuscular injection in oil, an early attempt to increase the duration of a bronchodilator response. Although Hyde Salter is better known for his contributions to the history of the use of xanthines in asthma, it is interesting to note that in the 1860s he had described an "instantaneous cure of asthma" by "violent emotions";[9] he may have been observing a beneficial bronchodilator effect of endogenous adrenaline.

C. SYMPATHOMIMETIC AMINES RELATED TO ADRENALINE ARE SYNTHESIZED

In 1910, after an extensive investigation of a large number of newly synthesized amines related to adrenaline, Barger and Dale[10] defined some basic structural requirements for pharmacological activity in these amines. They introduced the term "sympathomimetic" to describe the general effects of the group because the pharmacological effects of the compounds were similar to those observed when sympathetic autonomic nerves were stimulated. Over the next 40 years many sympathomimetic amine compounds were synthesized and many structure-activity studies carried out, for a spectrum of sympathomimetic responses. Subsequent research on one of these amines, tyramine, led to the suggestion that some sympathomimetic amines worked via a direct action on the effector cell receptors in the responding tissue, whereas others, such as tyramine, worked indirectly through an action on the sympathetic nerve endings. The effects of the latter group of compounds could be abolished by pretreatment of the animals with reserpine, which depleted the tissues of endogenous noradrenaline.[11]

A number of pharmaceutical companies undertook major research and development programs on sympathomimetic amines during the 1930s and 1940s. A large number of compounds were examined for their bronchodilator potency *in vivo* or *in vitro,* using inhibition of drug-induced bronchospasm in dogs or bronchodilatation in guinea pig isolated perfused lung preparations.[12-15] The bronchodilator potencies of the compounds were frequently compared with their potencies as pressor agents, but Tainter et al.[12-15] found no consistent correlation between these potencies. They suggested that these two effects were produced by different mechanisms. They also made an important early observation that the cardiac effects of these amines were more closely correlated with their bronchodilator effects than with their pressor effects. Many other compounds, such as 3,4-dihydroxyephedrine and some *N*-ethyl or *N*-methoxy derivatives of ephedrine and adrenaline, were later identified as also being more potent as bronchodilators and less potent as pressor agents than the parent compounds.[16-21] However, in general, there was less emphasis on the structural requirements necessary for adrenaline-like inhibitory effects (which included bronchial responses) than on those required for adrenaline-like excitatory, especially pressor, effects.

D. EPHEDRINE IS USED ORALLY IN ASTHMA

Ephedrine (Figure 1) was introduced for use in asthma 20 years after adrenaline and was widely used in the 1930s. Although it was less potent than adrenaline as a bronchodilator, its oral activity and its longer duration of action were considered to be advantageous. Ephedrine is a natural product that is found in a Chinese herbal medicine, Ma huang *(Ephedra vulgaris),* and it has been in use in China for more than 5000 years. As an herbal medicine it was reputed to improve the circulation, cause sweating, ease coughing, and reduce fever. On returning to China from the United States in the early 1920s, Chen took an interest in this herbal medicine and, with Schmidt, isolated and tested the active substance. They reported its potent adrenaline-like and tyramine-like activity and showed that, unlike adrenaline, it was active by mouth.[22,23] They also found that the substance that they identified had previously been isolated in Japan (in 1897) and called ephedrine.

Over the next few decades, the oral activity of ephedrine was explained by its resistance to breakdown by the enzymes monoamine oxidase (due to the presence of a methyl group on the alpha carbon of the side chain of the molecule) and catechol-O-methyltransferase (COMT) (because it lacked the catechol moiety). The major metabolic route of metabolism of ephedrine was shown to be by demethylation to norephedrine (later marketed as phenylpropanolamine in decongestants and cold cures). The sympathomimetic responses to ephedrine were also shown to be complex, comprising both direct and indirect sympathomimetic effects.

Ephedrine was not a potent bronchodilator by comparison with drugs that were to be introduced later, and it still had side effects associated with the use of adrenaline, for example, pressor effects and cardiac stimulation. In addition, patients were troubled by side effects due to stimulation of the central nervous system. Thus, tablets were produced which contained a barbiturate as well as ephedrine and also the xanthine drug, theophylline. These combination tablets were later severely criticized.

E. ISOPRENALINE IS SHOWN TO BE PROMISING IN ASTHMA

From the structure-activity studies carried out during the 1940s, it was clearly evident that for good bronchodilator activity in a sympathomimetic amine, the group substituted on the nitrogen atom should be greater in size than the methyl group present in the adrenaline molecule. In the early years of World War II, Konzett[24,25] in Boehringer-Ingelheim in Germany had recognized that the *N*-isopropyl derivative of adrenaline might be promising for the relief of bronchospasm in asthma and that this compound was more or less free of the troublesome pressor effects of adrenaline. After the war, clinical reports confirmed his predictions,[26,27] and the drug was introduced for use under the approved name of isoproterenol in the United States and isoprenaline elsewhere.

Isoprenaline (Figure 1), unlike ephedrine, did not cross the blood-brain barrier; hence, it lacked the central nervous system side effects of ephedrine, such as insomnia, as well as lacking the pressor effects of adrenaline. Isoprenaline was not active orally, and it was necessary to administer it either by sublingual lozenge or by inhalation to achieve its potent bronchodilator effects. Isoprenaline and adrenaline are both catecholamines, and it was subsequently shown that when these drugs are given by the oral route the phenolic hydroxyls are conjugated to inactive ethereal sulfates by enzymes present in the gut wall as well as the liver. The duration of action of inhaled isoprenaline was also short, and this was later shown to result from the O-methylation of the drug by COMT present in the lungs. Nevertheless, for 20 or more years isoprenaline was considered to be a drug of choice for the relief of acute asthmatic attacks with patients mainly reporting cardiac side effects and tremor. Problems arose when the drug was available in pressurized aerosols in the early 1960s. The duration of action of isoprenaline was too short for it to be useful for prophylaxis in asthma; thus, ephedrine was used for this purpose for quite some time.

F. ISOPRENALINE IS A KEY SUBSTANCE IN THE ALPHA-BETA RECEPTOR CONCEPT

Although research during the 1940s provided much information on the structural requirements for excitatory and inhibitory responses to sympathomimetic amines, many of the results on different test preparations were conflicting. A satisfactory explanation for qualitative differences in the effects of different compounds as sympathomimetic amines had not been formulated. At that time the terms ''adrenergic'' and ''sympathomimetic'' were virtually synonymous with vasoconstrictor, and pressor, effects. Thus, it was unclear why the bronchodilator sympathomimetic amine isoprenaline, in contrast to adrenaline, was only vasodilator, that is, inhibitory on blood vessels, but, like adrenaline, was a potent cardiac stimulant (excitatory).

In 1948 Ahlquist[28] published his now classic report on adrenotropic receptors (later called adrenergic receptors, adrenoreceptors, or adrenoceptors and referred to in this book as receptors). The availability of isoprenaline provided Ahlquist with a key substance in the formulation of his theory. Also, the ''adrenergic'' blocking agent dibenamine (dibenzyline) had just been described.[29]

Ahlquist proposed that sympathomimetic amines could act on two kinds of receptor, alpha and beta. In making this proposal he was diverting attention back to work carried out early in the 20th century. Ehrlich[30] (1900) had suggested that drugs could act on specific cellular substances, but Langley[31] (1905) was the first to suggest that a receptor was a structure on a cell that translated either electrical or chemical events into a measurable physiological response. He was of the opinion that there were two different ''receptive substances'' for adrenaline. Dale[32] (1906) observed that ergot extracts blocked the pressor effects in animals of the recently synthesized adrenaline but left intact the subsequent depressor effects. On various isolated smooth muscle preparations, the ergot extracts also blocked those responses to adrenaline, or sympathetic nerve stimulation, that were motor (excitatory) but not those that were inhibitory. To explain these observations Dale reinforced the "receptive mechanism for adrenaline" concept.

During the 1930s Cannon and Rosenblueth[33] developed their sympathin hypothesis to explain the anomalous findings of Dale with adrenaline. These researchers believed in the release of a single transmitter substance (probably adrenaline) after stimulation of sympathetic nerves. They proposed that this substance combined with, or was changed by, substances in the target tissue to produce either one or two new chemicals, which then circulated around the body as chemical transmitters. They proposed that one of these substances produced excitatory effects and the other inhibitory effects and named the substances sympathin E and I, respectively.

The view of Cannon and Rosenblueth was widely held, and it not only shifted research attention toward finding the nature of the chemical transmitter(s) in sympathetic nerves, but it also meant that the "receptor" concept that had been put forward much earlier by Langley[31] and by Dale[32] was largely ignored by the research community. When he reviewed his career 30 years after his 1948 article, Ahlquist[34] admitted that he proposed his dual receptor concept somewhat innocently at a time when receptors were still "figments of the imagination". By putting forward a "receptor" hypothesis, he was challenging the dogma of the time, i.e., the sympathin transmitters theory. In retrospect, the transmitter theory prevented the receptor concepts of the early 1900s from having any impact in experimental pharmacology until the early 1950s. Fortunately, Ahlquist's ideas were accepted by the teaching and pharmaceutical communities because they not only offered a rational explanation for the observed effect of the new drug, isoprenaline, but they opened up the potential to find new, more specific, therapeutic agents. One of the therapeutic areas to benefit was the drug treatment of asthma.

Ahlquist[35] reviewed how he came to postulate his theory. Briefly, as a result of some observations with a number of sympathomimetic amines, including the then new drug isoprenaline, he observed that for different sympathomimetic responses, the order of potency of the amines fell into two distinct groups. In particular, isoprenaline was a potent drug in producing certain responses (e.g., cardiac stimulation, vasodilatation) but was inactive for other responses (e.g., vasoconstriction, uterine contraction). Ahlquist recognized that the two groups of responses did not fit neatly into an excitatory and an inhibitory category; hence, he named the receptors alpha (associated with most, but not all, of the excitatory responses) and beta (associated with most of the inhibitory responses). The inhibition of bronchial smooth muscle was classified by Ahlquist with the beta receptor responses, although this conclusion was based not on his own data but by reference to the results of others.[18] Thus, it was now considered that future sympathomimetic bronchodilators should be specific agonists of beta, as opposed to alpha, receptors. However, the labeling of drugs as "beta agonists" did not occur until the hypothesis was finally fully accepted. Although Ahlquist had been able to block responses mediated by alpha receptors with dibenamine, it was not until the late 1950s that drugs were found that would block responses to isoprenaline. The first of these, dichloroisoprenaline, resulted from a research program in which substituted isoprenaline compounds were being screened for bronchodilator properties.[36] The first of the clinically tested beta receptor blocking drugs soon followed.[37,38] For a while the alpha-beta receptor concept did not go unchallenged and additional receptors were sometimes invoked to account for responses not effectively blocked by alpha or beta receptor blocking drugs.[39] Subsequently, most of these anomalies were accommodated within the alpha-beta receptor terminology.

III. SELECTIVE BETA RECEPTOR AGONIST DRUGS

A. DRUGS WITHOUT ALPHA RECEPTOR AGONIST SIDE EFFECTS ARE SOUGHT

The alpha-beta receptor hypothesis in 1948 now provided an explanation for differences between the side effects of the bronchodilator drugs isoprenaline and adrenaline. Both isoprenaline and adrenaline caused bronchodilatation and cardiac side effects through activation of beta receptors. But isoprenaline caused vasodilatation, also through an action on beta receptors, whereas adrenaline, because of its potent alpha receptor agonist effects, caused peripheral vasoconstriction and hence an increase in blood pressure.

Many new bronchodilators were found during the 1950s and early 1960s. Compounds that had been synthesized one or two decades earlier, during the extensive structure-activity studies on sympathomimetic amines, were now described as beta agonists with less alpha agonist side effects. Many of these compounds were catecholamine analogs of isoprenaline, and some of them had an alkyl group substituted on the alpha carbon in the side chain, for example, isoetharine[40] (Figure 1) and ethylnoradrenaline.[41] These drugs were orally active and had a longer duration of action than isoprenaline. They also lacked the central stimulant effects of ephedrine because the drugs could not enter the central nervous system.

Another important drug at that time was orciprenaline (metaproterenol in the United States; Figure 1), the resorcinolamine equivalent of the catecholamine isoprenaline.[42] This drug was active orally and was also widely used as an aerosol.[43,44] Because it lacked a catecholamine nucleus, it was not metabolized by COMT in the lung. Thus, orciprenaline had a longer duration of action than isoprenaline by the inhaled route. Orciprenaline was a less potent bronchodilator than isoprenaline, but it lacked alpha agonist side effects. It still caused tachycardia as a side effect, although in the aerosolized form this was considered to be less of a problem than with isoprenaline.

Many other compounds satisfying the requirements for good bronchodilatation with less side effects and better pharmacokinetic properties were studied. One of these was the compound soterenol (MJ 1992), in which the 3-hydroxyl group on the catechol nucleus of isoprenaline was substituted with

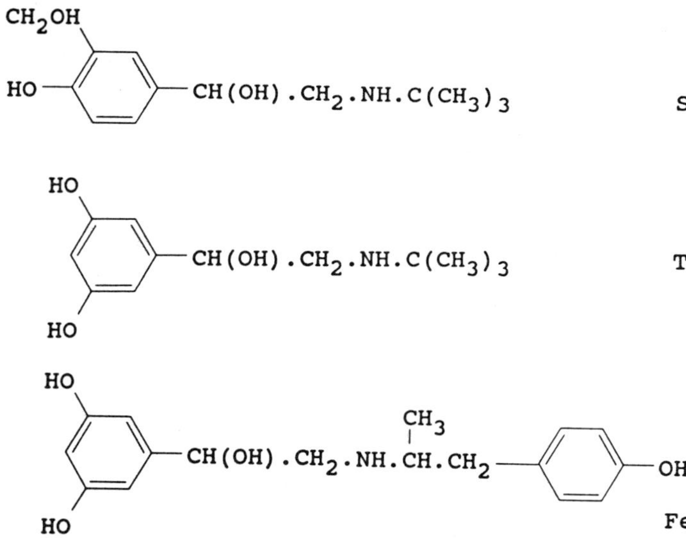

FIGURE 2. Chemical structures of the main $beta_2$ receptor selective agonist bronchodilator drugs.

a methane sulfonamide.[45] But only four beta agonist bronchodilator aerosols were available for use in asthma in the United States at the beginning of the 1970s, i.e., adrenaline, isoprenaline, isoetharine, and orciprenaline (Figure 1).[46]

B. DRUGS WITH REDUCED CARDIAC SIDE EFFECTS ARE DESCRIBED

In the United Kingdom, researchers at Allen and Hanburys (now part of the Glaxo Group) had replaced the 3-position hydroxyl group in isoprenaline with a bulkier hydroxymethyl group (a saligenin). As they predicted, this produced a beta agonist bronchodilator with a longer duration of action, due to resistance of the compound to the actions of COMT. The compound was active orally as well as by inhalation. By further increasing the bulk of the N-substituted alkyl group, that is, by replacing isopropyl with a *t*-butyl group, they obtained a compound with increased bronchodilator potency but fewer cardiac side effects. This was the compound salbutamol (AH 3365) (Figure 2).[47,48]

Independently, chemists at Draco (now part of the Astra group) in Sweden had synthesized a series of resorcinolamines with bulkier N-substituent groups. Replacement of the N-isopropyl group of orciprenaline with a N-t-butyl group also resulted in a potent beta agonist bronchodilator with less cardiac effects. The drug had the required oral activity and longer duration of action. This was the compound terbutaline (Figure 2).[49-51] The good bronchodilator effects of these drugs in asthma with lesser, although not absent, cardiac stimulant side effects were supported by many clinical studies.[52-55]

In Germany Boehringer-Ingelheim also produced a series of relatives of orciprenaline with bulkier N-substituted aralkyl groups. One of these was the compound fenoterol (Th 1165a) (Figure 2). This compound was shown to be a potent beta agonist with less cardiac potency and a longer duration of action.[56] Clinical studies supported its bronchodilator effectiveness and reduced side effect potential.[57,58]

It is interesting to note that the bronchodilator-cardiac selectivity of these sympathomimetic drugs was noted before general acceptance of the $beta_1$-$beta_2$ receptor subtype hypothesis. Hence, it was only later that salbutamol, terbutaline, and fenoterol became known as the $beta_2$-selective bronchodilators. Thus, while the beta receptor subtypes hypothesis provided an explanation for the effects of these drugs, the drugs also provided the tools with which to (1) confirm the beta receptor subtype hypothesis and (2) classify the beta receptor subtype(s) present in different tissues that responded to beta agonists.

Although these three drugs have been the main $beta_2$-selective agonist bronchodilators for asthma for more than two decades, many other compounds have been identified as $beta_2$ selective. The chemical structures of many of these compounds and the major differences in their pharmacological actions have been summarized by Brittain et al.[59] The more interesting compounds underwent extensive investigation especially after the dual beta receptor hypothesis was introduced.[60,61]

C. THE $BETA_1$-$BETA_2$ RECEPTOR SUBTYPES HYPOTHESIS IS PROPOSED

The researchers of Sterling Winthrop in the United States had been carrying out structure-activity studies on sympathomimetic amines throughout the 1930s and 1940s,[18-21] and they had accumulated evidence that compounds might show bronchodilator-cardiac selectivity. As early as 1949, Lands[62] had foreshadowed that the newly proposed receptors for sympathomimetic amines in the heart might prove to be different from those mediating contraction or relaxation of smooth muscle, but it was not until 1967 that Lands et al.[63,64] proposed that beta receptors should be divided into two distinct types, $beta_1$ and $beta_2$. Their proposal, like for the alpha-beta hypothesis, was based on the different order of potencies of a series of catecholamine-sympathomimetic amines on different pharmacological preparations. They classified beta responses on heart, adipose tissue, and small intestine with $beta_1$ receptors and on bronchioles, vasculature, diaphragm, and uterus with $beta_2$ receptors. They also observed that $beta_2$ receptors were more sensitive to adrenaline than noradrenaline and vice versa for $beta_1$. This dual beta receptor hypothesis gained widespread acceptance, despite some early controversies relating, for example, to the choice of beta agonists and use of experimental conditions that did not take into account the influence on beta receptor potencies of alpha receptor stimulation, uptake mechanisms, and metabolic enzymes. The rigid classification of beta responses into $beta_1$ or $beta_2$ was later relaxed when it was demonstrated that in some tissues, including airway preparations[65,66] and human isolated heart preparations, the response to beta agonists could be mediated by $beta_1$ and $beta_2$ receptors present in the same tissue. This indicated that the useful selectivity of $beta_2$ agonists would be dependent not only on the selectivity of the drug but also on the relative populations of each beta receptor subtype present in the target tissues. In an attempt to provide a physiological basis for the two subtypes of beta receptor, the hypothesis was explored that $beta_1$ receptors might be "innervated" receptors because of their preference for noradrenaline and $beta_2$ receptors might be "hormonal" receptors because of their preference for adrenaline.[67]

D. MANY $BETA_2$ RECEPTOR SELECTIVE BRONCHODILATORS ARE DESCRIBED

The beta receptor subtype hypothesis stimulated the search for compounds with better separation between their bronchodilator ($beta_2$) and cardiac stimulant ($beta_1$) potencies; such drugs were labeled as $beta_2$ selective. Many drugs were explored and some were tested clinically in asthma, but none really displaced the original $beta_2$ agonists in practice. Examples of drugs that were examined include salmefamol,[68] carbuterol,[69] pirbuterol,[70] clenbuterol,[71,72] rimiterol,[73,74] hexoprenaline,[75,76] quinprenaline,[77] and others.[46] Many drugs showed good $beta_2$ selectivity in animal studies but were never used commercially in asthma either because of toxicity or because they were unable to compete commercially with existing drugs.

E. ATTEMPTS ARE MADE TO REMOVE UNREQUIRED $BETA_2$ RECEPTOR AGONIST SIDE EFFECTS

The ready availability of $beta_2$-selective bronchodilators meant that the risk of direct cardiac ($beta_1$) side effects was now minimized, provided that the drugs were not used in excessive dosage. The available drugs were effective bronchodilators and, because they acted as functional antagonists of smooth muscle spasmogens, they provided symptomatic relief irrespective of the severity of the asthma or the provoking spasmogen. Nevertheless, attempts to improve on the existing drugs continued and studies followed a number of different directions.

Attempts to find drugs with increased separation between the bronchodilator and cardiac stimulant doses, i.e., with improved $beta_2$-$beta_1$ selectivity, were continued. The selectivity of the clinically used drugs was not great and, with the development of ligand-binding techniques, it was later shown that although salbutamol and fenoterol showed bronchodilator-cardiac selectivity *in vitro* and *in vivo,* there was no difference in their affinities for $beta_2$ and $beta_1$ receptors.[78] The functional selectivity of these drugs was attributed to their higher efficacy on $beta_2$ than $beta_1$ receptors. Fenoterol, unlike salbutamol but like isoprenaline, was a full agonist on guinea pig atria (rate) as well as on trachea (relaxation).[61] These properties made this drug a useful tool in studies designed to classify beta receptor subtypes in tissues.[66]

However, whether this difference is of relevance in the use of fenoterol in severe asthma has never been thoroughly explored.

Some of the newer $beta_2$-selective drugs, for example, procaterol (OPC-2009),[79,80] were shown to have significantly greater affinity for $beta_2$ than $beta_1$ receptors *in vitro,* but this was not paralleled by any major improvement in selectivity in *in vivo* experiments and the drug still caused cardiovascular side effects in clinical trials.[81] Nevertheless, procaterol, because of its potency and good $beta_2$-$beta_1$ selectivity *in vitro,* also proved to be a useful pharmacological tool. It was used in functional studies designed to detect small populations of $beta_2$ receptors in tissues containing predominantly $beta_1$ receptors.[80]

The more potent $beta_2$ agonist bronchodilators were also potent vasodilators because relaxation of bronchial and vascular smooth muscle were both $beta_2$ receptor responses. As a result, $beta_2$ agonist bronchodilators could still, in theory, produce tachycardia via a reflex response to the decrease in blood pressure even if the drug itself was bronchodilator-cardiac selective at the receptor level. Furthermore, occurrence of vasodilatation in pulmonary blood vessels supplying poorly ventilated areas of the lungs could result in ventilation-perfusion mismatch and arterial hypoxemia.[82] However, the side effect that proved to be most troublesome to asthma patients, especially those patients on oral preparations, was fine skeletal muscle tremor, which was also a $beta_2$ receptor effect.

Thus, various attempts were made to find good bronchodilators that were less effective as vasodilators and/or in producing tremor, that is, to remove undesired $beta_2$ receptor responses. It eventually became clear that both these objectives were difficult to achieve. No evidence could be found, in response studies on isolated tissues from animals, for a difference between $beta_2$ receptors in respiratory and vascular smooth muscle.[83] Also, although considerable effort was put into attempts to reduce the tremorigenic potency of $beta_2$ agonist bronchodilators, the effects of these agonists on airway smooth muscle relaxation were always well correlated with their effects on soleus muscle contraction (reflecting tremor) in animals, both *in vitro* and *in vivo.*[84] Nevertheless, some compounds were found to show bronchodilator-tremor selectivity in the animal models, but this occurred only under restricted experimental conditions; hence, these drugs, such as AH 7616, were never tested in humans.[85] Other compounds, such as D 2343, were tested clinically but did not improve on existing drugs.[86,87] Attempts to achieve bronchodilator-tremor selectivity by using compounds that were full agonists on airway smooth muscle but partial agonists on skeletal muscle were also unsuccessful.[81,88]

During the search for bronchodilators with less tremorigenic effects, some unexpected observations were followed up. For example, the compound KWD 2131 was an order of magnitude more potent *in vitro* in inhibiting antigen-induced release of histamine from mast cells in sensitized guinea pig lungs (also a $beta_2$ receptor effect), but this drug also had no advantages over the related drug terbutaline in clinical asthma provoked by antigen.[89]

Thus, after a decade or more of study, no $beta_2$ agonist bronchodilators were on the market that totally lacked cardiac side effects and/or had significantly reduced vasodilator and/or tremorigenic properties.

All the clinically used $beta_2$-selective agonists were available for inhalation as well as for oral use. The inhaled route allowed a small, but effective, dose of drug to be delivered directly to the airways and this produced a fairly prompt bronchodilator response. In addition, inhalation provided an indirect means of reducing the side effects of the drugs. Because the dose of drug was small, the amount of drug absorbed from the lungs, or the gastrointestinal tract (because up to 90% of an inhaled dose is swallowed) resulted in a negligible circulating plasma concentration. Hence, less drug was available to cause extrapulmonary side effects, such as cardiac stimulation and fine muscle tremor. The original inhalation devices for $beta_2$-selective agonists were pressurized metered dose inhalers, which use chlorofluorocarbon propellants. A variety of spacers were introduced to assist patients with any coordination difficulties in the use of these devices. Recently, $beta_2$ agonists have been provided in dry powder inhaler devices, the most recent of which is multidose and dispenses terbutaline.[90]

F. $BETA_2$ RECEPTOR SELECTIVE AGONISTS WITH A LONG DURATION OF ACTION ARE PROMOTED

For more than two decades salbutamol, terbutaline, and fenoterol have been the $beta_2$-selective bronchodilators most widely used in asthma. It is only in the last few years that any drugs have been introduced with the potential to provide physicians with additional, or alternative, $beta_2$ agonist bronchodilators. These newer drugs are all longer acting than the current drugs. The current drugs have a duration of action (of a single inhaled dose) of, at the most, 6 h. This is not adequate when prolonged protection from bronchoconstriction is required, for example, in nocturnal asthma. Recently, two drugs for use by the inhaled route, salmeterol and formoterol, and one drug for oral use, bambuterol, have been widely promoted. Salmeterol and formoterol resulted from structural modification to existing $beta_2$-selective agonists and bambuterol from a prodrug approach.

Formoterol (aformoterol, foradil) was first synthesized in the mid-1970s (BD 40A) by Japanese researchers.[91,92] In formoterol, the N-substituted aralkyl group is the same as in salmefamol, but a formamide moiety is present instead of the saligenin group (Figure 3). In humans the duration of action of salmefamol was not much different from that of salbutamol,[93] but the longer duration of formoterol has been clearly demonstrated in animals[94] and in humans.[95-97]

Formoterol is also a potent agonist, being at least ten times more potent than isoprenaline in relaxing airway smooth muscle *in vitro*. It has a high intrinsic activity, good $beta_2$ selectivity and a high affinity for $beta_2$ receptors.[94] The drug is lipophilic and appears to persist in airway tissue to cause airway smooth muscle relaxation *in vitro* over a prolonged period.[94] Other $beta_2$ agonists are also lipophilic, for example, salmeterol, the resorcinol

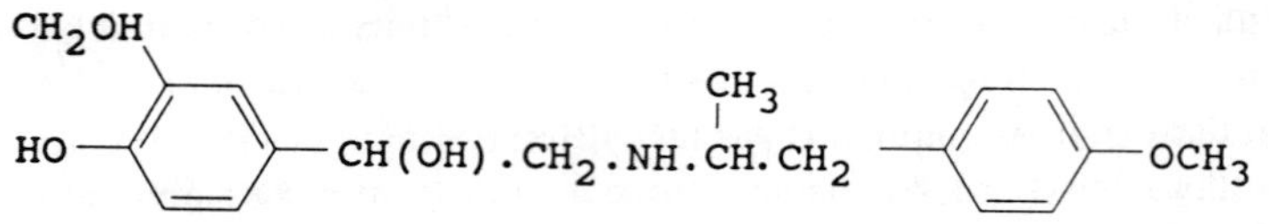

Salmefamol

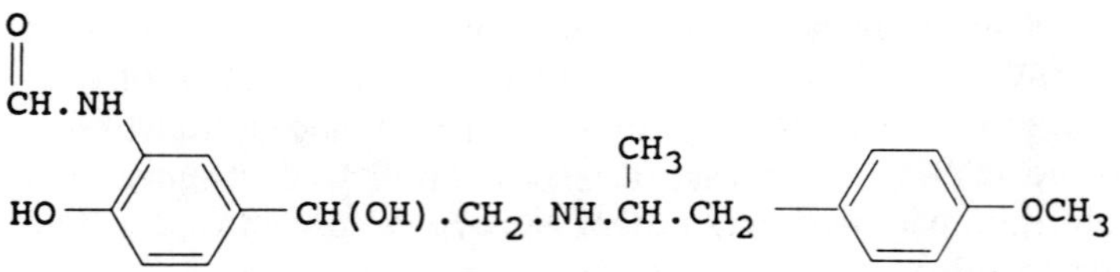

Formoterol

FIGURE 3. The chemical relationship between the long-acting beta$_2$ receptor selective bronchodilator drug formoterol and the earlier drug salmefamol.

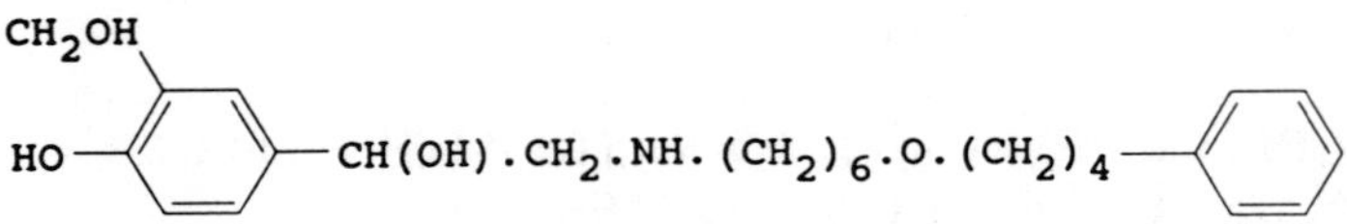

Salmeterol

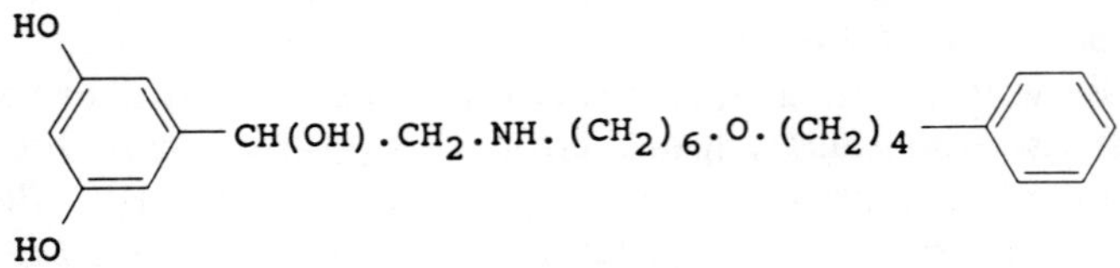

D 2489

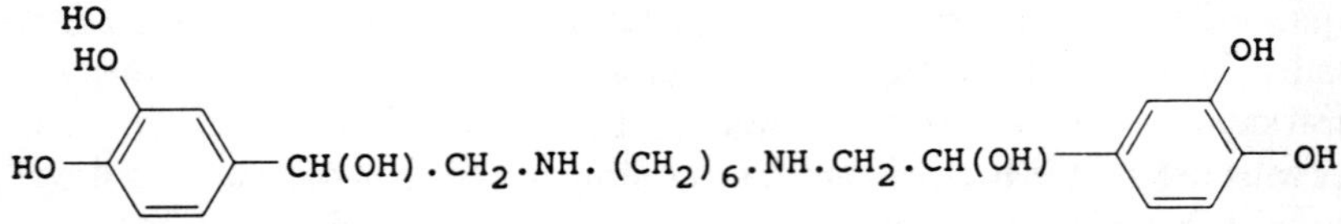

Hexoprenaline

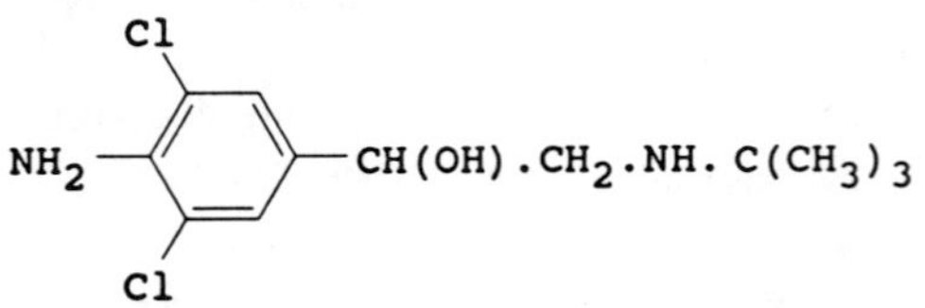

Clenbuterol

FIGURE 4. The chemical relationship of the long-acting beta$_2$ receptor selective bronchodilator drug salmeterol and some other lipophilic compounds.

analog of salmeterol (D 2489), clenbuterol (Figure 4), and some derivatives of terbutaline.[98]

Salmeterol is chemically related to salbutamol, and it has also been shown to be beta$_2$ selective and to have a long duration of bronchodilator action in animals[99,100] and in humans.[101,102] Like formoterol, its bronchodilator action in asthma lasts at least 12 h, but the onset of action of formoterol is quicker both in *in vitro* experiments[98] and in humans.[102]

Salmeterol has a large nonpolar (lipophilic) N-substituent group that comprises an oxyalkylphenyl group separated from the nitrogen of the salbutamol molecule by a 6-carbon chain "spacer". The drug resulted from a program designed to find compounds that might bind to "exosites" adjacent to the beta receptor sites in the cell membrane.[103] This principle was first expounded by Brittain et al.[59] in 1976, but a catecholamine compound, hexoprenaline, with some structural similarities to salmeterol had been studied in the early 1970s.[104] Hexoprenaline contains a second catechol nucleus that is separated from the amine group by the same 6-carbon "spacer" used in salmeterol (Figure 4). Hexoprenaline is a $beta_2$-selective agonist, and it also has a long duration of action in animals *in vivo,* but the definitive reason for the latter was not clarified.[75]

It has been proposed that the lipophilic side chain in salmeterol holds the active moiety of the molecule in the vicinity of the beta receptor and that this maintains the concentration of the drug in the receptor biophase for a considerable time. Other lipophilic $beta_2$ agonists that do not possess the long side chain of salmeterol also have properties *in vitro* that suggest they are retained in the tissue receptor biophase, for example, clenbuterol[71] (Figure 4) and D 2343,[98] but these drugs do not have a longer duration of action in humans.[94] This suggests that additional factors are also involved in explaining the duration of action in humans of the $beta_2$-selective drugs.[97]

An alternative approach to improving the bioavailability and duration of action of the $beta_2$ agonist bronchodilators was to form prodrugs. One of the therapeutic limitations of the available drugs was pharmacokinetic in nature (their conjugation prior to systemic availability and, for catecholamines, metabolism by COMT). The hydrophilic nature of many of the molecules also led to slow and/or incomplete absorption of the drugs and hence to variation in plasma levels between patients. The prodrug approach aimed to protect the vulnerable phenolic hydroxyl groups in the catechol or resorcinol nucleus with a suitably inert group. The objectives were to increase chemical stability, decrease metabolic inactivation, and increase lipophilicity. The protecting groups tended to result in an inactive molecule. Thus, it was also essential that the protective groups could be easily and specifically cleaved in the lungs because a bronchodilator action was required.

A number of catecholamine-derived ester prodrugs were initially described, and one of these was bitolterol, a *bis-p*-toluate prodrug of N-t-butyl noradrenaline (colterol, the catecholamine equivalent of terbutaline).[105] The drug was a good bronchodilator in animals and had a prolonged duration of action,[106] but it had no advantages over salbutamol in humans.[107] However, its relatively long duration of action was believed to reflect the high affinity of the lipophilic prodrug for lung tissue. This was thought to retain the drug in the lung where it was then hydrolyzed to the parent active $beta_2$ agonist.

The first prodrug bronchodilator in which the therapeutic side effects were reduced was ibuterol.[108] The usefulness of this bis-isobutyrate prodrug

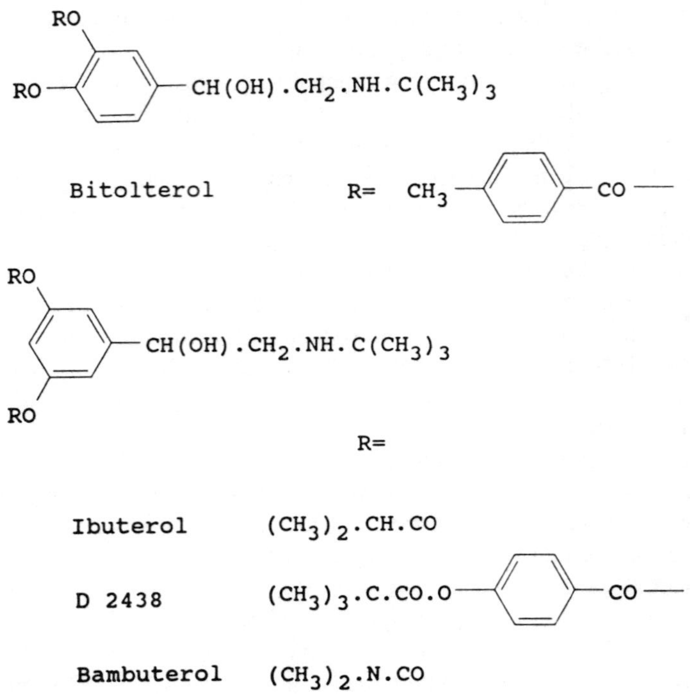

FIGURE 5. Chemical structures of bitolterol, a catecholamine prodrug, and of three prodrugs of the resorcinolamine, terbutaline, including the drug bambuterol.

of terbutaline (Figure 5) was limited by its short duration of action after oral administration. Nevertheless, the studies with this drug indicated that a satisfactory prodrug of terbutaline would need to possess greater resistance to presystemic metabolism and preferential retention in the lung tissue where hydrolysis would then release active drug. In this way bronchodilator selectivity, that is, a reduction of systemic side effects, would be achieved.

Two terbutaline ester prodrugs were designed with these goals in mind. One of these, D 2438, in which the ester is derived from *p*-pivaloyloxybenzoic acid[109] (Figure 5), had the required properties in dogs but not when tested in humans (esterase activity is higher in humans than in dogs). A more satisfactory drug was the *bis-N,N*-dimethylcarbamate ester prodrug, bambuterol (Figure 5).[110,111] The dimethylcarbamate groups in this compound provided a built-in esterase inhibitory function, that is, bambuterol slowed down its own rate of hydrolysis by reversibly inhibiting pseudocholinesterase. In addition, through oxidative metabolism of the carbamate groups, the drug was metabolized to various additional lipophilic, inactive, metabolite prodrugs. These could then be spontaneously broken down to terbutaline. This feature contributed to the prolonged duration of action of the drug when it was given orally to asthmatic patients. Bambuterol also had the required lung specificity in that both the drug and its metabolites were retained in the lung tissue. The latter may be the explanation why an increased ratio of bronchodilatation to side effects is seen in patients despite low plasma concentrations of terbutaline; the drug may be generating therapeutic levels of terbutaline only in the lungs. Thus, bambuterol provided a new orally active bronchodilator for asthma with a long duration of action and with a favorable bronchodilator:side effects ratio.

G. ADDITIONAL BETA$_2$ RECEPTOR AGONIST EFFECTS OF THE BRONCHODILATOR DRUGS ARE EMPHASIZED

It was shown in the early 1970s that sympathomimetic amines could inhibit antigen-induced release of histamine in a variety of experimental models of sensitized lung[112] and that this was a beta receptor response.[113] Beta$_2$ agonists, such as terbutaline, also produced this effect.[114] Studies with highly purified human lung mast cell populations have recently confirmed that beta$_2$ agonists are more potent than sodium cromoglycate in stabilizing mast cells and that the receptor subtype involved is beta$_2$.[115] Clinical studies have supported the view that beta$_2$ agonists can prevent the release of mast cell mediators when the drugs are used in asthmatics sensitized to allergen.[116,117] Hence, until the hypothesis was recently challenged by Page,[118] the ability of sympathomimetic bronchodilator drugs to inhibit the release of mast cell mediators was considered to be an advantage especially when treating asthma where allergen was involved.

Mast cell mediators can undoubtedly contribute not only to acute bronchospasm but to inflammatory events in the airways, e.g., bronchial microvascular leakage and plasma exudation[119,120] and infiltration of airway tissue with proinflammatory cells.[121] Beta$_2$ agonists have been shown to attenuate the microvascular leakage effects of mediators in the tracheobronchial airways in animal models,[122,123] but more studies are needed to clarify their effects on proinflammatory cells, such as eosinophils. Also, the relevance of these observations in animals to clinical asthma has not yet been established. Thus, the recent promotion of salmeterol as a bronchodilator with anti-inflammatory properties when used in asthmatics, the latter being based on the ability of the drug to stabilize mast cells, inhibit eosinophil infiltration, and attenuate microvascular leakage in the airways in animal models, has been criticized.[124]

IV. CONCLUSIONS

The sympathomimetic bronchodilators have been used throughout this century to provide asthmatic patients with relief from their symptoms. Until the early 1950s most of the available drugs could not be given orally and they caused troublesome, and sometimes dangerous, side effects. The only orally active drug of note was ephedrine, which caused insomnia as an additional side effect.

There is no doubt that success in finding drugs with a more favorable profile of bronchodilator effects to cardiovascular side effects, first in the 1950s with the specific beta agonists and then in the 1970s with the beta$_2$-selective agonists, were significant milestones in the history of antiasthma drug therapy. Considerable effort and expenditure on basic and clinical research into beta agonist drugs continued throughout the 1970s and 1980s, the objective being to achieve a beta$_2$ agonist bronchodilator with ideal pharmacokinetic properties and no unwanted side effects. Yet 20 years after the development of salbutamol, terbutaline, and fenoterol, these drugs are still the main bronchodilator drugs being used for asthma. It is only in the last few years that any additional drugs in this pharmacological group have been commercialized, and these drugs have novel pharmacokinetic properties rather than any new pharmacological actions or side effect profiles.

Ever since their introduction into clinical use the beta receptor agonist drugs have been the subject of controversy, especially in relation to their safety in asthmatics, and in the 1990s this is still so. However, until the primary defects underlying asthma are fully understood, there will always be a need for bronchodilator drug therapy. At present, it is difficult to see how any of the alternative airway smooth muscle relaxant mechanisms that are being investigated could provide more effective and/or safer bronchodilators than beta$_2$ agonists considering the variety of spasmogens that are almost certainly released in asthmatic lungs. The need for beta$_2$ receptor agonist bronchodilators at the present time is thus not in doubt, but the way in which they are prescribed and used in asthma needs to be continually reassessed as our knowledge increases. In common with all the drug groups currently being used in the treatment of asthma, continuing basic and clinical research is needed if we are to define in detail the mechanisms responsible for the beneficial effects of beta$_2$ receptor agonists in the lungs of asthmatic patients.

ACKNOWLEDGMENTS

The research carried out by my group on beta receptor agonist drugs has received financial support for many years from the National Health and Medical Research Council of Australia. I gratefully acknowledge this financial support together with that of the many pharmaceutical companies that have also supported our research programs. I am especially grateful to my colleague, Dr. Janet Wanstall, who made significant contributions to our original research work with beta receptor agonist drugs. I would also like to thank Kellie Mundie for secretarial assistance.

REFERENCES

1. **Oliver, G. and Schäfer, E. A.,** The physiological effects of extracts of the suprarenal capsules, *J. Physiol.,* 18, 230, 1895.
2. **Takamine, J.,** The blood-pressure-raising principle of the suprarenal glands: a preliminary report, *Ther. Gazette,* 27, 221, 1901.
3. **Hartung, W. H.,** Epinephrine and related compounds: influence of structure on physiological activity, *Chem. Rev.,* 9, 389, 1931.
4. **Elliott, T. R.,** The action of adrenalin, *J. Physiol. (Lond.),* 32, 401, 1905.
5. **Von Euler, U. S.,** A specific sympathomimetic ergone in adrenergic nerve fibres (sympathin) and ergone in adrenergic nerve fibres (sympathin) and its relations to adrenaline and noradrenaline, *Acta Physiol. Scand.,* 12, 73, 1946.
6. **Solis-Cohen, S.,** The use of adrenal substance in the treatment of asthma, *JAMA,* 34, 1164, 1900.
7. **Bullowa, J. G. M. and Kaplan, D. M.,** On the hypodermic use of adrenalin chloride in the treatment of asthmatic attacks, *Med. News,* 83, 787, 1903.
8. **Goodman, L. S. and Gilman, A.,** *The Pharmacological Basis of Therapeutics,* 2nd ed., Macmillan, New York, 1958, 497.
9. **Persson, C. G. A.,** On the medical history of xanthines and other remedies for asthma: a tribute to HH Salter, *Thorax,* 40, 881, 1985.
10. **Barger, G. and Dale, H. H.,** Chemical structure and sympathomimetic action of amines, *J. Physiol.,* 41, 19, 1910.
11. **Burn, J. H. and Rand, M. J.,** The action of sympathomimetic amines in animals treated with reserpine, *J. Physiol. (London),* 144, 314, 1958.
12. **Tainter, M.,** Comparative actions of sympathomimetic compounds; phenyl and substituted phenyl derivatives; nonphenylic ring compounds and aliphatic amines, *Arch. Int. Pharmacodyn. Ther.,* 46, 192, 1933.
13. **Tainter, M. L., Pedden, J. R., and James, M.,** Comparative actions of sympathomimetic compounds: bronchodilator actions in perfused guinea pig lungs, *J. Pharmacol. Exp. Ther.,* 51, 371, 1934.
14. **Peddon, J. R., Tainter, M. L., and Cameron, W. M.,** Comparative actions of sympathomimetic compounds: bronchodilator actions in experimental bronchial spasm of parasympathetic origin, *J. Pharmacol. Exp. Ther.,* 55, 242, 1935.
15. **Cameron, W. M. and Tainter, M. L.,** Comparative actions of sympathomimetic compounds: bronchodilator actions in bronchial spasm induced by histamine, *J. Pharmacol. Exp. Ther.,* 57, 152, 1936.
16. **Becker, T. J., Warren, M. R., Marsh, D. G., Thompson, C. R., and Shelton, R. S.,** Pharmacological and toxicological studies on 1-N-ethylephedrine hydrochloride, *J. Pharmacol. Exp. Ther.,* 75, 289, 1942.
17. **Graham, B. E. and Cartland, G. F.,** Some comparative pharmacological actions of beta-hydroxy and methoxy phenyl-n-propylamines, *J. Pharmacol. Exp. Ther.,* 81, 360, 1944.
18. **Lands, A. M., Nash, V. L., McCarthy H. M., Granger, H. R., and Dertinger, B. L.,** The pharmacology of N-alkyl homologues of epinephrine, *J. Pharmacol. Exp. Ther.,* 90, 110, 1947.
19. **Lands, A. M., Nash, V. L., Dertinger, B. L., Granger, H. R., and McCarthy, H. M.,** The pharmacology of compounds structurally related to hydroxytyramine, *J. Pharmacol. Exp. Ther.,* 92, 369, 1948.

20. **Marsh, D. F., Pelletier, M. H., and Ross, G. A.,** The comparative pharmacology of the N-alkylarterenols, *J. Pharmacol. Exp. Ther.,* 92, 108, 1948.
21. **Siegmund, O. H., Granger, H. R., and Lands, A. M.,** The bronchodilator action of compounds structurally related to epinephrine, *J. Pharmacol. Exp. Ther.,* 90, 254, 1947.
22. **Chen, K. K. and Schmidt, C. F.,** The action of ephedrine: the active principle of the Chinese drug Ma Huang, *J. Pharmacol. Exp. Ther.,* 24, 339, 1924.
23. **Chen, K. K. and Schmidt, C. F.,** The action and clinical use of ephedrine, *JAMA,* 87, 836, 1926.
24. **Konzett, H.,** Neues zur Asthmatherapie, *Klin. Wochenschr.,* 19, 1303, 1940.
25. **Konzett, H.,** Neue broncholytisch hochivirksame Körper der Adrenalinreihe, *N.S. Arch. Exp. Path. Pharmak.,* 19, 629, 1940.
26. **Segal, M. S. and Beakey, J. F.,** Management of bronchial asthma: the use of 1-(3,4,dihydroxyphenyl)-2 isopropylaminoethanol, *Ann. Allergy,* 5, 317, 1947.
27. **Gay, L. N. and Long, J. W.,** Clinical evaluation of isopropyl-epinephrine in management of bronchial asthma, *JAMA,* 139, 452, 1949.
28. **Ahlquist, R. P.,** A study of the adrenotropic receptors, *Am. J. Physiol.,* 153, 586, 1948.
29. **Nickerson, M. and Goodman, L. S.,** Pharmacological properties of a new adrenergic blocking agent: N, N-dibenzyl-β-chloroethylamine (dibenamine), *J. Pharmacol. Exp. Ther.,* 89, 167, 1947.
30. **Ehrlich, P.,** On immunity with special reference to cell life, *Proc. R. Soc. London Ser. B,* 66, 424, 1900.
31. **Langley, J. N.,** On the reaction of cells and of nerve-endings to certain poisons, chiefly as regards the reaction of striated muscle to nicotine and to curari, *J. Physiol. (London),* 33, 374, 1905.
32. **Dale, H. H.,** On some physiological actions of ergot, *J. Physiol.,* 34, 163, 1906.
33. **Cannon, W. B. and Rosenblueth, A.,** Studies on conditions of activity in endocrine organs. XXIX. Sympathin E and Sympathin I, *Am. J. Physiol.,* 104, 557, 1933.
34. **Ahlquist, R. P.,** Adrenoceptors: from figment to fact, *Trends Auton. Pharmacol.,* 2, 3, 1982.
35. **Ahlquist, R. P.,** The adrenergic receptor, *J. Pharm. Sci.,* 55, 359, 1966.
36. **Powell, C. E. and Slater, I. H.,** Blocking of inhibitory adrenergic receptors by a dichloroanalog of isoproterenol, *J. Pharmacol. Exp. Ther.,* 122, 480, 1958.
37. **Black, J. W. and Stephenson, J. S.,** Pharmacology of a new adrenergic beta-receptor-blocking compound (nethalide), *Lancet,* 2, 311, 1962.
38. **Black, J. W., Crowther, A. F., Shanks, R. G., Smith, L. H., and Dornhorst, A. C.,** A new adrenergic beta-receptor antagonist, *Lancet,* 1, 1080, 1964.
39. **Furchgott, R. F.,** The receptors for epinephrine and norepinephrine (adrenergic receptors), *Pharmacol. Rev.,* 11, 429, 1959.
40. **Herschfus, J. A.,** A new sympathomimetic amine (''Neosupril'') in the treatment of bronchial asthma, *Ann. Allergy,* 9, 769, 1951.
41. **Christensen, J. M., Valasek, F. E., and Tainter, M. L.,** Ethylnorepinephrine: a unique bronchodilator, *Am. Pract. Dig. Treat.,* 9, 916, 1958.
42. **Engelhardt, A., Hoefke, W., and Wick, H.,** Zum pharmakologie des sympathomimeticums 1-(3,5-dihydroxyphenyl)-1-hydroxy-2-isopropylaminoäthan, *Arzneim. Forsch.,* 11, 521, 1961.
43. **Gunther, W.,** Experimental spirographic studies with 1-(3,5-dihydroxyphenyl)-2-isopropylaminoethanol sulphate as a therapeutic aerosol, *Arzneim. Forsch.,* 12, 1127, 1962.
44. **Kennedy, M. C. S.,** A new bronchodilator drug: Alupent (Th 152), *Br. J. Clin. Pract.,* 17, 563, 1963.
45. **Dungan, K. W., Cho, Y. W., Gomoll, A. W., Aviado, D. M., and Lish, P. M.,** Pharmacologic potency and selectivity of a new bronchodilator agent: soterenol (MJ 1992), *J. Pharmacol. Exp. Ther.,* 164, 290, 1968.
46. **Leifer, K. N. and Wittig, H. J.,** The beta-2 sympathomimetic aerosols in the treatment of asthma, *Ann. Allergy,* 35, 69, 1975.

47. **Brittain, R. T., Farmer, J. B., and Jack, D. J.,** α-(t-butylamino)-methyl-4-hydroxy-m-xylene-α^1, α^3-diol (AH 3365): a selective β-adrenergic stimulant, *Nature,* 219, 862, 1968.
48. **Hartley, D., Jack, D., Lunts, L. H. T., and Ritchie, A. C.,** New class of selective stimulants of β-adrenergic receptors, *Nature (London),* 219, 861, 1968.
49. **Wetterlin, K. I. L. and Svensson, L.-Å.,** Belgium patent No. 704932, 1968.
50. **Bergman, J., Persson, H., and Wetterlin, K.,** Two new groups of selective stimulants of adrenergic β-receptors, *Experientia,* 25, 899, 1969.
51. **Persson, H. and Olsson, T.,** Some pharmacological properties of terbutaline (INN), 1-(3,5-dihydroxyphenyl)-2-(t-butylamino)-ethanol, a new sympathomimetic β-receptor-stimulating agent, *Acta Med. Scand.* [Suppl.], 512, 11, 1970.
52. **Kennedy, M. C. S. and Simpson, W. T.,** Human pharmacological and clinical studies on salbutamol: a specific β-adrenergic bronchodilator, *Br. J. Dis. Chest,* 63, 165, 1969.
53. **Cullum, V. A., Farmer, J. B., Jack, D., and Levy, G. P.,** Salbutamol: a new, selective β-adrenoreceptive receptor stimulant, *Br. J. Pharmacol.,* 35, 141, 1969.
54. **Formgren, H.,** A clinical comparison of the effect of oral terbutaline and orciprenaline, *Scand. J. Respir. Dis.,* 51, 195, 1970.
55. **Freedman, B. J.,** Trial of new bronchodilator, terbutaline, in asthma, *Br. Med. J.,* 1, 633, 1971.
56. **O'Donnell, S. R.,** A selective β-adrenoreceptor stimulant (Th1165a) related to orciprenaline, *Eur. J. Pharmacol.,* 12, 35, 1970.
57. **Powles, A. C. P.,** The bronchodilator effect of fenoterol (Berotec), *N.Z. Med. J.,* 81, 249, 1975.
58. **Blackhall, M. I., Dauth, M., Mahoney, M., and O'Donnell, S. R.,** Inhalation of fenoterol (Berotec) by asthmatic children: a clinical comparison with salbutamol, orciprenaline and isoprenaline, *Med. J. Aust.,* 2, 439, 1976.
59. **Brittain, R. T., Dean, C. M., and Jack, D.,** Sympathomimetic bronchodilator drugs, *Pharmacol. Ther.,* 2, 423, 1976.
60. **O'Donnell, S. R.,** An examination of some β-adrenoreceptor stimulants for selectivity using the isolated trachea and atria of the guinea-pig, *Eur. J. Pharmacol.,* 19, 371, 1972.
61. **O'Donnell, S. R. and Wanstall, J. C.,** Potency and selectivity *in vitro* of compounds related to isoprenaline and orciprenaline on β-adrenoceptors in the guinea-pig, *Br. J. Pharmacol.,* 52, 407, 1974.
62. **Lands, A. M.,** The pharmacological activity of epinephrine and related dihydroxyphenylalkylamines, *Pharmacol. Rev.,* 1, 279, 1949.
63. **Lands, A. M., Arnold, A., McAuliff, J. P., Ludena, F. P., and Brown, T. G.,** Differentiation of receptor systems activated by sympathomimetic amines, *Nature (London),* 214, 597, 1967.
64. **Lands, A. M., Luduena, F. P., and Buzzo, H. J.,** Differentiation of receptors responsive to isoproterenol, *Life Sci.,* 6, 2241, 1967.
65. **Furchgott, R. F.,** Postsynaptic adrenergic receptor mechanisms in vascular smooth muscle, in *Vascular Neuroeffector Mechanisms, 2nd International Symposium,* Bevan J. A., Ed., Karger, Basel, 1976, 131.
66. **O'Donnell, S. R.,** β-adrenoceptor classification in the respiratory tract, *Trends Auton. Pharmacol.,* 3, 1, 1985.
67. **Bryan, L. J., Cole, J. J., O'Donnell, S. R., and Wanstall, J. C.,** A study designed to explore the hypothesis that *beta*-1 adrenoceptors are "innervated" and *beta*-2 adrenoceptors are "hormonal" receptors, *J. Pharmacol. Exp. Ther.,* 216, 395, 1981.
68. **Kennedy, M. C. S. and Dash, C. H.,** The bronchodilator effect of a new adrenergic aerosol — salmefamol, *Acta Allergy,* 27, 22, 1972.
69. **Wardell, J. R., Colella, D. F., Shetline, A., and Fowler, P. J.,** Studies on carbuterol (SK&F 40383-A), a new selective bronchodilator agent, *J. Pharmacol. Exp. Ther.,* 189, 167, 1974.

70. **Steen, S. N., Ziment, I., and Thomas, J. S.,** Pyrbuterol: a new bronchodilator. Phase I — single dose study. *Curr. Ther. Res.,* 16, 1077, 1974.
71. **O'Donnell, S. R.,** Selectivity of clenbuterol (NAB 365) in guinea-pig isolated tissues containing β-adrenoceptors, *Arch. Int. Pharmacodyn. Ther.,* 224, 190, 1976.
72. **Baronte, A., Gireco, A., and Vibelli, C. A.,** A comparison between inhaled clenbuterol and salbutamol in chronic bronchitis with reversible airways obstruction, *Eur. J. Respir. Dis.,* 61, 143, 1980.
73. **O'Donnell, S. R. and Wanstall, J. C.,** Some aspects of the trachea-heart selectivity of rimiterol *in vitro* and *in vivo* in guinea-pigs, *Arch. Int. Pharmacodyn. Ther.,* 226, 214, 1977.
74. **Eriksson, N. E. and Lindgren, S. B.,** The rapidity of bronchodilatation: a comparison of isoprenaline, terbutaline and rimiterol, *Scand. J. Respir. Dis.,* 59, 30, 1978.
75. **O'Donnell, S. R. and Wanstall, J. C.,** Hexoprenaline: β-adrenoreceptor selectivity in isolated tissues from the guinea-pig, *Clin. Exp. Pharmacol. Physiol.,* 2, 541, 1975.
76. **Schonell, M., Harris, M., McMiken, D., Jenne, H., and Evers, R.,** Bronchodilator effects of hexoprenaline aerosol in bronchial asthma and chronic bronchitis, *Med. J. Aust.,* 2, 828, 1977.
77. **Scriabine, A., Moor, P. F., Ioro, L. C., Goldman, I. M., McShane, W. K., and Booker, K. D.,** Quinterenol, a new beta adrenergic stimulant, *J. Pharmacol. Exp. Ther.,* 162, 60, 1968.
78. **Minneman, K. P., Hedberg, A., and Molinoff, P. B.,** Comparison of *beta* adrenergic receptor subtypes in mammalian tissues, *J. Pharmacol. Exp. Ther.,* 211, 502, 1979.
79. **Yabuuchi, Y.,** The β-adrenoceptor stimulant properties of OPC-2009 on guinea-pig isolated tracheal, right atrial and left atrial preparations, *Br. J. Pharmacol.,* 61, 513, 1977.
80. **O'Donnell, S. R. and Wanstall, J. C.,** Responses to the β2-selective agonist procaterol of vascular and atrial preparations with different functional β-adrenoceptor populations, *Br. J. Pharmacol.,* 84, 227, 1985.
81. **Waldeck, B., Olsson, O. A. T., and Svensson, L.-Å.,** New possibilities for the β-adrenoceptor agonist bronchodilator drugs, in *New Anti-asthma Drugs,* O'Donnell, S. R. and Persson, C. G. A., Eds., Birkhäuser-Verlag, Basel, *Agents and Actions,* Suppl. 23, 1988, 55.
82. **Harris, L.,** Comparison of the effects on blood gases, ventilation and perfusion of isoproterenol, phenylephrine and salbutamol in chronic bronchitis with asthma, *J. Allergy Clin. Immunol.,* 49, 63, 1972.
83. **O'Donnell, S. R. and Wanstall, J. C.,** The contribution of extraneuronal uptake to the trachea-blood vessel selectivity of β-adrenoceptor stimulants *in vitro* in guinea-pigs, *Br. J. Pharmacol.,* 57, 369, 1976.
84. **Olsson, O. A. T., Swanberg, E., Svedinger, I., and Waldeck, B.,** Effects of β-adrenoceptor agonists on airway smooth muscle and on slow-contracting skeletal muscle: *in vitro* and *in vivo* results compared, *Acta Pharmacol. Toxicol.,* 44, 272, 1979.
85. **Apperley, G. H. M., Daly, M. J., and Levy, G. P.,** Selectivity of β-adrenoceptor agonists and antagonists on bronchial, skeletal, vascular and cardiac muscle in the anaesthetized cat, *Br. J. Pharmacol.,* 57, 235, 1976.
86. **Anderson, P., Olsson, O. A. T., and Waldeck, B.,** Some problems encountered in the evaluation of new bronchodilating β-adrenoceptor agonists, *Acta Pharmacol. Toxicol.,* 51, 358, 1982.
87. **Lofdahl, C.-G., Bengtsson, B., Svedmyr, K., and Svedmyr, N.,** Two new β2-adrenoceptor agonists, D 2343 and QH 25, studied in asthmatic patients, *Allergy,* 37, 351, 1982.
88. **Waldeck, B., Jeppsson, A.-B., and Widmark, E.,** Partial agonism and functional selectivity: a study on β-adrenoceptor mediated effects in tracheal, cardiac and skeletal muscle, *Acta Pharmacol. Toxicol.,* 58, 209, 1986.

89. **Hegardt, B., Pauwels, R., and Van der Streten, M.,** Inhibitory effect of KWD 2131, terbutaline and DSCG on the immediate and late allergen-induced bronchoconstriction, *Allergy,* 36, 115, 1981.
90. **Newman, S. P., Moren, F., Trofast, E., Talaee, N., and Clarke, S. W.,** Deposition and clinical efficacy of terbutaline sulphate from Turbuhaler, a new multi-dose powder inhaler, *Eur. Respir. J.,* 2, 247, 1989.
91. **Ida, H.,** Comparison of the action of BD 40A and some other β-adrenoceptor stimulants on the isolated trachea and atria of the guinea pig, *Arzneim. Forsch.,* 26, 839, 1976.
92. **Ida, H.,** Cardiorespiratory activities of 3-formylamino-4-hydroxy-α(N-1-methyl-2-p-methoxyphenylethylaminomethyl)-benzyl alcohol-hemifumarate (BD 40A) and some other β-adrenoceptor stimulants in conscious guinea pigs, *Arzneim. Forsch.,* 26, 1337, 1976.
93. **Campbell, I. A., Dash, C. H., McHardy, G. J. R., and Shoffer, M. W.,** Comparison of salmefamol and salbutamol in patients with chronic airways obstruction, *Br. J. Clin. Pharmacol.,* 3, 151, 1971.
94. **Anderson, G. P.,** Pharmacology of formoterol: an innovative bronchodilator, in *New Drugs for Asthma Therapy,* Anderson, G. P., Chapman, I. D., and Morley, J., Eds., Birkhäuser-Verlag, Basel, *Agents and Actions,* Suppl. 34, 1991, 97.
95. **Lofdahl, C.-G. and Svedmyr, N.,** Formoterol fumarate, a new β_2-adrenoceptor agonist, *Allergy,* 44, 264, 1989.
96. **Sykes, A. P. and Ayres, J. G.,** A study of the duration of the bronchodilator effect of 12μg and 24μg of inhaled formoterol and 200μg inhaled salbutamol in asthma, *Respir. Med.,* 84, 135, 1990.
97. **Wallin, A., Melander, B., Rosenhall, L., Sandström, T., and Wåhlander, L.,** Formoterol, a new long acting $beta_2$ agonist for inhalation twice daily, compared with salbutamol in the treatment of asthma, *Thorax,* 45, 259, 1990.
98. **Jeppson, A.-B., Löfdahl, C.-G., Waldeck, B., and Widmark, E.,** On the predictive value of experiments in vitro in the evaluation of the effect duration of bronchodilator drugs for local administration, *Pulm. Pharmacol.,* 2, 81, 1989.
99. **Johnson, M.,** Salmeterol, a novel drug for the treatment of asthma, in *New Drugs for Asthma Therapy,* Anderson, G. P., Chapman, I. D., and Morley, J., Eds., Birkhäuser-Verlag, Basel, *Agents and Actions,* Suppl. 34, 1991, 79.
100. **Ball, D. I., Brittain, R. T., Coleman, R. A., Denyer, L. H., Jack, D., Johnson, M., Lunts, L. H. C., Nials, A. T., Sheldrick, K. E., and Skidmore, I. F.,** Salmeterol, a novel long-acting β_2-adrenoceptor agonist: characterization of pharmacological activity *in vitro* and *in vivo, Br. J. Pharmacol.,* 104, 665, 1991.
101. **Ullman, A. and Svedmyr, N.,** Salmeterol, a new long acting inhaled β_2-adrenoceptor agonist: comparison with salbutamol in adult asthmatic patients, *Thorax,* 43, 674, 1988.
102. **Löfdahl, C.-G. and Chung, K. F.,** Long-acting β_2-adrenoceptor agonists: a new perspective in the treatment of asthma, *Eur. Respir. J.,* 4, 218, 1991.
103. **Brittain, R. T.,** Approaches to a long-acting selective β2-adrenoceptor stimulant, *Eur. Respir., J.,* 2, 200, 1989.
104. **Turkheim, K. and Kraupp, O.,** Pulmonary and systemic circulatory effects and β-adrenergic selectivity of hexoprenaline, salbutamol, oxyfedrine and isoproterenol, *Eur. J. Pharmacol.,* 15, 231, 1971.
105. **Kass, I. and Mingo, T. S.,** Bitolaterol mesylate (WIN 32784) aerosol: a new long acting bronchodilator with reduced chronotropic effects, *Chest,* 78, 283, 1980.
106. **Minatoya, H.,** Studies on Bitolterol, Di-*p*-toluate ester of N-*tert.*-butylarterenol: a new long-acting bronchodilator with reduced cardiovascular effects, *J. Pharmacol. Exp. Ther.,* 206, 515, 1978.
107. **Svensson, L.-Å.,** Sympathomimetic bronchodilators: increased selectivity with lung-specific prodrugs, *Pharmaceutical Res.,* 4, 156, 1985.
108. **Hornblad, Y., Ripe, E., Magnusson, P. O., and Tegner, K.,** The metabolism and clinical activity of terbutaline and its prodrug ibuterol, *Eur. J. Clin. Pharmacol.,* 10, 9, 1975.

109. **Olsson, O. A. T. and Svensson, L.-Å.,** New lipophilic terbutaline ester prodrugs with long effect duration, *Pharmaceutical Res.,* 1, 19, 1984.
110. **Svensson, L.-Å.,** Bambuterol, a bronchodilator prodrug with sustained action, enhances delivery of active drug to the lung, in *Directions for New Anti-Asthma Drugs,* O'Donnell, S. R. and Persson, C. G. A., Eds., Birkhäuser-Verlag, Basel, *Agents and Actions,* Suppl. 23, 1988, 271.
111. **Svensson, L.-Å.,** Mechanism of action of bambuterol: a β-agonist prodrug with sustained lung affinity, in *New Drugs for Asthma Therapy,* Andersson, G. P., Chapman, I. D., and Morley, J., Eds., Birkhäuser-Verlag, Basel, *Agents and Actions,* Suppl. 34, 1991, 71.
112. **Assem, E. S. K.,** Adrenergic mechanisms and immediate-type allergy, *Clin. Allergy,* 4, 185, 1974.
113. **Assem, E. S. K. and Schild, H. O. J.,** Antagonism by β-adrenoceptor blocking agents of the antianaphylactic effect of isoprenaline, *Br. J. Pharmacol.,* 42, 620, 1971.
114. **Sörenby, L.,** Inhibition of the antigen-induced release of histamine from guinea-pig lung by terbutaline, *Acta Pharmacol. Toxicol.,* 34, 267, 1974.
115. **Church, M. K. and Hiroi, J.,** Inhibition of IgE dependent histamine release from human dispersed mast cells by anti-allergic drugs and salbutamol, *Br. J. Pharmacol.,* 90, 421, 1987.
116. **Howarth, P. H., Durham, S. R., Lee, T. H., Kay, B., Church, M. K., and Holgate, S. T.,** Influence of albuterol, cromolyn sodium and ipratropium bromide on the airway and circulatory mediator responses to allergen bronchial provocation in asthma, *Am. Rev. Respir. Dis.,* 132, 986, 1985.
117. **Sheinman, B. D., Moran, D. J. R., Cundell, D. R., Smart, W., and Davies, R. J.,** Effects of inhaled salbutamol and sodium cromoglycate on mediator release in immediate asthma, in *Asthma and Bronchial Hyperreactivity,* Herzog, H. and Perruchoud, A. P., Eds., Karger, Basel, 1985, 56.
118. **Page, C. P.,** One explanation of the asthma paradox: inhibition of natural anti-inflammatory mechanism by β_2-agonists, *Lancet,* 337, 717, 1991.
119. **O'Donnell, S. R.,** Airway microvascular permeability in asthma: a target for drug action?, in *New Anti-Asthma Drugs,* O'Donnell, S. R. and Persson, C. G. A., Eds., Birkhäuser-Verlag, Basel, *Agents and Actions,* Suppl. 23, 1988, 217.
120. **Persson, C. G. A.,** Leakage of macromolecules from the tracheobronchial microcirculation, *Am. Rev. Respir. Dis.,* 135, S71, 1987.
121. **Sanjar, S., Colditz, I., Aoki, S., Boubekeur, K., and Morley, J.,** Pharmacological modulation of eosinophil accumulation in guinea-pig airways, in *Eosinophils in Asthma,* Morley, J. and Colditz, I., Eds., Academic Press, London, *Perspectives in Asthma,* Vol. 4, 1989, 201.
122. **Erjefält, I. and Persson, C. G. A.,** Pharmacologic control of plasma exudation into tracheobronchial airways, *Am. Rev. Respir. Dis.,* 143, 1008, 1991.
123. **O'Donnell, S. R.,** Pharmacology of β-adrenoceptors in lung disease, in *Adrenoceptors: Structure, Mechanisms, Function,* Szabadi, E. and Bradshaw, C. M., Eds., Birkhäuser-Verlag, Basel, *Advances in Pharmacological Science,* 1991, 265.
124. **Crompton, G. K.,** β_2 agonists in asthma (Letter to the editor), *Lancet,* 337, 45, 1991.

Section 2
Studies of Time Trends in Asthma Mortality

Chapter 2

A CENTURY OF ASTHMA MORTALITY

Rodney T. Jackson

TABLE OF CONTENTS

0-8493-6761-1/93/$0.00 + $.50

This is the first of two chapters that discuss international time trends in asthma mortality and their relationship to sales of beta agonist drugs. In this chapter, the time trends in asthma mortality over the past century are examined, which include gradual changes in mortality and asthma mortality epidemics. The validity of the data is discussed, and possible explanations for the trends are examined. In Chapter 3, Stolley focuses on the epidemiological approach to studying asthma mortality epidemics, and shows how this can give rise to hypotheses about the hazards of specific beta agonists, such as isoprenaline and fenoterol. The methodology of analytical epidemiological studies to investigate such hypotheses is discussed in Chapters 4 and 5.

I. INTRODUCTION

Studies of time trends in asthma mortality have been stimulated by two recent epidemics of asthma death: one reported in several countries during the mid-1960s[1] and a second isolated to New Zealand during the late 1970s.[2] National and international mortality trend data have been used to generate hypotheses subsequently tested in analytic studies. These data have also directly influenced government policy;[3] for example, over-the-counter sales of aerosolized isoprenaline were banned in the United Kingdom in the mid-1960s after reports associated sales of these drugs with national trends in asthma mortality.[1]

Associations based on ecological data, such as national mortality trends and drug sales, are not considered strong evidence for judging causality given the considerable potential for confounding and other methodological problems when data come from groups rather than individuals. Nevertheless, the usefulness of ecological data is often underestimated. When mortality rates differ substantially between populations and over time within populations, useful causal inferences can often be made. Moreover, ecological data may be the only data available when policy decisions have to be made. This is particularly the case for relatively uncommon events, such as asthma death, when studies in individuals may not be easy or even feasible.

Throughout the chapter emphasis is placed on data restricted to younger age groups (typically 5 to 34 years) because the diagnosis of asthma death is considered to be most clear-cut in this group and therefore less susceptible to misclassification and changes in diagnostic fashion over time.

II. ASTHMA MORTALITY TIME TRENDS

A. GENERAL TRENDS

Most recent epidemiological reviews of asthma mortality have restricted their period of observation to the last 30 or so years. There are a number of methodological issues that arise when longer-term trends are examined. In

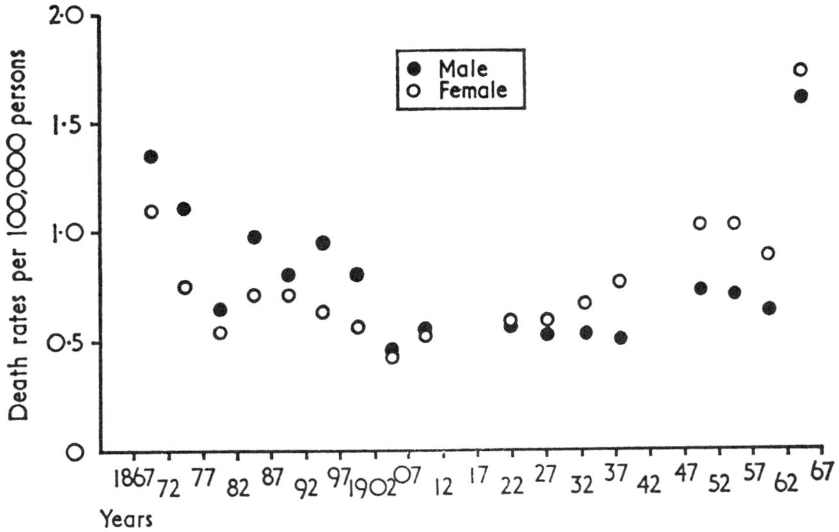

FIGURE 1. Death rates from asthma for England and Wales, 1867–1967, in males and females 5 to 34 years of age. (From Speizer, F. E. and Doll, R., *Br. Med. J.*, 3, 245, 1968. With permission.)

particular, changes in diagnostic fashions and death classification criteria over time can seriously affect the validity of trend data based on routinely collected national and international mortality statistics. Nevertheless, several authors have reviewed asthma mortality trends before 1960 and although these data need to be interpreted with particular caution, they help to place recent mortality changes in a historical perspective.

Speizer and Doll examined asthma mortality in the 5–34 year age group in England and Wales for the period 1867–1967 (Figure 1).[4] Data for the years covered by World War I and World War II were omitted because of the possible effect on mortality of selection of young people for the armed forces. Reported asthma mortality declined substantially between 1867 and 1902 followed by a period of relative stability until the late 1930s. Rates in the 1950s were consistently higher than in the 1940s; however, the most striking feature this century was the sudden dramatic increase in deaths in the mid-1960s. The authors also noted that male rates were higher than female rates before 1920, but subsequently female rates were consistently higher than for males until the 1960s epidemic.

Burney also reviewed asthma deaths in 5–34 year olds in England and Wales, but for the period 1931–1985.[5] Figure 2 illustrates even more clearly than Figure 1 the unusual character of mortality trends in the mid-1960s. After a 30-year period of relative stability, reported asthma mortality increased approximately threefold in 3 years and then subsided at a similarly dramatic rate. Between 1970 and 1976, reported asthma mortality continued to decline,

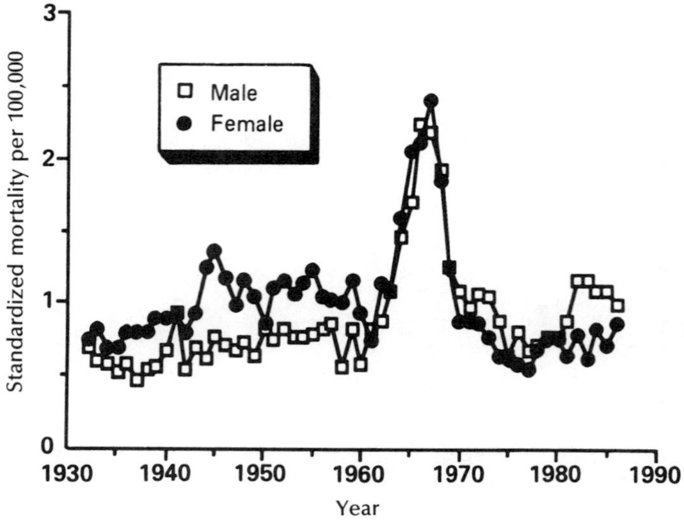

FIGURE 2. Age standardized mortality from asthma among 5–34 year olds in England and Wales 1931–1985. (From Burney, P., *J. Epidemiol. Community Health,* 42, 316, 1988. With permission.)

but at a slower rate. However, since then there appears to have been a slow but steady increase in deaths, particularly in males. Figure 2 also shows the sex differences in mortality described by Speizer and Doll,[4] as well as a new pattern emerging after the 1960s epidemic, with male mortality again predominating. Although mortality in the period before the mid-1960s was relatively stable, there is some indication of an increase in reported asthma deaths during the 1940s and 1950s, particularly in females.

Trends in asthma mortality in Australia between 1908 and 1965 were reported by Gandevia for the age group 5–54 years and for all ages (Figure 3).[6] These data are not strictly comparable with the data from Figures 1 and 2 because of the different age groups examined. The importance of defining the appropriate age group is highlighted by the differences in trends between the restricted and unrestricted age groups shown in Figure 3. Asthma mortality increases with age and as reported by Gandevia,[6] mortality in the older age groups are more susceptible to the effects of disease-coding changes. This is well illustrated in Figure 3, which shows an apparent abrupt threefold increase in mortality for the all ages category about 1950 followed by a sudden decline in the late 1950s. Gandevia[6] attributed this apparent epidemic to coding changes. In the 5–54 year age group there was a steady increase in reported mortality between about 1940 and 1962 followed by the more dramatic increase in 1964. The sex differences are consistent with the English data; male rates are higher before 1930, followed by a female predominance until the 1960s.

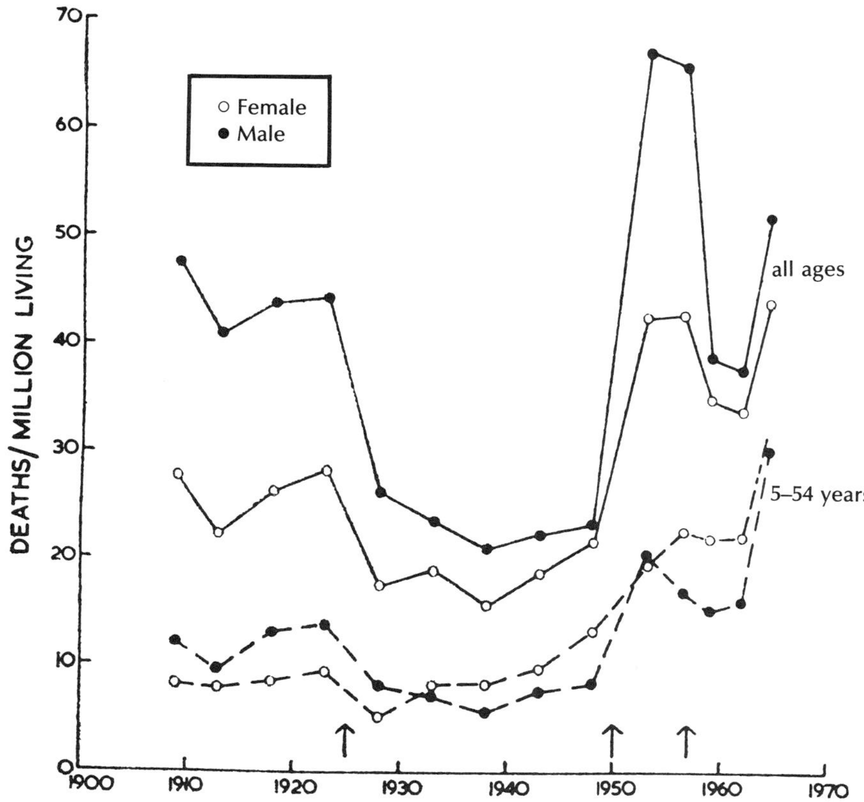

FIGURE 3. Mortality from asthma for the period 1908–1965 in Australia. (From Gandevia, B., *Med. J. Aust.*, 1, 747, 1968. With permission.)

The most recent review of long-term national trends in reported asthma mortality is based on New Zealand data. Beasley et al. examined reported asthma deaths in 5–34 year old non-Maori New Zealanders for the period 1908–1986 (Figure 4).[7] As in the United Kingdom and Australia, the mortality rate in the first 35 to 40 years of this century was relatively stable. Reported asthma mortality increased steadily through the 1940s and early 1950s following the Australian pattern, but then peaked in 1955–1956 at a level approximately three times the 1940 rate. The death rate subsequently declined, reaching a plateau in the late 1950s, which was still twice the 1940 rate. Between 1959 and 1965, mortality remained relatively stable and then, following the pattern that had occurred in the United Kingdom and Australia several years earlier, albeit more dramatically, mortality almost tripled in one year. This was by far the largest short-term increase in asthma mortality observed in New Zealand over a 60-year period. The subsequent decline in mortality was also dramatic, but New Zealand later experienced a second epidemic in the late 1970s.

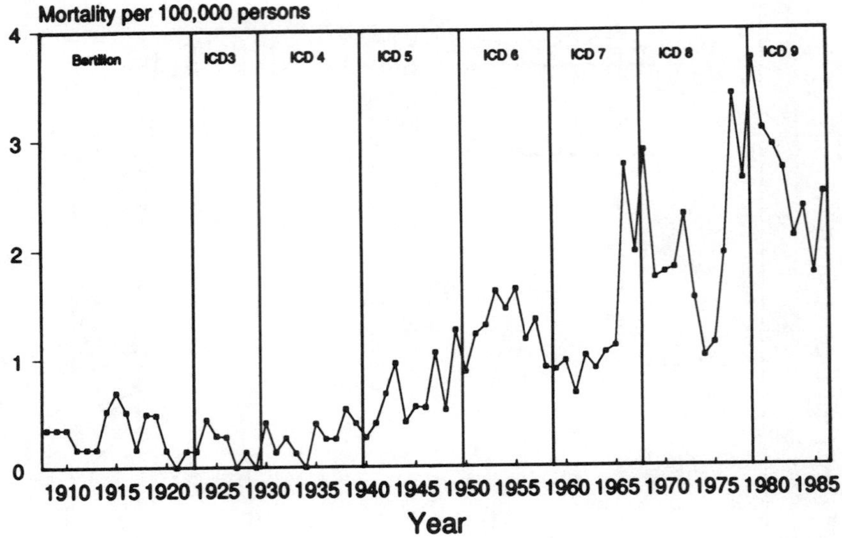

FIGURE 4. Asthma mortality in non-Maori 5–34 year olds in New Zealand, 1910–1985. (From Beasley, R., Smith, K., Pearce, N., Crane, J., and Burgess, C., *Med. J. Aust.*, 157, 570, 1990. With permission.)

B. THE 1960s EPIDEMICS

The striking increase in asthma mortality in the United Kingdom in the early 1960s, followed by similar trends in Ireland, Australia, New Zealand, and to a lesser extent in Norway, has been reviewed in numerous publications. The most comprehensive examination of international trends in asthma mortality through the 1960s and early 1970s was conducted by Stolley and Schinnar.[8,9] Figure 5 compares asthma mortality rates in the 5–34 year age group in six countries between 1959 and 1979, illustrating the different mortality patterns in epidemic and nonepidemic countries. As previously indicated, a substantial increase in asthma mortality during the 1960s also occurred in the Republic of Ireland and Norway. Stolley reviewed mortality rates in a total of 14 countries and showed that the epidemic appeared to have been limited to those aforementioned countries.[8]

C. THE SECOND NEW ZEALAND EPIDEMIC

By the early 1970s the epidemics had waned in most countries except perhaps New Zealand where mortality remained about twice the pre-epidemic level. Then in 1981, Wilson et al. reported a possible increase in asthma mortality in Auckland, New Zealand,[10] which stimulated a comprehensive update of international trends in asthma deaths.[2] The increase in New Zealand deaths was confirmed (Figure 5) and showed that after a downward trend in mortality from the late 1960s until the mid-1970s, an even more dramatic increase in asthma deaths than in the 1960s epidemic occurred. The death

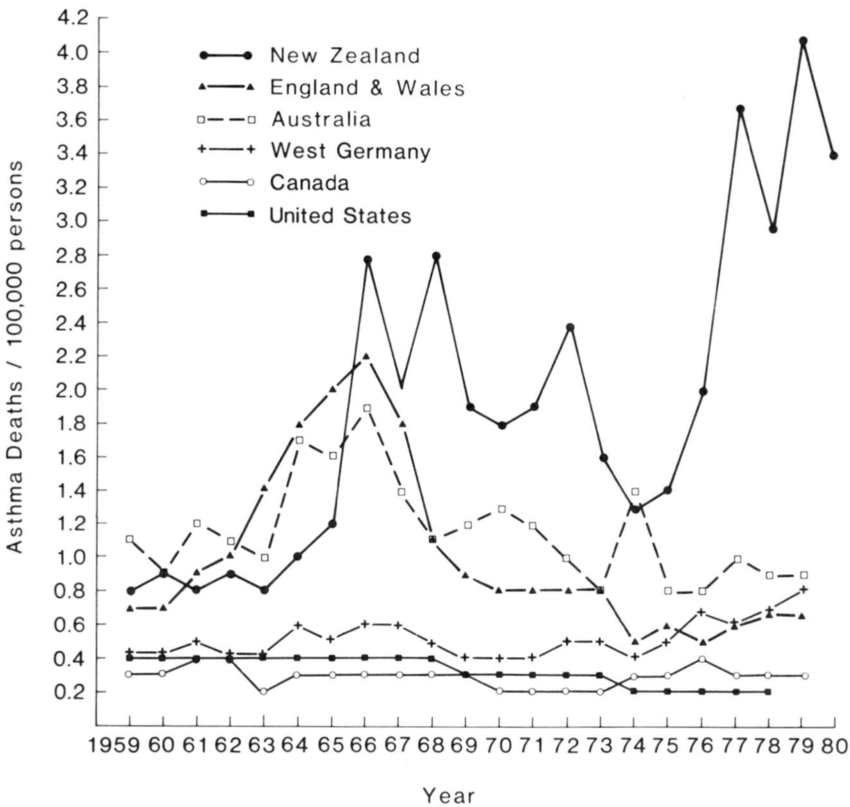

FIGURE 5. Asthma mortality in 5–34 year olds in six countries during 1959–1979. (From Jackson, R. T., Beaglehole, R., Rea, H. H., and Sutherland, D. C., *Br. Med. J.*, 285, 771, 1982. With permission.)

rate in 5–34 year olds in New Zealand increased more than 3-fold between 1974–1975 and 1977. The peak occurred in 1979 (Figure 4) at 4.1 deaths per 100,000 and (as in the 1960s epidemic) subsided rapidly, although until 1989 mortality remained between 2 and 3 deaths per 100,000, which was more than twice the pre-1960 level.[7]

D. RECENT GENERAL TRENDS

Although no other country appeared to experience a similar epidemic, slow and steady increases in mortality have been reported. A review of international trends in reported asthma mortality between 1970 and 1985 among 5–34 year olds in 14 countries demonstrated an increase in most countries examined.[11] Increases of more than 15% between 1976–1978 and 1982–1984 were seen in 10 of the 14 countries. A recent update of these data for five countries (Figure 6) shows the gradual increase in reported mortality

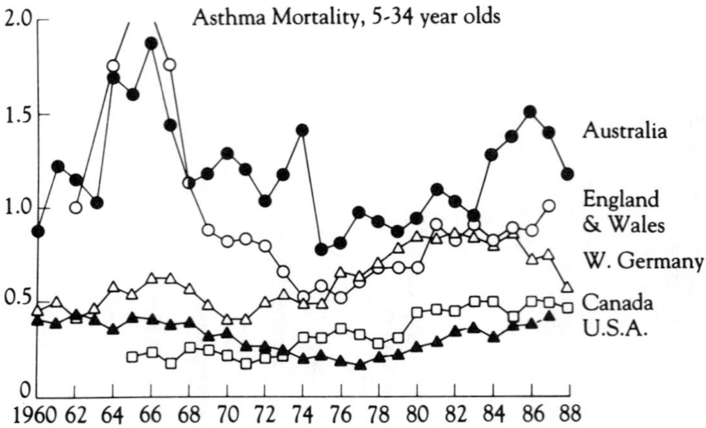

FIGURE 6. Trends in asthma mortality in 5–34 year olds in five countries during 1960–1988. (From Sears, M. R., *Proc. 2nd Natl. Asthma Epidemiology Workshop,* Ruffin, R. E., Ed., *Excerpta Medica,* Sydney, 1990. With permission.)

in the United States and Canada, and more substantial increases in Australia, West Germany, and England and Wales.[12]

It should be noted that most of the mortality data presented herein refers to 5–34 year olds because of issues relating to accuracy of diagnosis (see Figures 3 and 7). However, asthma mortality increases with age and despite the overdiagnosis of asthma death in older age groups, the major public health burden of asthma death will be among those older than 35 years. The epidemics of the mid-1960s and late 1980s did occur in all age groups,[12] although the relative increase in mortality during the epidemics was much greater in the younger age groups. In the mid-1980s asthma mortality in 5–34 year olds in New Zealand was approximately 2 to 3 per 100,000, whereas for all ages the mortality was 6 to 7 per 100,000.[12]

III. VALIDITY OF MORTALITY DATA

The validity and, therefore, the usefulness of examining trends based on routinely collected national mortality statistics depend primarily on the accuracy of death certificate diagnoses, changes in disease classification, and changes in diagnostic fashions.

A. ACCURACY OF DEATH CERTIFICATES

Several studies have examined the accuracy of the diagnosis of asthma on death certificates. This is generally done by formal review of information on the medical history and circumstances of death in individuals certified as having died of asthma. The New Zealand National Asthma Study reviewed all deaths certified as due to asthma in New Zealand for the 2-year period

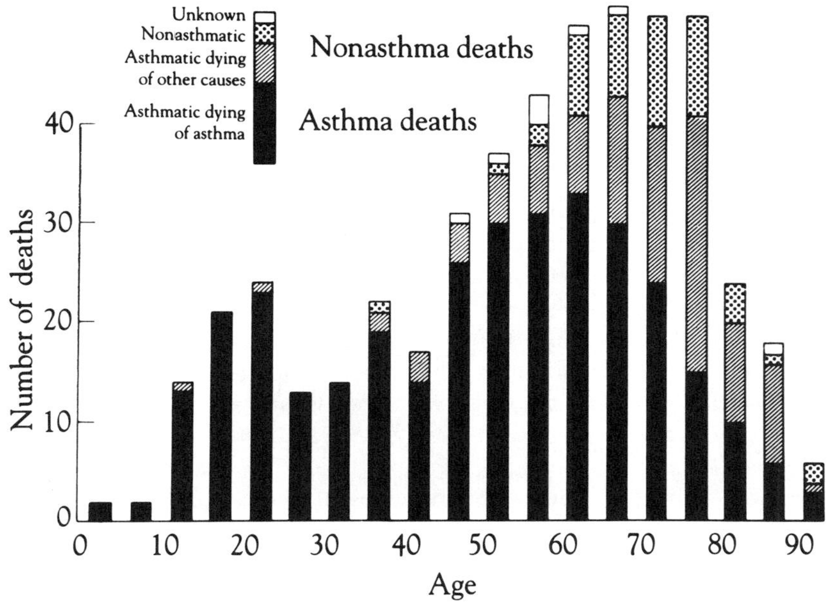

FIGURE 7. Accuracy of certification of asthma deaths as judged by a review panel of physicians, of 492 cases with asthma in Part 1 of the death certificate or on the coroner's report of cause of death. (From Sears, M. R., *Proc. 2nd Natl. Asthma Epidemiology Workshop,* Ruffin, R. E., Ed., *Excerpta Medica,* Sydney, 1990. With permission.)

1981–1983.[13] The findings are summarized in Figure 7 and show that accuracy was high in 5–34 year olds but was much less satisfactory in the older age groups, particularly over age 55. This study suggested that asthma was overdiagnosed as the cause of death in the older age groups. The New Zealand study used similar criteria to a British study that had found a similar degree of accuracy.[14]

The studies described herein, however, only examined false-positive reporting and give no indication of false-negative reporting, that is, people who died of asthma but were certified as dying of other causes. There appears to be only one published study that has examined false-negative reporting.[2] This New Zealand study identified all deaths over a 6-month period in Auckland, in people younger than 55 years, who were certified as dying of conditions that could possibly be confused with asthma. Information from a variety of sources was examined by two physicians, and only 1 of 66 deaths reviewed were thought to be due to asthma. Therefore, false-negative reporting did not appear to be an important problem, at least in New Zealand. These various studies provide support for the decision by many investigators to restrict their investigations of asthma mortality to the younger age groups.

B. CHANGES IN DISEASE CLASSIFICATION

Since the early 1900s, the International Classification of Diseases (ICD), which has been used to classify national mortality statistics, has undergone several major alterations in coding practices and classification procedures with regard to asthma.[15] The timing of the introduction of new ICD revisions is shown for New Zealand in Figure 4.[7] In most other countries, ICD revisions occurred at or about the same time. Speizer and Doll stated that the most important revision occurred in 1940 when the method of coding the underlying cause of death was changed,[4] although in the United Kingdom, New Zealand, and Australia (Figures 2 to 4) no major changes in mortality rates were observed at this time. From 1950 to 1958 (ICD 6) deaths certified as due to asthma and bronchitis or asthmatic bronchitis were classified as asthma rather than bronchitis as in the previous revision. This would be expected to increase the reported asthma mortality rate, and indeed as illustrated in Figures 1 to 4, mortality was generally higher throughout the 1950s than the previous 20 years. As reported by Gandevia[6] and illustrated in Figure 3, this effect was much greater in the older age groups among whom bronchitis mortality is considerably more prevalent. In 1958 the ICD classification procedures for asthma reverted to the pre-1950 definition when deaths due to asthma with mention of bronchitis were removed from the asthma category. This change was reflected in lower asthma mortality rates in the United Kingdom, Australia, and New Zealand. Therefore, it is likely that the observed increases in reported asthma mortality in the early and mid-1950s followed by a decrease in deaths in the late 1950s were at least in part related to classification changes. However, as Beasley et al.[7] noted, a moderate increase in deaths in New Zealand occurred within the period of the 6th ICD revision (Figure 4).

The classification of asthma was similar in the 7th (1959–1967) and 8th (1968–1978) ICD revisions except that cases with coexistent emphysema were excluded in the latter revision. However, this change is unlikely to have affected the mortality rates in the 5–34 year age group to any measurable degree because death from emphysema rarely occurs in this age group.[2] Changes in the 9th revision in 1979 were more significant as bronchitis unspecified as acute or chronic, with mention of asthma, was now coded as asthma rather than bronchitis. A bridge-coding exercise was undertaken in the United Kingdom and indicated that in people younger than 45 years of age, a 9% increase in asthma mortality could be attributed to the revision.[16] For the age group 5–34 years, this reported increase is likely to lead to an overestimate given that death from bronchitis is consistently much lower than in 35–44 year olds.

Although the various revisions in ICD coding appear to have had measurable effects on reported national asthma mortality statistics, the two major epidemics, in the mid-1960s and the late 1970s, are clearly unrelated to these changes for several reasons. Most importantly, both epidemics started within the period of one revision. Second, none of the changes could account for two- to threefold increases in reported mortality.

C. CHANGES IN DIAGNOSTIC FASHION

There can be little doubt that diagnostic fashions change with time and vary by country. The question is, however, whether these changes could account for the observed international differences and trends in asthma mortality. Table 1 and Figure 6 show up to sixfold differences in asthma mortality between countries, even during nonepidemic periods. Asthma mortality in the United States, for example, has been consistently low, and Sears[12] noted that American doctors probably underreport asthma death. A recent American study suggested that 30% of asthma deaths were unreported, and this study was conducted at a time when reported deaths had been increasing.[17] It is possible that the reason asthma deaths are underreported in the United States is because of fear of litigation, given that asthma death is considered to be largely preventable. The reasons for the substantial differences in asthma mortality between countries in nonepidemic periods, however, remain unclear and require further investigation.

A number of attempts have been made to assess the degree of changes in diagnostic fashions over time.[2,7,11] If reciprocal changes in mortality trends for diseases that could be confused with asthma were observed, this would suggest a change in diagnostic fashion. Figure 8 shows both asthma mortality and mortality from all other respiratory disease in New Zealand, the United States, and England and Wales for the period 1970–1985 in 5–34 year olds. There has been a relatively steady decline in respiratory disease mortality other than asthma throughout the period examined and indeed throughout most of this century.

It is not possible from these data to exclude changes in diagnostic fashions as an explanation for the slow increase in reported asthma mortality observed in many western countries in recent years. Because asthma is most likely to be misdiagnosed as bronchitis or emphysema, a more appropriate comparison is probably between asthma and bronchitis/emphysema. Data on mortality from asthma and bronchitis/emphysema for the United States in the 5–34 year age group for the period 1970–1984 do not show reciprocal changes and suggest that the steady increase in asthma mortality in the United States since 1977 is real.[11]

It is possible to be more confident in excluding diagnostic changes as an explanation for the second New Zealand epidemic in the late 1970s. There is no evidence of a reciprocal decrease in nonasthma respiratory deaths during the epidemic, which could account for the observed trends (Figure 8). Similarly, no reciprocal decrease in nonasthma mortality was observed in epidemic countries during the 1960s epidemic.[1]

The moderate increase in asthma deaths reported by Beasley et al. in New Zealand in the 1950s[7] could, however, be partly due to changes in diagnostic fashions. Figure 9 shows asthma mortality and mortality from bronchitis/emphysema in 5–34 year olds between 1910 and 1985 in New Zealand. This clearly illustrates the lack of reciprocal changes in mortality during the 1960s and 1970s epidemics but suggests such changes could account in part for the

TABLE 1
Asthma Mortality at Ages 5–34 Years in 14 Countries by 3-Year Periods between 1970 and 1984

Country (annual no. of deaths)	1970–72	1973–75	1976–78	1979–81	1982–84	Percentage increase between: 1976–78 and 1982–84	Percentage increase between: 1979–81 and 1982–84
New Zealand (21–68)	1.93	1.38	2.86	3.63	2.67	−7	−28
Singapore (6–24)	1.27	0.60	0.78	0.62	0.91	17	47
Australia (54–106)	1.18	1.13	0.91	0.97	1.09	20	12
Japan (180–532)	0.84	0.49	0.40	0.36	0.42	5	17
England/Wales (113–199)	0.82	0.59	0.60	0.76	0.86	43	13
West Germany (108–227)	0.44	0.51	0.66	0.82	0.83	26	1
Israel (0–8)	0.35	0.41	0.15	0.15	0.38	153	153
Finland (1–11)	0.32	0.26	0.24	0.13	0.16	−33	23
Sweden (8–25)	0.32	0.32	0.37	0.66	0.46	24	−30
Switzerland (5–13)	0.30	0.26	0.37	0.25	0.23	−38	−8

United States (183–408)	0.29	0.22	0.19	0.26	0.34	78	31
Netherlands (6–25)	0.21	0.24	0.18	0.25	0.30	67	20
Canada (21–62)	0.20	0.28	0.32	0.40	0.48	50	20
France (33–91)	0.20	0.20	0.25	0.25	0.29	16	16

Note: Rates are per 100,000 population per year.

From Jackson, R., Sears, M. R., Beaglehole, R., Rea, H. H., *Chest,* 94, 914, 1988. With permission.

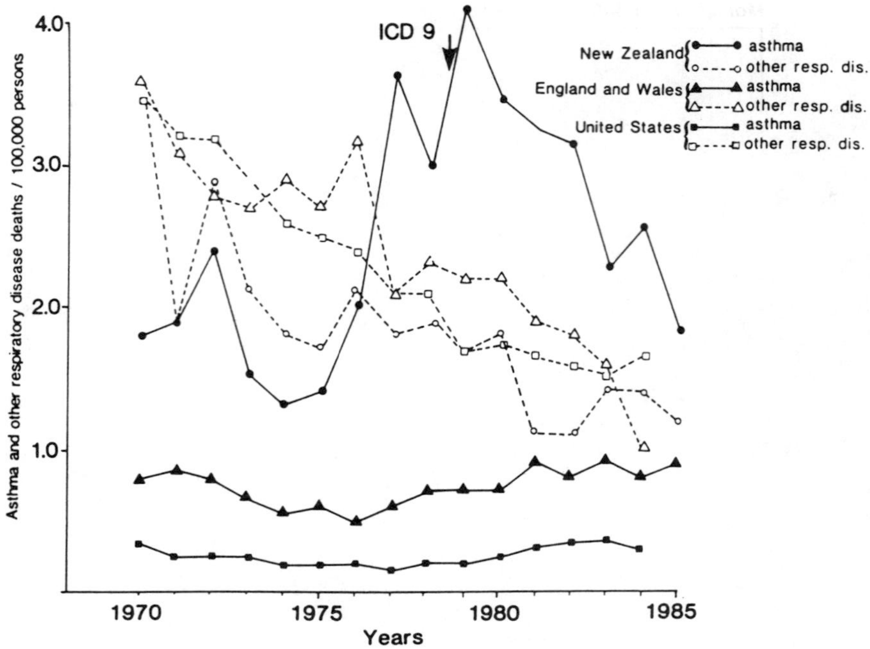

FIGURE 8. Asthma mortality and mortality from all other respiratory diseases in 5–34 year olds in three countries in 1970–1985. (From Jackson, R., Sears, M. R., Beaglehole, R., and Rea, H. H., *Chest,* 94, 914, 1988. With permission.)

increase in asthma mortality in the 1940s and 1950s. Although both asthma and bronchitis/emphysema mortality increased around 1940, this initial increase may have been due to the change in the method for choosing the underlying cause of death.

Changes in diagnostic fashions are likely to happen slowly and therefore are more likely to account for slow increases than for rapid increases in reported mortality rates. However, arguments have also been advanced to explain more rapid changes in diagnostic fashions. The introduction of a new treatment, such as a bronchodilator, could act almost as a diagnostic test. Esdaile et al. pointed out that asthma could be defined as bronchodilator-reversible airway obstruction.[3] Given the massive increase in sales of aerosolized bronchodilators in the early 1960s, they suggest this could have accounted for a substantial increase in the diagnosis of asthma and thus reported deaths. However, they also noted that there are a number of arguments that can be raised against this hypothesis. The most important is that it cannot account for the subsequent rapid decline in mortality despite increasing total beta agonist sales. In addition, aerosolized bronchodilator sales were high in many countries that did not experience the 1960s epidemic.[9]

The introduction of new therapy for asthma is nevertheless likely to have increased the diagnosis of asthma and may account in part for the gradual

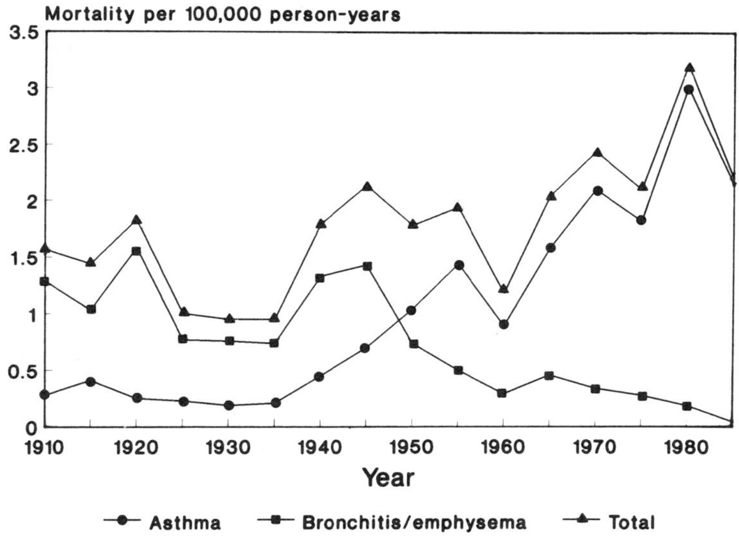

FIGURE 9. Mortality from obstructive airway disease (asthma, bronchitis, emphysema) in non-Maori 5–34 year olds in New Zealand in 1908–1986. (From Beasley, R., Smith, K., Pearce, N., Crane, J., and Burgess, C., *Med. J. Aust.*, 157, 570, 1990. With permission.)

increases in reported asthma mortality during the 1940s and 1950s and more recently. Beasley et al. noted that in the United Kingdom isoprenaline first became available as a sublingual preparation or as an atomizer spray in 1948; corticosteroids came into use for asthma in the 1950s.[7] The first aerosolized beta agonists were introduced in the late 1950s, and sales of these and newer preparations increased dramatically throughout the following 20 years.[18]

IV. INTERPRETATION OF THE TIME TRENDS

As indicated in the introductory section, ecological data, such as time trends in routinely reported national mortality statistics, must be interpreted with considerable caution. Nevertheless, a number of inferences can be drawn from these data.

There have been two superimposed patterns of reported asthma mortality during this century. The first is a slow but steady increase in mortality throughout the period, best illustrated in Figure 4, which shows long-term New Zealand data. The limited early data available indicate a somewhat similar pattern in the United Kingdom and Australia. Since 1960 various reviews have examined trends in a large number of western countries and, as illustrated in Figure 6 and Table 1, this slow increase in mortality has become more universal since the mid-1970s. Although some data suggest these trends are real, it remains a real possibility that these trends are an artifact due to changes in disease classification and diagnostic fashions.

Burney attempted to address this issue by using age/period/cohort analyses on asthma mortality data in England and Wales between 1931 and 1985.[5] This approach allows the effect of age to be separated from a cohort effect and also an effect related to time (period) of death. He found independent cohort and period effects as well as the well-described age effect. The cohort effect was most apparent before 1920 and since 1940. The cohort effect since 1940 suggests that at least part of the increase in mortality observed since the 1940s is real and not due to changes in reporting practices, which would have affected all ages.

The second pattern, characterized by sudden and substantial increases in mortality followed by equally dramatic decreases in death rates, was observed in a number of countries in the mid-1960s and in New Zealand for a second time in the late 1970s. It is possible to state with confidence that these reported epidemics were real. No plausible alternative arguments have been advanced to explain these sudden increases in asthma deaths. They occurred within the periods of single ICD coding revisions, and there is no evidence that sudden changes in diagnostic fashions could account for the reported rates.

A possible explanation for a decrease in mortality after an epidemic increase is that susceptible individuals die out. This would also account for a subsequent increase in mortality, as was seen in many countries in the mid-1970s, even if there were no underlying change in asthma mortality, because a particular age group would be replenished with individuals unaffected by the earlier epidemic. However, Markowe showed a similar pattern of declining and then increasing mortality in age groups both affected and unaffected by the 1960s epidemic, which negates this hypothesis.[19]

Several additional inferences can be drawn from the epidemic patterns. Countries at opposite ends of the world coincidentally experienced the 1960s epidemic, whereas countries geographically adjacent to epidemic countries were spared (for example, Norway had an epidemic, but Sweden did not). This makes it extremely unlikely that climatic or other major environmental factors could have caused the epidemic. These international patterns also rule out a dramatic natural increase in prevalence as an explanation because again it would require an exposure that would coincidentally affect countries at opposite ends of the globe but not adjacent countries. Stolley's hypothesis, that is, the introduction of isoprenaline forte, a high-dose beta agonist aerosol, into epidemic countries caused the epidemic,[8] is the only explanation put forward to date that is consistent with the international patterns observed in the 1960s. The epidemics receded after the issuing of warnings about the overuse of beta agonist inhalers and the banning of over-the-counter sales.

The second reported epidemic, in New Zealand, followed an identical pattern to the first, as shown in Figure 4, which suggests a similar etiology. The hypothesis that this epidemic was related to the introduction of fenoterol,[20-22] also a high-dose beta agonist, is also consistent with mortality patterns. The epidemic receded, with mortality declining by one half, after warnings were issued about the safety of fenoterol in mid-1989.

The large differences observed in reported mortality between countries, even in nonepidemic years (Figures 5 and 6, Table 1), have not been adequately explained. As noted, mortality may be underreported in some countries for litigation reasons. The limited international comparisons of asthma prevalence suggest that the mortality differences cannot be explained on this basis.[11] This suggests either that the international mortality differences in nonepidemic periods are artifactual or that mortality may be related to treatment.

The sex differences in asthma mortality, which have changed several times this century, are consistent between countries, suggesting the observations are real. However, no adequate explanation has been advanced to explain these patterns. The early excess in males before 1900 may have been related to greater occupational exposure to sensitizing agents in males, but the reasons for the subsequent crossovers are unknown.

V. CONCLUSIONS

It can be stated with confidence that the two reported epidemics of asthma death in young people during the mid-1960s in a number of countries and then in New Zealand alone during the late 1970s were real. The epidemics also occurred in older age groups but to a lesser extent. Moreover, problems with diagnostic accuracy and susceptibility to changes in disease classification in older age groups make it difficult to assess the magnitude of the epidemics in older people. No other similar epidemics of asthma death occurred earlier this century. A reported increase in deaths in the 1950s, particularly in New Zealand, may have been related to changing coding practices and diagnostic fashions. The patterns of the two epidemics were identical, suggesting a similar etiology. Further, the geographic pattern of the first epidemic indicates that climatic or other major environmental factors could not have caused the epidemic. The hypothesis that the introduction of new therapies into some countries and not others caused the epidemics is consistent with the trend data, as is the evidence that the epidemics receded after warnings were issued about the safety of these therapies.

Although it is gratifying that both epidemics subsided, the apparent gradual increase in asthma mortality in many western countries in recent years requires further investigation. It is not clear whether these recent trends are real or artifactual, although on balance, at least part of the increase is probably real. Recent reports[23] that regular beta agonist therapy may adversely affect control of asthma need further investigation in the light of these apparent trends.

However, a central issue is the validity of the mortality data. It will be important to establish a uniform international protocol to examine the accuracy of death certificates in terms of both false-positive and -negative coding. In addition, standardized prevalence studies in adults, similar to those carried out in children in New Zealand, Australia, and Canada, may help to clarify whether validated international mortality differences are a function of asthma prevalence, severity, or variations in management.[11]

REFERENCES

1. **Speizer, F. E., Doll, R., and Heaf, P.,** Observations on recent increases in mortality from asthma, *Br. Med. J.*, 1, 335, 1968.
2. **Jackson, R. T., Beaglehole, R., Rea, H. H., and Sutherland, D. C.,** Mortality from asthma: a new epidemic in New Zealand, *Br. Med. J.*, 285, 771, 1982.
3. **Esdaile, J. M., Feinstein, A. R., and Horwitz, R. I.,** A reappraisal of the United Kingdom epidemic of fatal asthma, *Arch. Intern. Med.*, 147, 543, 1987.
4. **Speizer, F. E. and Doll, R.,** A century of asthma deaths in young people, *Br. Med. J.*, 3, 245, 1968.
5. **Burney, P.,** Asthma death in England and Wales 1931–85: evidence for a true increase in asthma mortality, *J. Epidemiol. Community Health,* 42, 316, 1988.
6. **Gandevia B.,** The changing pattern of mortality from asthma in Australia, *Med. J. Aust.*, 1, 747, 1968.
7. **Beasley, R., Smith, K., Pearce, N., Crane, J., and Burgess, C.,** Trends in asthma mortality in New Zealand, 1908–1986, *Med. J. Aust.*, 157, 570, 1990.
8. **Stolley, P. D.,** Asthma mortality. Why the United States was spared an epidemic of deaths due to asthma, *Am. Rev. Respir. Dis.*, 105, 883, 1972.
9. **Stolley, P. D. and Schinnar, R.,** Association between asthma mortality and isoproterenol aerosols: a review, *Prev. Med.*, 7, 519, 1978.
10. **Wilson, P. D., Sutherland, D. C., and Thomas, A. C.,** Has the change to beta-agonists combined with oral theophylline increased cases of fatal asthma, *Lancet,* 1, 1235, 1981.
11. **Jackson, R., Sears, M. R., Beaglehole, R., and Rea, H. H.,** International trends in asthma mortality: 1970 to 1985, *Chest,* 94, 914, 1988.
12. **Sears, M. R.,** Trends in asthma mortality: New Zealand and international experience, in *Proc. 2nd Natl. Asthma Epidemiology Workshop,* Ruffin, R. E., Ed., *Excerpta Medica,* Sydney, 1990.
13. **Sears, M. R., Rea, H. H., de Boer, G., Beaglehole, R., Gillies, A. J. D., Holst, P. E., O'Donnell, T. V., and Rothwell, R. P. G.,** Accuracy of certification of deaths due to asthma: a national study, *Am. J. Epidemiol.*, 124, 1004, 1986.
14. British Thoracic Association, Accuracy of death certificates in bronchial asthma, *Thorax,* 39, 505, 1984.
15. World Health Organization, *International Classification of Diseases,* 3rd revision, 1920; 4th revision, 1929; 5th revision, 1939; 6th revision, 1948; 7th revision, 1955; 8th revision, 1965; 9th revision, 1975. World Health Organization, Geneva, 1923, 1931, 1940, 1948, 1957, 1967, 1977.
16. **Lambert, P. M.,** "Oral Theophylline and Fatal Asthma" (letter), *Lancet,* 2, 200, 1981.
17. **Hunt, L. W., Mair, J. E., Laplante, J. M., Anderson, H. M., Notermann, M. L., Reed, C. E., O'Connell, E. J., Melton, L. J., O'Fallon, W. M., and Yunginger, J. W.,** Accuracy of the death certificate in reporting asthma, *Abstracts Annual Meeting, American Academy Allergy and Immunology,* 1989, 20.
18. **Jackson, R. T. and Mitchell, E. A.,** Trends in hospital admission rates and drug treatment of asthma in New Zealand, *N.Z. Med. J.*, 96, 727, 1983.
19. **Markowe, H. L. J.,** Asthma mortality in England and Wales, *Lancet,* 2, 636, 1986.
20. **Crane, J., Pearce, N., Flatt, A., Burgess, C., Jackson, R., Kwong, T., Ball, M., and Beasley, R.,** Prescribed fenoterol and death from asthma in New Zealand, 1981–83: case-control study, *Lancet,* 1, 917, 1989.

21. **Pearce, N., Grainger, J., Atkinson, M., Crane, J., Burgess, C., Culling, C., Windom, H., and Beasley, R.,** Case-control study of prescribed fenoterol and death from asthma in New Zealand 1977–1981, *Thorax,* 45, 170, 1990.
22. **Grainger, J., Woodman, K., Pearce, N., Crane, J., Burgess, C., Keane, A., and Beasley, R.,** Prescribed fenoterol and death from asthma in New Zealand, 1981–7: a further case-control study, *Thorax,* 46, 105, 1991.
23. **Sears, M. R., Taylor, D. R., Print, C. G., Lake, D. C., Li, Q., Flannery, E., Yates, D. M., Lucas, M. K., and Herbison, G. P.,** Regular inhaled beta-agonist treatment in bronchial asthma, *Lancet,* 336, 1391, 1990.

Chapter 3

ASTHMA MORTALITY EPIDEMICS: THE PROBLEM APPROACHED EPIDEMIOLOGICALLY

Paul D. Stolley and Tamar Lasky

TABLE OF CONTENTS

0-8493-6761-1/93/$0.00 + $.50

In the previous chapter, Jackson examined long-term time trends in asthma mortality and identified two distinct patterns: a slow but steady increase in asthma mortality since the middle of this century and a superimposed pattern of asthma mortality epidemics that occurred in six countries in the 1960s and again in New Zealand in the late 1970s. In this chapter the focus is on the epidemiological approach to studying asthma mortality epidemics.

I. THE EPIDEMIOLOGICAL APPROACH TO INVESTIGATING AN INCREASE IN MORTALITY

When the epidemiologist examines the problem of the increase in mortality attributed to a certain disease, he or she follows an orderly and systematic pathway of reasoning that the clinician may not appreciate. The questions the epidemiologist attempts to answer are listed next and are illustrated by historical examples:

1. Is the increase in death rates real or an artifact of reporting practices or nosologic changes? Has there been a change in nosology, nomenclature, or coding practices over the course of the presumed epidemic and what is the possible effect of such changes?

An example is the change of the coding of diabetes as the "underlying" cause of death in the 1957 revision of the WHO coding manual, which led to a sudden increase in diabetes death rates worldwide, which could be "corrected" mathematically when secular trends were examined.[1] Sudden infant death syndrome (SIDS), if traced over time, seems to have risen markedly in the United States beginning shortly after World War II. However, this same condition used to have other names, such as "status thymo-lymphaticus", and it may well be that the mortality has been fairly constant but only the name has changed.

2. Has there been a change in the denominator so that the population at risk in calculation of the rate is either undercounted or overcounted?

In following death rates attributed to cancer of the uterus over time, the rates were falsely low because the denominator included women who had had hysterectomies and thus were really not at risk, not having the organ in which the cancer could develop. These rates were then corrected for the high hysterectomy rate in the U.S. population, and although the slope of the upward trend was similar, the corrected rates were shown to be higher than before the adjustment procedure.[2]

3. Has a new diagnostic tool been introduced that could lead to improved diagnosis or detection of the disease of interest, thus artifactually elevating death rates compared with earlier periods?

The introduction of noninvasive and accurate imaging devices such as the computed axial tomograph (CAT) scan or magnetic resonance imaging (MRI) has improved the accuracy of diagnosis of previously hard to diagnose diseases, such as ovarian or pancreatic cancer. Any attempt to interpret the increase in death rates would have to take into account these improved diagnostic tools.

4. Has there been a change in the incidence or prevalence of the disease that could account for the change in the death rates?

Infectious disease incidence rates can have extreme volatility from year to year, thus causing changes in the mortality rates. This is less often seen with so-called "chronic" diseases. However, the decline in death rates due to coronary heart disease has been shown to be partly due to a decline in the incidence rates since about 1965.[3,4] Distinguishing between changes in incidence as contrasted to changes in the case:fatality ratio is an important step in the unraveling of the sequence of events when mortality rates change over time and a possible epidemic increase is suspected.

5. Is the increase in death rates uniform in all groups at risk or concentrated among particular groups?

Mortality from cancer of the anus was noted to concentrate in adult males listed as "single" or "unmarried". This suggested that the disease might be largely one of homosexual males who practiced anal intercourse and thereby transmitted a virus leading to the cancer. Subsequent case-control investigations tended to support this hypothesis.[5]

6. If the deaths are plotted on a "spot map", do they cluster geographically?

Spotmapping was used successfully in plotting bladder cancer mortality in the United States, and geographic clustering around known areas where chemical manufacturing plants were located led to a series of subsequent investigations to further define this relationship.[6]

7. If deaths are examined month by month, do they cluster or concentrate seasonally or temporally in any pattern?

Influenza mortality is a classic example of a mortality pattern that is clearly seasonal, as expected (Figure 1).[7] Unexpected and unexplained seasonality has also been noted for certain noninfectious diseases, such as stroke.

8. Has a new treatment been introduced that could lead to an improved or worsened outcome for affected persons?

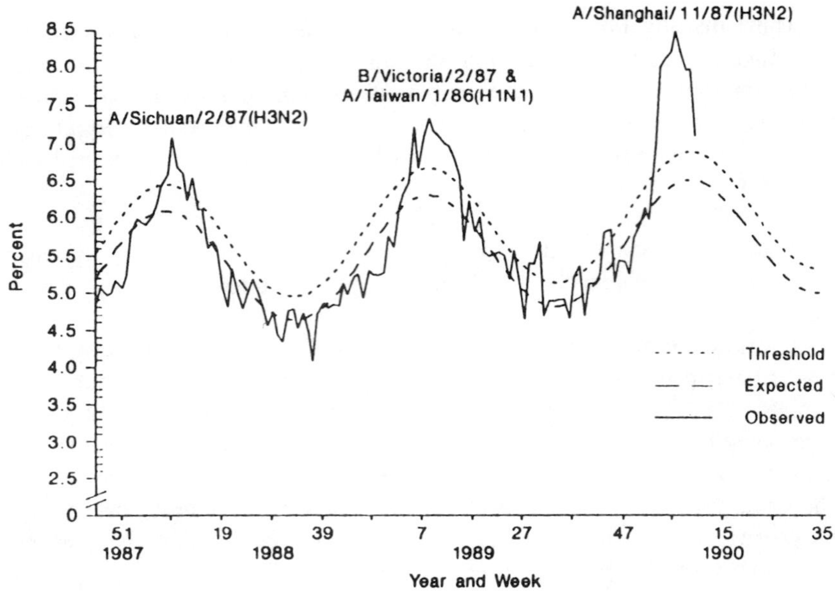

FIGURE 1. Pneumonia and influenza (P&I) deaths as a percentage of total deaths in the United States from October 1988 to March 3, 1990. Reported to CDC from 121 U.S. cities. P&I deaths include all deaths for which pneumonia is listed on the death certificate as a primary or underlying cause or for which influenza is listed on the death certificate. The predominant strains are shown above the peak of mortality for each season. The epidemic guideline (threshold) for each season is 1.645 standard deviations above the expected baseline estimated using a periodic regression model applied to observed percentages since 1983. This baseline was estimated using a robust regression procedure. (From Center for Disease Control, M.M.W.R., 39, 158, 1990.)

Occasionally, dramatic worsening or improvement of mortality rates can be due to the introduction of a new and efficacious therapy or preventative measure or due to a new but toxic therapy. Poliomyelitis incidence and mortality dropped markedly the year after the mass immunization campaign was completed in the United States, for example. In contrast, the incidence and mortality rate of cancer of the vagina rose about 20 years after the widespread use of diethylstilbestrol (DES) in pregnancy. The decline in these same rates followed the decline in use of this synthetic nonsteroidal estrogen by pregnant women.[8] Phocomelia appeared shortly after the introduction of thalidomide to the market and disappeared after its withdrawal,[9,10] and subacute myelo-optic neuropathy (SMON) declined in Japan after the suspect halogenated hydroxyquinolone (Enterovioform®) was withdrawn.

9. If the death rate increases are real and represent the true picture of mortality, what working hypotheses can explain this unusual phenomenon?

In the investigation of any epidemic, such as one due to an infectious agent, working hypotheses are proposed and then investigations mounted to explore these hypotheses. As an example, when the small epidemic of vaginal cancer in young women was detected, the two working hypotheses explored in greatest detail were that of prenatal X-ray exposure and prenatal and/or postnatal drug exposure. The latter hypothesis was clearly supported in case-control investigations, and subsequently an animal model was developed in which pregnant rodents were exposed to DES and their progeny developed genital tumors as adults.[11-13]

II. THE 1960s EPIDEMIC OF ASTHMA MORTALITY

These steps and reasoning can be applied to the problem of increases in asthma mortality, as experienced by certain countries around the world in the decade of the 1960s. The most striking aspect of the epidemic of the 1960s was its abrupt onset, but only in certain countries. Adjacent countries in Europe had different asthma experiences in the 1960s, and this peculiar pattern must be explained by any who propose explanatory hypotheses. Why certain countries were spared the epidemic while other countries, similar in most other respects, had severe epidemics is a crucial question. A striking increase in asthma mortality was first noticed in England and Wales in the 1960s when asthma mortality showed a sevenfold increase in certain age-groups.[14] Twofold or threefold (or greater) increases were observed in several other countries, such as Ireland, Scotland, Australia, New Zealand, and Norway, peaking in 1965–1967 and then declining. For example, the asthma mortality rate rose from 0.66 to 2.18 per 100,000 for the age group 5–34 years during 1959–1966 in England and Wales, and from 0.81 to 2.87 in New Zealand during the same years (Figure 2).[15]

Other countries (Germany, The Netherlands, Belgium, the United States) showed no changes in mortality during the same period of time, staying between 0.37 and 0.43 per 100,000 in the United States during 1959–1966 and between 0.39 to 0.63 in Germany during the same years. Japan, Denmark, and Sweden showed mild and inconsistent increases in asthma mortality or fluctuations due to a small denominator during these years. Japan's rate rose from 0.71 to 1.01 per 100,000, while Denmark's rate fluctuated from 0.15 to 0.66 during 1959–1966. However, Japan's rate was close to 1.0 during the 1950s, also (Table 1).[15]

III. THE ISOPRENALINE FORTE HYPOTHESIS

The observations about these international time trends in asthma mortality led to discussion of a number of hypotheses. It was established in the United Kingdom that the mortality rate changes were real and not artifactual results of changes in coding, nomenclature, diagnosis, the size of the denominator

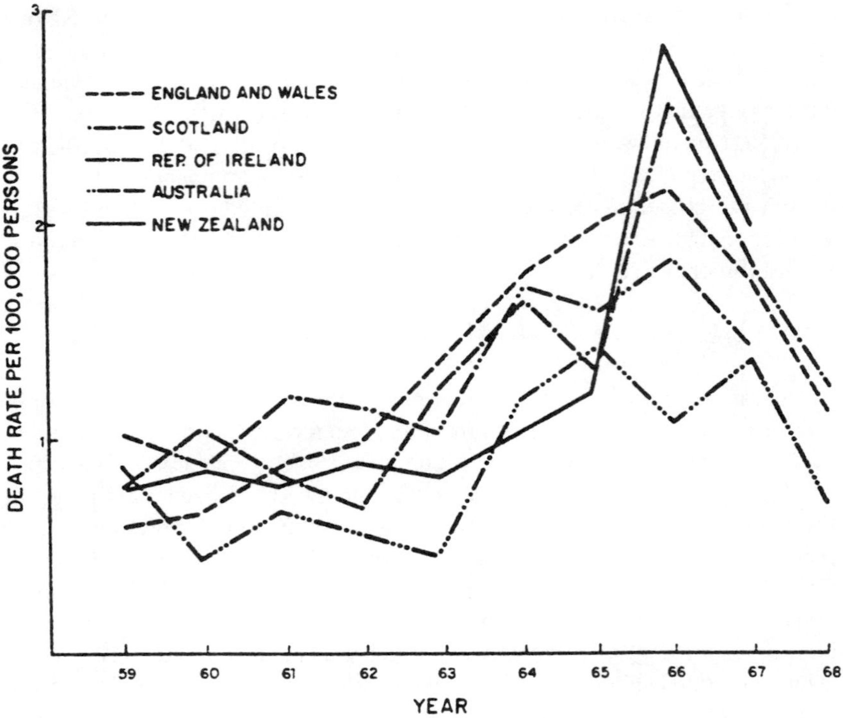

FIGURE 2. Annual mortality from asthma during 1959–1968 for persons 5–34 years of age in England and Wales, Scotland, Ireland, Australia, and New Zealand. (From Stolley, P. D., *Am. Rev. Respir. Dis.*, 105, 883, 1972. With permission.)

at risk population, or the incidence and prevalence of asthma. There appeared to be no seasonality to the mortality trends. Hypotheses were then generated regarding treatments that were introduced in the 1960s and varied from country to country. Speizer and Doll examined the asthma mortality patterns in the United Kingdom and determined that the increase in England and Wales was large and concentrated in younger age groups (sevenfold to eightfold in age group 10–14 years over a 7-year period and threefold to fourfold in age group 5–34 years during the same period).[14] They produced evidence that the increase in mortality was not due to an increase in asthma incidence but rather due to an increase in the case: fatality ratio. These same authors pointed out that the abrupt increase in mortality coincided with the introduction of a new therapy, the handheld pressurized nebulizer containing a potent nonselective beta agonist, isoprenaline (called isoproterenol in the United States). Subsequent work by Inman and Adelstein, plotting sales of these nebulizers against deaths over time, showed such excellent correspondence in England and Wales that further case-control studies of this matter were not completed, although they had been initiated (Figure 3).[16] However, epidemics of asthma

TABLE 1
Mortality from Asthma at Ages 5 to 34 Years in 14 Countries

	1959	1960	1961	1962	1963	1964	1965	1966	1967	1968
England and Wales	0.66	0.68	0.89	1.00	1.40	1.76	2.05	2.18	1.76	1.13
Scotland	0.82	1.08	0.79	0.70	1.23	1.63	1.32	2.59	1.77	1.22
Republic of Ireland	0.90	0.45	0.71	0.55	0.47	1.18	1.42	1.06	1.36	0.66
Australia	1.06	0.89	1.23	1.15	1.03	1.70	1.60	1.88	1.44	—
New Zealand	0.81	0.88	0.78	0.92	0.82	1.03	1.24	2.87	1.99	—
Sweden	—	—	0.64	0.48	0.51	0.76	0.31	0.62	0.55	—
Denmark	0.15	0.15	0.24	0.19	0.34	0.24	0.28	0.66	0.42	—
Federal Republic of Germany	0.39	0.41	0.53	0.42	0.45	0.59	0.54	0.63	0.56	—
The Netherlands	0.42	0.68	0.35	0.42	0.52	0.42	0.55	0.51	0.59	0.38
Belgium	0.24	0.42	0.24	0.36	0.46	0.38	0.65	0.37	—	—
United States	0.37	0.41	0.40	0.43	0.41	0.36	0.42	0.41	0.38	—
Japan	0.71	0.86	0.84	0.89	0.99	1.03	1.00	1.01	1.01	—
Norway	0.13	0.13	0.00	0.26	0.51	0.76	1.26	1.00	0.68	0.49
Canada	0.30	0.34	0.41	0.37	0.24	0.33	0.32	0.31	0.26	0.35

Note: Dash indicates that data were not available.

From Stolley, P. D., *Am. Rev. Respir. Dis.*, 105, 883, 1972. With permission.

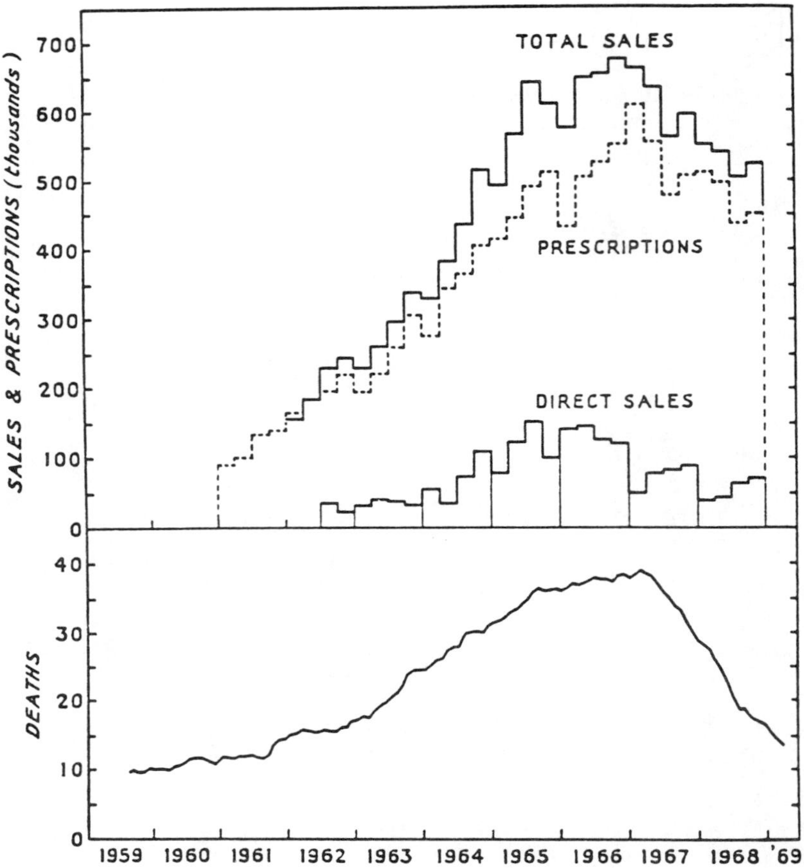

FIGURE 3. Asthma deaths of persons aged 5–34 compared with sales and prescriptions of asthma preparations in England and Wales for 1959–1968. (From Inman, W. H. W. and Adelstein, A. M., *Lancet,* 2, 279, 1969. With permission.)

mortality were detected in other countries in addition to England and Wales. Scotland, Australia, New Zealand, and Denmark showed increases during the same years as the English epidemic. Other countries reported no increase in asthma mortality, notable among these being the United States, Canada, and Sweden, but these latter countries, spared the epidemic, also had introduced and marketed the beta agonist nebulizers at the same time as the countries experiencing the epidemic (Figure 4). Here was an exception to the nebulizer theory that had to be explained by any causal hypothesis advanced, if it were to be credible.

The exceptions to the original nebulizer hypothesis were studied by Stolley and the results published in an article entitled, ''Asthma mortality: why the United States was spared an epidemic of asthma mortality''. Stolley sum-

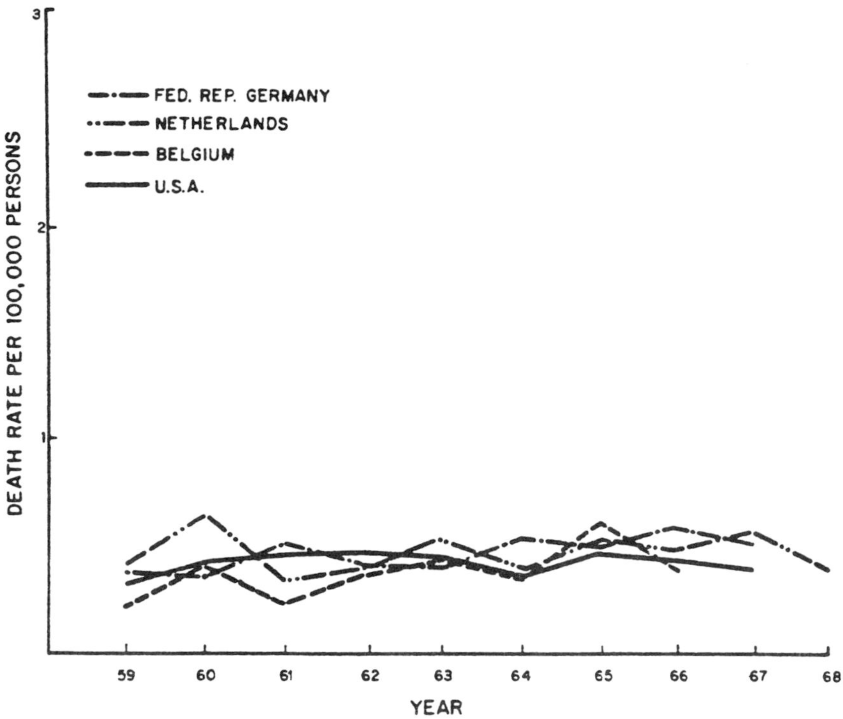

FIGURE 4. Annual mortality from asthma during 1959–1968 for persons 5–34 years of age in Germany, The Netherlands, Belgium, and the United States. (From Stolley, P. D., *Am. Rev. Respir. Dis.*, 105, 883, 1972. With permission.)

marized asthma mortality rates by year and by country and also summarized per capita sales of bronchodilator aerosol nebulizers for the same years.[15] Whereas per capita sales were generally higher in England and Wales (an epidemic country) than in the United States (a nonepidemic country), the United States (nonepidemic) and New Zealand (epidemic) had similar consumption rates. Therefore, differences in nebulizer constituents were examined.

It turned out that all countries experiencing an epidemic had licensed and used an extremely potent form of the isoprenaline nebulizer (Table 2). The countries experiencing an epidemic of asthma deaths had all licensed a dosage form that was fivefold more potent than the next strength. This dosage form was much more potent than the dosage forms licensed in the nonepidemic countries. In the United States and Canada the common dosage form contained 0.08 mg isoprenaline per "puff". This dosage form was commonly used in the epidemic countries, but there was also a next higher strength dosage form available and it was *five times* the strength of the usual dose. This stronger dose, called "forte" by the manufacturer, contained 0.40 mg per puff. If an

TABLE 2
Asthma Death Rates and Per Capita Sales[a] of Highly Concentrated Isoproterenol Nebulizers, by Country, for 1965–1967

Country	Asthma death rate for ages 5–34 years (averaged for 1965–1967)	Index of highly concentrated isoprenaline nebulizer sales[b]
New Zealand	2.03	8.8
England and Wales	2.00	Estimated 13–20
Scotland	1.89	On market[c]
Australia	1.64	On market[c]
Republic of Ireland	1.28	12.1
Norway	0.98	2.1
Japan	1.01	0
Federal Republic of Germany	0.58	0
The Netherlands	0.55	1.3
Belgium	0.51[d]	Introduced in 1966[c]
Sweden	0.49	0
Denmark	0.45	0
United States	0.40	0
Canada	0.30	0

[a] Source is the sales estimates from manufacturer.
[b] (average number of units sold in 1965–1967/total population in 1966) × 1000.
[c] Number of units sold was not available.
[d] Average is for 1965–1966 because rate was not available.

From Stolley, P. D., *Am. Rev. Respir. Dis.*, 105, 883, 1972. With permission.

asthmatic child were doing poorly, the physician might write a prescription for the "next strength" nebulizer, the forte form, never realizing it was fivefold stronger than the currently used nebulizer. This was like giving a child five of the usual strength nebulizers all going off simultaneously — a potentially dangerous situation. Shortly after the forte data were published, the *British Medical Journal* editorially supported the high-dose nebulizer hypothesis with a lead editorial entitled, "Asthma deaths: a question answered".[17]

The most definitive test of this high dosage form hypothesis would have been either a case-control study or an experiment in prevention in which this dosage form was removed from the market and the death rates tracked. By the time the high-dose hypothesis was advanced, however, the isoprenaline nebulizers had been largely replaced by more selective beta agonists and by cromolyn (Intal®) and other forms of therapy. Nevertheless, a regression analysis could be carried out tracking the decline of the epidemic in relation to sales of nebulizers, and this analysis tended to support the high-dose hypothesis.

A 1978 article by Stolley and Schinnar presented an analysis of aggregate data in an effort to quantify the strength of association between bronchodilator use and asthma mortality.[18] The sales figures for bronchodilator pressurized aerosols were used as a proxy for consumption, summarized by country, and expressed as per capita sales. The figures were also presented broken down into two isoprenaline groups: regular and forte. Asthma mortality per 100,000 persons age 5–34 years was used as the outcome measure. Regression analysis was carried out with data from the United States, England and Wales, New Zealand, Germany, Australia, and Canada, and the use of isoprenaline forte was found to be significantly associated with mortality. This analysis gave additional support for the isoprenaline forte hypothesis.

IV. HISTORY IS REWRITTEN

During the next two decades following the mortality epidemic of the 1960s, other explanatory hypotheses were advanced. Some speculated that the nebulizers led to delays in treatment or other changes in care or diagnosis. Another hypothesis attributed mortality to the over-the-counter prescription status of some nebulizers in some countries. Two major critiques questioned the process leading from ecological studies to regulatory action.[19,20] Lanes and Walker criticized the evidence supporting any type of association between bronchodilators and asthma mortality, preferring the hypothesis that asthma incidence, prevalence, or severity had changed.[19] It is not clear how this could also explain the decline in asthma mortality that followed the epidemic. The critique of Esdaile et al.[20] was broader, reminding scientists of the inherent weaknesses of ecological studies and cautioning against what they regarded as precipitous regulatory action. They presented alternative hypotheses that might also explain the ecological data. They hypothesized that (1) bronchodilators allowed better diagnosis of asthma and (2) the increase in asthma mortality in the United Kingdom was a result of "increased confidence of physicians in citing asthma as an underlying cause of death." To accept this hypothesis, one would have to ignore the geographic variability of the data (why did a change in diagnosis occur in the United Kingdom and not in the United States?), and ignore the decline in mortality that followed removal of isoprenaline from the market (did physicians change their patterns of assessment of asthma as an underlying cause of death *twice* in a 7- or 8-year time frame?). The ecological data do not support such a hypothesis, and there are no data suggesting that patterns of asthma diagnosis are subject to such fluctuations. Indeed, there is no evidence that physician behavior changes this rapidly in two different directions in a less than 10-year time period.

Esdaile et al.[20] presented four shortcomings of the diagnostic-exchange explanation and acknowledged that the major value of their concept is an example of another hypothesis that could be supported by the ecological data. Although they presented this hypothesis as a demonstration concept, and probably not as a serious explanation of the epidemic, it has defects even as a demonstration concept. Their hypothesis did not explain the geographic variability in mortality patterns, the decrease in mortality, or the short time frame in which such shifts in behavior are postulated to have occurred.

The isoprenaline forte hypothesis was critiqued on the basis that ecological studies have inherent limitations. To counter the isoprenaline forte hypothesis, less plausible hypotheses were put forward, which did not explain the time trend data, were not supported by any body of knowledge (do physicians change their patterns of diagnosis every few years?), and were not even taken seriously by the proponents themselves. Both groups of critics called for hypothesis testing studies, such as randomized trials, controlled cohort, or case-control studies.

This peculiar phenomenon of rewriting history occurred in the absence of any new data. One group of investigators hypothesized a diagnostic exchange wherein asthma deaths were suddenly misclassified; no data were presented to substantiate this claim.[20] Another group denied that the increase in case-fatality ever occurred and that, instead, an increase in prevalence or incidence occurred; again no substantive data were produced.[19] It became commonplace to refer to the epidemic of the 1960s as having been due to undertreatment with steroids, but when the references were traced, there were articles making the same claim without any data to support it.[21] Case studies of the circumstances surrounding the death of asthmatics in nonepidemic countries or after the epidemic had receded were applied to the earlier epidemic period, even though it was clear that they were studying the baseline pre-epidemic or post-epidemic period.

V. REQUIREMENTS OF A CREDIBLE EXPLANATORY HYPOTHESIS

Any viable hypothesis about the cause of the 1960s epidemic must explain a number of different facts:

1. That the epidemic of deaths among asthmatics began abruptly;
2. That the epidemic affected only some countries and spared others;
3. That asthma mortality had been remarkably constant in most countries until the epidemic began;
4. That beta agonist nebulizers were widely used in all Western countries during the 1960s.

The only hypothesis proposed that can simultaneously explain all four of these conditions is the high-dosage (forte) nebulizer hypothesis. That this hypothesis was never as adequately tested or subjected to potential falsification as one would like does not justify adhering to a less plausible and less testable alternative hypothesis, such as the "failure to treat with steroids" hypothesis or diagnostic exchange explanation. To explain the 1960s asthma mortality epidemic, the high-dose (isoprenaline forte) hypothesis must rely on what some have labeled "circumstantial evidence". The American philosopher Henry David Thoreau wrote (at a time when it was commonplace to adulterate commercially sold milk with river water): "Some circumstantial evidence is very strong, as when you find a trout in your milk."[22] This author believes the evidence clearly shows a "trout in the milk" and that the isoprenaline forte hypothesis is still the best explanation of the 1960s epidemic.

VI. ANOTHER EPIDEMIC OCCURS

In 1976 a second asthma mortality epidemic began in New Zealand.[23] Several hypotheses were put forth relating to delay in treatment, interaction of medications, changes in management of asthma, and delay in seeking medical care.[23-25] Finally, the hypothesis was proposed that associated the inhaled beta agonist fenoterol with asthma fatality. Time trend data showed that the epidemic began the same year that fenoterol was introduced and that fenoterol was being dispensed in what was effectively a "forte" preparation.[26]

The second New Zealand epidemic had many similar features to the 1960s epidemics, in that it occurred abruptly with mortality more than doubling within a few years, and it was established that the mortality changes were real and were not artifactual results of changes in coding, nomenclature, diagnosis, the size of the denominator at risk population, or the incidence and prevalence of asthma.[24] As for the 1960s epidemics, the epidemic was associated with a particular beta agonist (fenoterol) rather than beta agonists in general, the epidemic occurred only in the country (New Zealand) with a high per capita usage, and mortality fell sharply once warnings were issued about the safety of the drug. After the association of fenoterol with asthma deaths was first published in mid 1989 and warnings were issued about the overuse of fenoterol, the mortality rate fell by 50% and the epidemic receded.[27] This experiment in prevention is thus consistent with the hypothesis that fenoterol was a major factor in the epidemic. However, a key difference between the 1960s epidemics and the second New Zealand epidemic was that in the latter instance, case-control studies of asthma deaths were performed to investigate the fenoterol hypothesis.[28-30] As noted, this is one of the definitive approaches for investigating hypotheses of this type. The methodology and results of such studies is discussed in Chapters 4 and 5.

REFERENCES

1. **Harriss, M. I. and Entmacher, P. S.,** Mortality from diabetes, in *Diabetes in America,* U.S. Department of Health and Human Services, NIH, National Institute of Arthritis, Diabetes, and Digestive and Kidney Diseases. NIH Publication No. 85-1468, 1985.
2. **Lyon, J. L. and Gardner, J. W.,** The rising frequency of hysterectomy: its effect on uterine cancer rates, *Am. J. Epidemiol.,* 105, 439, 1977.

3. **Havlik, R. J. and Feinleib, M.,** *Proceedings of the Conference on the Decline in Coronary Heart Disease Mortality,* DHEW No. (NIH) 79-1610. U.S. Government Printing Office, Washington, D.C., 1979.
4. **Kannel, W. B., Thom, T. J., and Hurst, J. W.,** Incidence, prevalence, and mortality of cardiovascular diseases, in *The Heart,* 6th ed., McGraw-Hill, New York, 1986.
5. **Daling, J. R., Weiss, N. S., Hislop, T. G., Maden, C., Coates, R. J., Sherman, K. J., Ashley, R. L., Beagrie, M., Ryan, J. A., and Corey, L.,** Sexual practices, sexually transmitted diseases and the incidence of anal cancer, *N. Engl. J. Med.,* 317, 973, 1987.
6. **Pickle, L. W., Mason, T. J., Howard, N., Hoover, R., and Fraumeni, J. F.,** *Atlas of U.S. Cancer Mortality among Whites: 1950–1980,* U.S. Health and Human Services, Public Health Service, NIH, DHHS Publication No. (NIH) 87-2900, U.S. Government Printing Office, Washington, D.C., 1987.
7. Center for Disease Control, *M. M. W. R.,* 39, 158, 1990.
8. **Herbst, A. L., Ulfelder, H., and Poskanzer, D. C.,** Adenocarcinoma of the vagina: association of maternal stilbestrol therapy with tumor appearances in young women, *N. Engl. J. Med.,* 284, 878, 1971.
9. **McBride, W. G.,** Thalidomide and congenital abnormalities (letter to the editor), *Lancet,* 2, 1358, 1961.
10. **Sjostrom, H. and Nilsson, R.,** *Thalidomide and the Power of the Drug Companies,* Penguin, London, 1972.
11. **Shapiro, S. and Slone, D.,** The effects of exogenous female hormones on the fetus, *Epidemiol. Rev.,* 1, 110, 1979.
12. **Herbst, A. L.,** The epidemiology of vaginal and cervical cell adenocarcinoma, in *Developmental Effects of Diethylstilbestrol (DES) in Pregnancy,* Herbst, A. L. and Bern, H. A., Eds., Thieme-Stratton, New York, 1981.
13. **McLachlan, J. A.,** Rodent models for perinatal exposure to diethylstilbestrol and their relation to human disease in the male, in *Developmental Effects of Diethylstilbestrol (DES) in Pregnancy,* Herbst, A. L. and Bern, H. A., Eds., Thieme-Stratton, New York, 1981.
14. **Speizer, F. E. and Doll, R.,** A century of asthma deaths in young people, *Br. Med. J.,* 3, 245, 1968.
15. **Stolley, P. D.,** Asthma mortality: why the United States was spared an epidemic of deaths due to asthma, *Am. Rev. Respir. Dis.,* 105, 883, 1972.
16. **Inman, W. H. W. and Adelstein, A. M.,** Rise and fall of asthma mortality in England and Wales in relation to use of pressurized aerosols, *Lancet,* 2, 279, 1969.
17. Editorial. Asthma deaths: a question answered, *Br. Med. J.,* 4, 443, 1972.
18. **Stolley, P. D. and Schinnar, R.,** Association between asthma mortality and isoproterenol aerosols: a review, *Prev. Med.,* 7, 519, 1978.
19. **Lanes, S. F. and Walker, A. M.,** Do pressurized bronchodilator aerosols cause death among asthmatics?, *Am. J. Epidemiol.,* 125, 755, 1987.
20. **Esdaile, J. M., Feinstein, A. R., and Horwitz, R. I.,** A reappraisal of the United Kingdom epidemic of fatal asthma, *Arch. Intern. Med,.* 147, 543, 1987.
21. **Benatar, S. R.,** Fatal asthma, *N. Engl. J. Med.,* 314, 423, 1986.
22. **Evans, B.,** *Dictionary of Quotations,* Avenel, New York, 1978. (As quoted in Thoreau's Journal, November 11, 1854.)
23. **Wilson, J. D., Sutherland, D. C., and Thomas, A. C.,** Has the change to beta-agonists combined with oral theophylline increased cases of fatal asthma? *Lancet,* 1, 1235, 1981.
24. **Jackson, R. T., Beaglehole, R., Rea, H. H., and Sutherland, D. C.,** Mortality from asthma: a new epidemic in New Zealand, *Br. Med. J.,* 285, 771, 1982.
25. **Grant, I. W. B.,** Asthma in New Zealand, *Br. Med. J.,* 286, 374, 1983.
26. **Pearce, N. E., Crane, J., Beasley, R., and Burgess, C.,** Beta agonists and asthma mortality "déjà vu". *Clin. Exp. Allergy,* 21, 401, 1991.

27. **Crane, J., Pearce, N. E., Beasley, R., and Burgess, C.,** Asthma deaths in New Zealand, *Br. Med. J.,* 304, 1307, 1992.
28. **Crane, J., Pearce, N., Flatt, A., Burgess, C., Jackson, R., Kwong, T., Ball, M., and Beasley, R.,** Prescribed fenoterol and death from asthma in New Zealand, 1981–83: case-control study, *Lancet,* 1, 917, 1989.
29. **Pearce, N., Grainger, J., Atkinson, M., Crane, J., Burgess, C., Culling, C., Windom, H., and Beasley, R.,** Case-control study of prescribed fenoterol and death from asthma in New Zealand, 1977–81, *Thorax,* 45, 170, 1990.
30. **Grainger, J., Woodman, K., Pearce, N. E., Crane, J., Burgess, C., Keane, A., and Beasley, R.,** Prescribed fenoterol and death from asthma in New Zealand, 1981–1987: a further case-control study, *Thorax,* 46, 105, 1991.

Section 3

Analytical Epidemiological Studies of Beta Receptor Agonist Therapy and Asthma Mortality

Chapter 4

EPIDEMIOLOGICAL METHODS FOR STUDYING THE ROLE OF BETA RECEPTOR AGONIST THERAPY IN ASTHMA MORTALITY

Neil E. Pearce and Julian Crane

TABLE OF CONTENTS

0-8493-6761-1/93/$0.00 + $.50

I. INTRODUCTION

Until recently, epidemiological studies of the role of beta agonists in asthma mortality had been primarily descriptive. These largely involved calculating annual mortality rates from asthma (in persons 5–34 years of age) and comparing the time trends in mortality with the time trends in beta agonist sales in various countries. The initial descriptive studies were conducted in response to the epidemics of asthma mortality (discussed in Chapters 2 and 3), which occurred in several countries in the 1960s.[1-3] An association with use of the newly developed high-dose isoprenaline aerosols was the most plausible, and contentious, hypothesis. In particular, Stolley[2,3] showed that there was a close international and temporal association between sales of a high-dose preparation of isoprenaline, known as isoprenaline forte, and the mortality epidemics.

Unfortunately, a cohort or case-control study of asthma mortality was never conducted because the epidemic declined before there was time to commence such a study. However, most protagonists agreed that the case-control design was most appropriate for addressing this issue. For example, Stolley[2] noted, "Ideally, the most conclusive manner of investigating this question would entail a retrospective study of the products used by young asthmatic patients dying suddenly and unexpectedly at the peak of the epidemic." This viewpoint has been echoed by several critics who have disputed Stolley's conclusions, largely on the basis that the evidence was merely descriptive and that case-control studies (or other formal epidemiological studies) were never conducted. For example, one review (in response to the FDA decision to rescind the over-the-counter availability of orciprenaline[4]) stated, "It is surprising that there has not been a study designed to measure the effect of the use of certain bronchodilator drugs on the occurrence of death while controlling for other causes of death (especially asthma severity)."[5]

Similarly, Esdaile et al.[6] argued, "To be tested with scientific evidence, the hypothesis requires a randomized trial, controlled cohort, or case-control study that can investigate individuals, while linking the agent and the outcome in a correct temporal sequence . . . the recent epidemic of asthma deaths in New Zealand provides an opportunity to employ appropriate study designs for reassessing the role of therapeutic agents used to treat asthma."

The second New Zealand asthma mortality epidemic, referred to in the aforementioned quotation, was confined to New Zealand, commenced in 1976, and peaked during 1979–1981.[7] A series of national case-control studies of asthma deaths in the 5–45 year age group was eventually conducted[8-10] and found that an increased risk of mortality was associated with the prescription of fenoterol. These New Zealand case-control studies have been strongly criticized by a group of Boehringer Ingelheim reviewers.[11] These criticisms mostly involved hypothetical biases that would apply to any epidemiological study design, rather than specifically to case-control studies.

However, these studies have also been criticized in more general terms, i.e., that case-control studies are supposedly an inherently unreliable approach.

This is the first of two chapters that discuss the role of analytical epidemiological studies, and particularly that of case-control studies, in investigating the role of beta agonists in asthma mortality. In the current chapter the general study design principles involved are discussed, whereas, in Chapter 5 Elwood reviews the substantive knowledge from the case-control studies that have been conducted to date.

This chapter is divided into two main sections: in the first section, the importance of case-control studies in epidemiological research is discussed, and in the second section, their specific application to studies of the role of beta agonist therapy in asthma mortality is discussed. Concentration is given to the situation in which one particular beta agonist (for example, fenoterol) is especially hazardous (in comparison with other beta agonists). However, the more difficult task of investigating a possible class effect of beta agonists concludes the discussion.

II. CASE-CONTROL STUDIES

In a case-control study, a group of persons with a disease (or an event, such as asthma death) is compared with a control group of persons without the disease (or event) with respect to their past exposure to a particular factor. The first modern case-control study was published in 1926,[12,13] and this method is now perhaps the predominant form of epidemiological research. It is thus surprising that the first case-control study of asthma deaths was not published until 1986[14] and that the first case-control study of the role of asthma drugs in asthma deaths was not published until 1989.

Most of the major epidemiological findings since World War II were initially discovered in case-control studies and were later confirmed using other study designs.[15] The most noteworthy example is the association between cigarette smoking and lung cancer, which was discovered in the early 1950s in case-control studies conducted by Sir Richard Doll[16] and others.[17] These findings were subsequently supported by prospective cohort studies, which achieved similar findings but were considerably more expensive and took more than 20 years to complete.[18,19]

Other major causal associations that have recently been discovered using the case-control method include oral contraceptives and thromboembolism, tampon use and toxic shock syndrome, estrogens and endometrial cancer, *in utero* exposure to diethylstilbestrol and vaginal cancer, and aspirin and Reye's syndrome.[20] All of these discoveries have been greeted by controversy, most involving the same group of critics who also criticized such well-established associations as cigarette smoking and lung cancer.[20] All have essentially been resolved with the vindication of the original case-control findings.[20]

This conflict over case-control studies has also been reflected in the methodological literature. Some epidemiological texts have presented case-control studies as inherently different from cohort (follow-up) studies, in that causal inference supposedly proceeds from effect to cause, rather than from cause to effect. However, at least one critic of the case-control approach has now conceded, "I now realize that my main objections to backward-directed case-control studies were provoked by their relatively low level of scientific standards, rather than their backward temporal orientation . . . I now believe that such studies are valuable, important, and indispensable for certain research questions."[21]

More modern texts go much farther in rejecting this earlier view, and present the case-control design as involving only minor differences to the cohort study design.[22] At least one prominent epidemiologist has questioned whether the case-control approach should be regarded as a separate study design at all.[23]

The case-control approach developed as a logical progression from daily clinical practice. It starts with a group of patients with a particular disease (the effect) and then attempts to discover the cause. It thus appears to be different from the prospective approach (whether experimental or observational), which starts with exposure to a particular factor (a cause) and follows its effects over time. Some commentators have presented the case-control approach in this light and therefore concluded that it is inherently inferior. This negative view was encouraged (and to some extent justified) by some of the early case-control studies, which often involved a researcher simply assembling a group of cases of disease at a particular clinic and an arbitrarily chosen control group of persons who did not have the disease.

All this has now changed. Modern epidemiology texts now emphasize that the case-control design proceeds from cause to effect (just as for cohort studies) and is not inherently more prone to bias, or even inherently different.[22] The modern perspective was implicit in some of the earliest case-control studies,[16,17] but this perspective was reinforced with the development of the nested case-control design in the 1970s.[24] This design arose out of large cohort studies of occupational cancer. Such studies might typically involve 100,000 workers (perhaps 50,000 exposed to a particular chemical and 50,000 not exposed) who would be followed for 20 years or more to yield sufficient cases of a rare tumor (for example, 100 cases of bladder cancer). Such studies involved a massive undertaking, particularly because each worker's exposure had to be estimated by combining information from personnel records and industrial hygiene monitoring data.

Eventually, it was realized that such studies could be conducted more efficiently by enumerating the entire cohort, but only collecting exposure histories on the *cases* of disease (the 100 cases of bladder cancer) and a similar number of randomly sampled *controls* who did not develop the disease.[25] Such a *nested case-control study* would only involve collecting exposure histories on several hundred workers instead of the entire cohort.

This approach revolutionized the understanding of case-control studies because it showed that they did not involve an inherently different approach, but could actually be incorporated within cohort studies as a more efficient manner of achieving the same findings. This nested case-control approach only differed from the full cohort approach in one respect: that cases were compared with a sample of the cohort rather than the complete cohort. All of the other supposed shortcomings of case-control studies did not apply: there was no need for a "rare-disease" assumption; there was no greater tendency to bias (providing the control sample was genuinely random); and causal inference proceeded from cause to effect, just as in a full cohort study.[22] Furthermore, the case-control approach had several important advantages; in particular, when the outcome under study was rare, it was considerably more efficient. This increase in efficiency usually meant that a much larger study (in terms of the number of cases) could be conducted.

III. EPIDEMIOLOGICAL APPROACHES TO STUDYING ASTHMA MORTALITY

These considerations imply that the case-control design will usually be the optimal approach for studying asthma mortality (because it is a rare event) and suggest a general strategy for designing such studies. Suppose we wish to investigate the hypothesis that prescription of a particular drug (for example, fenoterol) increases the risk of asthma mortality compared with prescription of other beta agonists (such as salbutamol). A general strategy for designing a case-control study to investigate this hypothesis is as follows: first, design a (hypothetical) clinical trial to compare the mortality rate in patients prescribed fenoterol with that in patients prescribed salbutamol; next, design a (hypothetical) cohort study to achieve the same objective; finally, design a case-control study to achieve the same objective more efficiently than the full cohort study.[26] This approach will be illustrated in the following sections.

A. A CLINICAL TRIAL OF ASTHMA MORTALITY

In a clinical trial of fenoterol, salbutamol, and asthma mortality, it is most appropriate to study the effects of beta agonists in the clinical setting in which they are most commonly used.[27] There would be major practical problems with conducting a study involving randomization at the time of acute attacks, and in any case, asthma patients tend to also use their regular prescribed beta agonist for relief in acute attacks. Thus, the most reasonable approach would be to randomize patients to receive either fenoterol or salbutamol as their regular prescribed beta agonist therapy. This approach is most feasible and appropriate irrespective of whether the hypothesis under study involves chronic or acute side effects.

Figure 1 shows the design of such a hypothetical study. Patients would be identified at the time of hospitalization for asthma and would be randomized to receive either fenoterol or salbutamol. They would then be followed over time, and any subsequent deaths from asthma would be identified from national death registrations. (Some deaths would be identified because they

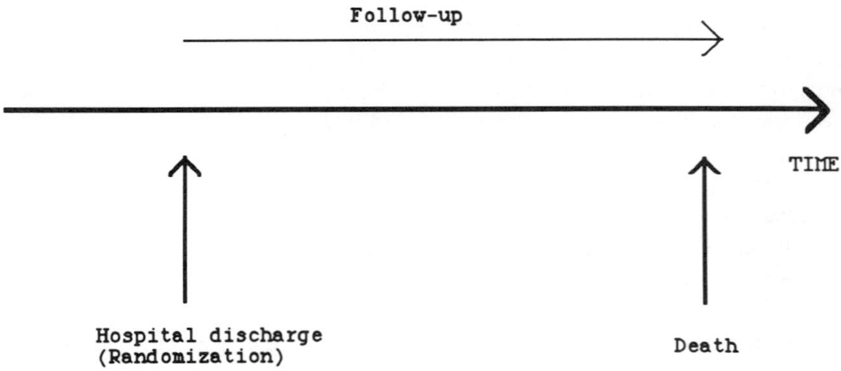

FIGURE 1. A hypothetical clinical trial or cohort study of asthma mortality.

occurred in hospital, but most would occur outside of hospital.) There would be two major methodological issues. First, for a variety of reasons, some patients would subsequently have changes to their beta agonist therapy. In particular, patients who were experiencing acute attacks with an increasing frequency or severity might have changes to their medication, including changes to their beta agonist. However, in analyzing such a study, it would be incorrect to take such changes into account because these might result in serious bias. The correct approach would be to analyze the data according to the "intention to treat" principle, that is, the study subjects would be classified according to the regular prescribed medication to which they were originally randomized, and subsequent changes to their medication would be ignored.

The second methodological problem is that although randomization should generally ensure that the two groups under study are similar with respect to their average chronic asthma severity, this cannot be guaranteed in every instance. Thus, it would be important to gather information on recognized markers of chronic asthma severity at the time of randomization, such as frequency of previous hospital admissions for asthma, and recent prescription of oral corticosteroids. (There has been some debate about the validity of these severity markers,[11] but this issue has been discussed extensively elsewhere[8-10] and is not relevant here.) The two groups would then be compared with respect to their average chronic asthma severity, and if they were found to differ in this respect, then the analysis would be split into subgroups defined by these severity markers. In other words, the study might be split into two groups: those that had chronically severe asthma according to a particular severity marker and those that did not. The comparison between the fenoterol and salbutamol groups would then be conducted within each of these two subgroups defined by the severity marker. (An overall effect estimate adjusted for chronic severity would also be derived if this were appropriate.)

It is important to note that only the baseline severity at the time of randomization would be relevant in this regard. It would be incorrect to

TABLE 1
Findings from a Hypothetical Clinical Trial or Cohort Study of Asthma Mortality

	Treatment	
	Fenoterol	Salbutamol
Deaths	50	25
Survivors	49,950	49,975
Total	50,000	50,000
Risk	50/50,000	25/50,000
Relative risk	2.0	

consider subsequent changes in acute or chronic severity because these could be a result of treatment. In particular, it appears that regular use of fenoterol increases chronic asthma severity.[28] Similarly, if fenoterol were primarily hazardous when overused in an acute attack, then one would expect the fenoterol group to show an increase in acute asthma severity, reflected in an increased frequency of severe or life-threatening attacks even if the overall frequency of attacks did not change. Thus, whichever mechanism by which fenoterol increased the risk of death, one would expect this to be reflected in an increase in either chronic severity or acute severity prior to death. Thus, only the baseline severity (at time of randomization) should be used when considering the potential for bias due to severity.

Table 1 shows data from such a hypothetical clinical trial. This involved enrolling 100,000 patients 5 to 34 years of age who had been admitted to hospital with asthma over a 5-year period. The study subjects were randomized to receive either fenoterol and salbutamol in equal numbers, and each study subject was followed for a period of 1 year after randomization (or up until the time of their next admission if this occurred within 1 year). If there were 50 deaths in the fenoterol group and 25 deaths in the salbutamol group, then the relative risk of death would be 2.0.

B. A COHORT STUDY OF ASTHMA MORTALITY

There would be considerable problems with conducting a clinical trial of the aforementioned type. In particular, although some notable clinical trials have been conducted of beta agonists and nonfatal hazardous outcomes,[28] it would be unethical and impractical to conduct such a trial involving a fatal outcome. Thus, an epidemiological (observational) rather than an experimental approach would be required; that is, it would be necessary to conduct a cohort (follow-up) study[29] rather than a clinical trial. The design of such a hypothetical cohort study would be identical to that of the hypothetical clinical trial shown in Figure 1, except that the subjects would not be randomized into treatment groups. Instead, their regular prescribed medication (either fenoterol or salbutamol) would be ascertained (rather than randomly allocated) at time of discharge. Once again, they would be followed for 1 year (or until their next admission) to ascertain subsequent asthma deaths.

The two major methodological concerns of the hypothetical clinical trial would also apply to this hypothetical cohort study. First, some patients would change their medication after leaving hospital, particularly if their asthma subsequently became more troublesome or severe, but it would be inappropriate to take such changes into account in the analysis. Although the "intention to treat" principle does not apply as a general principle to nonrandomized studies, the specific biases discussed in the context of clinical trials would also apply to a cohort study, and it would once again be necessary to analyze the data according to the regular prescribed medication at time of discharge. Second, the fenoterol and salbutamol groups might differ according to their chronic asthma severity at time of discharge. This problem would be of potentially greater concern in the cohort study because patients had not been randomized to treatments. However, the solution would be the same: to gather information on various markers of chronic asthma severity at time of hospitalization and to conduct analyses of subgroups defined by these severity markers. Once again, only the severity at the time of commencement of follow-up (at time of hospitalization) would be relevant, and it would be incorrect to consider subsequent changes in severity. In particular, subsequent changes in acute or chronic asthma severity could be a result of treatment, and it would be incorrect to control for this.

Assuming that there was little difference in the chronic asthma severity of those prescribed fenoterol and those prescribed salbutamol in this group of hospitalized patients (an assumption that is supported by available evidence in New Zealand[30]), the findings of the hypothetical cohort study would be similar to those of the hypothetical clinical trial shown in Table 1. If there were differences in chronic severity between the fenoterol and salbutamol groups, then this could be controlled for with the severity subgroup analyses described herein; however, this issue is not important in the current context, and only the simpler situation will be considered here.

Thus, a hypothetical cohort study might involve enrolling 100,000 patients 5 to 34 years of age who had been admitted to hospital with asthma over a given period and recording their regular prescribed medication from hospital notes at the time of discharge. Assume for simplicity that when this was done, it was found that 50% of patients had been prescribed fenoterol and 50% prescribed salbutamol. Each study subject was followed for a period of 1 year after randomization (or up until the time of their next admission if this occurred within 1 year). Once again, if there were 50 deaths in the fenoterol group and 25 deaths in the salbutamol group, then the relative risk would be 2.0 (Table 1).

C. A CASE-CONTROL STUDY OF ASTHMA MORTALITY

The cohort study described herein would have two major advantages over a clinical trial: (1) it would not have the same ethical problems, and (2) it

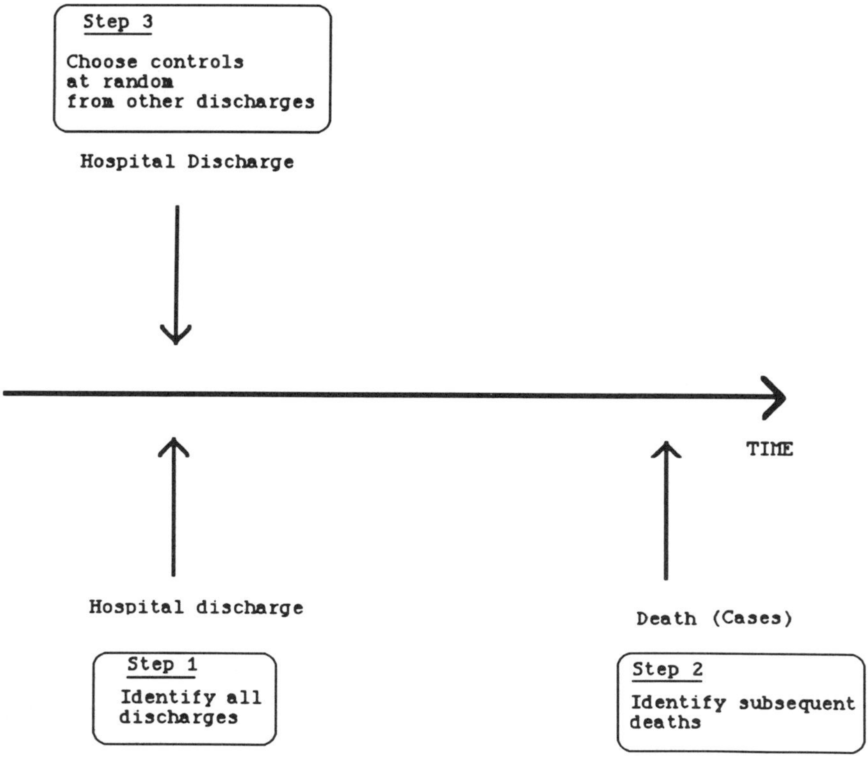

FIGURE 2. A hypothetical case-control study of asthma mortality.

could be conducted historically rather than prospectively. However, it would still have one major problem: the need to enroll 100,000 patients and to collect information on prescribed medication for all of them. Figure 2 shows the design of a case-control study intended to achieve the same results as the cohort study in a more efficient manner. This involves studying all of the cases of asthma mortality generated by the cohort and a control group sampled at random from the same cohort.

Once again, the same major methodological considerations would apply as in the clinical trial and cohort study. First, the data would be analyzed according to the regular prescribed medication at time of discharge, and changes in medication that occurred after discharge from hospital would not be considered.[15] Second, the potential for bias due to differences in chronic asthma severity would be exactly the same as in the full cohort study. The solution would also be exactly the same: to collect information on chronic asthma severity at time of hospitalization. Once again, it would be incorrect to control for subsequent changes in acute or chronic severity because these might be a result of treatment. It should also be noted that the subsequent acute severity of the controls would, by design, be different from that of the

TABLE 2
Findings from a Hypothetical Case-Control Study of Asthma Mortality

	Treatment			
	Fenoterol		**Salbutamol**	**Odds**
Deaths (cases)	50		25	50/25
Controls	150		150	150/150
Odds	50/150		25/150	
Relative risk (odds ratio)		2.0		

cases because the cases died and the controls did not. In this context, it should be emphasized that the controls are, in general, intended to be representative of the cohort that generated the cases and are not required to be identical with the cases in every respect.

It is also important to note the appropriate approach to assessing whether fenoterol was selectively prescribed to patients with more severe asthma. In a full cohort study (or clinical trial), this would be assessed by examining the full cohort (not just those who died) and comparing the average chronic severity of the fenoterol group and the salbutamol group. Because the control group (in the case-control study) is a sample of the full cohort, the same conclusions can be drawn (as would have been drawn from examining the full cohort) by comparing the average chronic severity of the controls prescribed fenoterol to the average chronic severity of the controls prescribed salbutamol. The cases are not relevant in this context, and biased results will be obtained if they are considered.[31]

Table 2 shows the data from a hypothetical case-control study. This hypothetical study involved studying the 75 asthma deaths that would have been identified in the full cohort study and a sample of 300 controls (four for each case). As before 50 deaths were in the fenoterol group and 25 deaths were in the salbutamol group. The controls were distributed in the same proportions as the cohort from which they were sampled: 150 (50%) were prescribed fenoterol and 150 (50%) were prescribed salbutamol. (The proportion will not be exactly 50:50 if the controls were sampled from the survivors [Table 1], but this bias is trivial if the disease is rare and is completely avoided if controls are selected by density sampling rather than cumulative incidence sampling.[24])

In case-control studies, the relative risk measure is the odds ratio. This can be calculated as the ratio of the odds of being a case in the fenoterol group (50/150) to the odds of being a case in the salbutamol group (25/150). This, once again, yields a relative risk of 2.0. Exactly the same answer can be obtained by taking the ratio of the odds of being prescribed fenoterol in the case group (50/25) to that of being prescribed fenoterol in the control group (150/150).

It should be emphasized that such a case-control study would achieve the same findings as the full cohort study but would be considerably more efficient because it would involve ascertaining the prescribed medication of 375 patients (75 cases and 300 controls) rather than 100,000 patients. This remarkable gain in efficiency is achieved with only a minimal reduction in the precision of the relative risk estimate. This may also make it possible to do a much larger case-control study, perhaps involving 150 cases and 600 controls. Because the number of cases is of crucial importance in determining the statistical power of a study, such a case-control study, involving 750 patients, would actually be much more powerful than a cohort study involving 100,000 patients, without any increase in bias.

A case-control study of this type could be nested within a formal cohort, created by listing all hospital admissions for asthma in a country or state over a period of time. However, the same result could be achieved more efficiently in the manner illustrated in Figure 3. This shows a study in which the first step is to identify asthma deaths from national death registration records. For each death, the records of hospitals to which the patient was likely to have been admitted in an acute attack were then searched to identify any admission for asthma in the previous 12 months. If such an admission were identified, the death was included in the study, and the admission closest to death was used. For each death, one or more controls was then selected at random from patients discharged from the same hospital with the diagnosis of asthma at the time that the case's discharge occurred. The prescribed medication at discharge was then ascertained for cases and controls. This approach would yield the same findings as the case-control design shown in Figure 2 (and the cohort/clinical trial design shown in Figure 1), but would have the advantage that it would not be necessary to enumerate the entire cohort before selecting controls.

It should also be noted that in some situations, the control group might not be chosen as a completely random sample. For example, it is common to ensure that the control group has a similar age distribution to the cases (that is, age matching) to make it easier to control for potential confounding by age. Similarly, it might be considered desirable to ensure that the control group had a similar average chronic severity to the cases at the time of hospitalization. (It would be impossible for the controls to have the same acute severity at the time of the final attack because the cases died and the controls did not.) This would not be necessary if there were no tendency for fenoterol to be selectively prescribed to more severe asthmatics. However, if this were not known with certainty, then it might be considered appropriate to match for chronic asthma severity, either directly or indirectly. A direct match for severity (pair matching) would involve taking each case and ensuring that the matched controls were identical to the case with respect to certain markers of chronic asthma severity. An indirect approach (analogous to frequency matching) might involve requiring potential controls to have had another hospital admission within a 1-year period, so that the cases had had

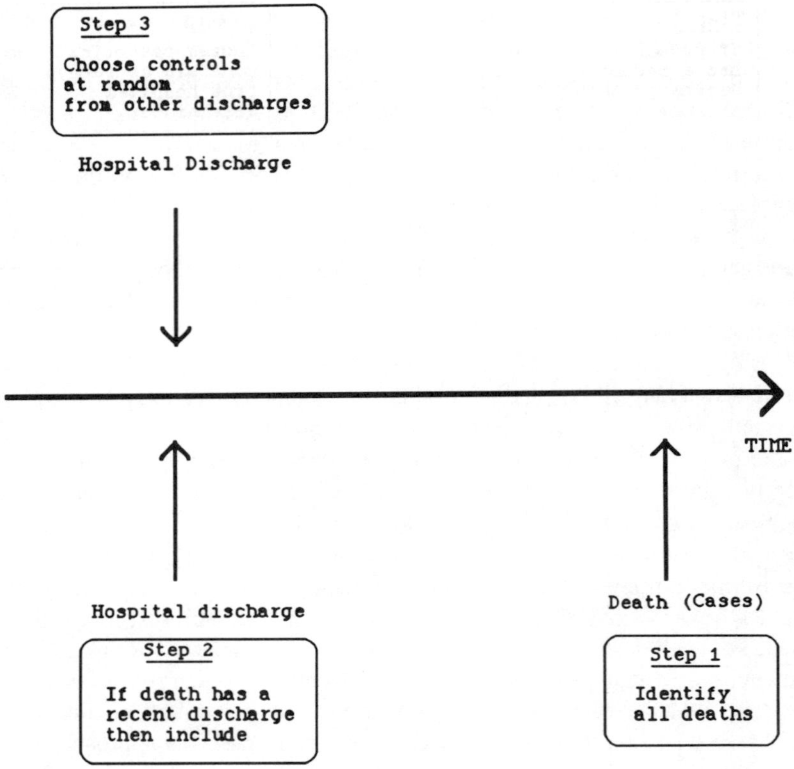

FIGURE 3. Alternative design for a hypothetical case-control study of asthma mortality.

an admission followed by death within 1 year and the controls had had an admission followed by another admission within 1 year (Figure 4).

The latter two approaches (Figures 3 and 4) have been followed in the most recent New Zealand asthma mortality case-control studies.[9,10] These studies can be viewed as examples of case-control studies nested within cohort studies. Full cohort studies (comprising all patients 5 to 45 years of age admitted to a major New Zealand hospital with asthma over a given period) would yield the same findings, but would be much more expensive and time-consuming.

IV. STUDYING CLASS EFFECTS OF BETA RECEPTOR AGONISTS

The previous discussion has concentrated on the situation in which one particular beta agonist (for example, fenoterol) may be especially hazardous (in comparison with other beta agonists, such as salbutamol). Although most attention has focused on the role of particular beta agonists (isoprenaline forte

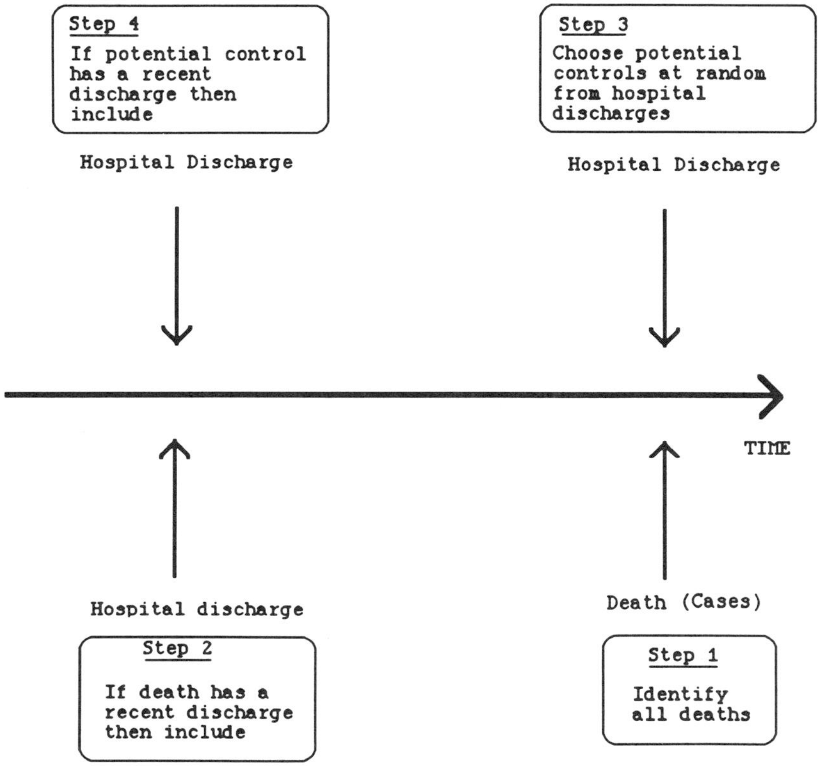

FIGURE 4. Another alternative design for a hypothetical case-control study of asthma mortality.

and fenoterol) in the mortality epidemics of the 1960s and 1970s, attention has more recently shifted to the possible role of a class effect of beta agonists in the gradual increase in asthma mortality, which has been occurring in many countries around the world.[32,33] In addition, one study[34] reported that although fenoterol appears to be especially hazardous, prescription of other beta agonists may also be associated with an increased risk of death.

In most developed countries, it is considerably more difficult to investigate a class effect of beta agonists using epidemiologic studies because virtually all asthmatics are using beta agonists and there is no appropriate comparison group. (This is analogous to a clinical trial in which there is no valid placebo group.) This situation is illustrated in Figure 5, which shows a typical situation in which virtually all asthmatics use either of two particular beta agonists (fenoterol or salbutamol) and there is only a very small group of asthmatics who do not use beta agonists at all.

There are at least three questions that could be addressed in studies of this type: (1) Is the death rate of those prescribed fenoterol higher than those

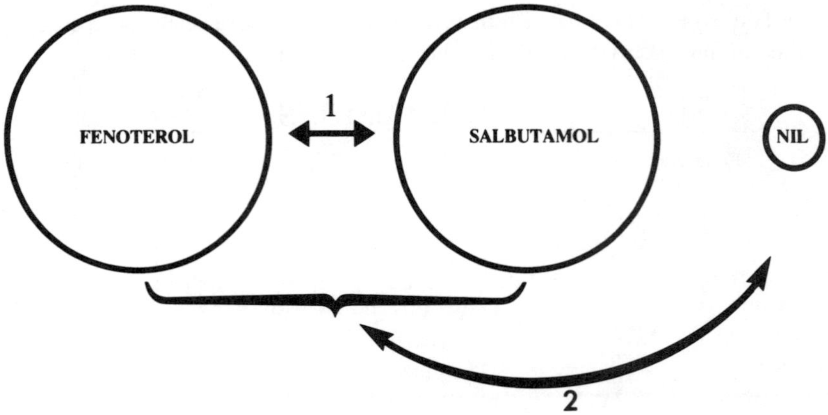

FIGURE 5. Comparisons involved in analyses of case-control studies of fenoterol, salbutamol, and asthma deaths.

prescribed other beta agonists? (2) Is the death rate of those prescribed beta agonists higher than those not prescribed beta agonists? (3) Is there a dose-response according to the number of units prescribed on a regular basis?

Previous studies of fenoterol and asthma mortality[8-10] and the previous discussion relate to question 1 and essentially involved a comparison of fenoterol with other drugs within the same class (Figure 5). It is much more difficult to determine whether all beta agonists (including salbutamol) are hazardous (question 2). Spitzer et al.,[34] in the recent Saskatchewan study, attempted to do this by entering salbutamol and fenoterol simultaneously into a logistic regression model. However, this procedure essentially involves the questionable comparison of the fenoterol and salbutamol groups with the small group that was not prescribed either drug (Figure 5). This approach depends on the relatively strong (and unlikely) assumption that there are no significant differences in asthma severity between patients using beta agonists and the small group of asthmatics who do not use beta agonists. Although it is possible to control for differences in severity, the problems in this respect are likely to be greater, and more intractable, when attempting to study a class effect, than when comparing two drugs within a class. The comparison problems are even more intractable when attempting to ascertain whether there is a dose-response according to the amount prescribed on a regular basis (question 3) because patients prescribed several units per month are likely to have more severe asthma.

Thus, it would appear that epidemiologic methods are most appropriate for making comparisons within the class of beta agonists (question 1) and that randomized controlled trials[28] are more appropriate when attempting to identify class effects of beta agonists (question 2) or a dose-response according to the amount prescribed on a regular basis (question 3).

V. CONCLUSIONS

Case-control studies are the most practicable and efficient form of epidemiological research when studying rare outcomes, and for this reason alone case-control studies are the optimal approach for investigating the causes of asthma mortality. As a result of their great efficiency, new (and therefore often unexpected and controversial) results are usually first shown in case-control studies.[15] However, the methodological issues are often complex, and some relatively poor case-control studies have been conducted, particularly in the years when this technique was first being developed. Partly as a consequence, case-control studies were initially regarded as an inherently inferior form of formal epidemiological research. However, it is now recognized that a well-designed case-control study only differs from a full cohort study in one respect: that cases are compared with a sample of the cohort rather than the full cohort. In all other respects, the case-control approach has all the advantages (and disadvantages) of the cohort approach. In addition, the case-control design has one important advantage: it is considerably more efficient. This increase in efficiency usually means that a much larger study (in terms of the number of cases) can be conducted.

It is surprising that the first case-control studies of asthma mortality have only been published recently because it was generally agreed that this would have been the definitive approach for investigating the asthma mortality epidemics of the 1960s. It is even more surprising that these recent case-control studies have been heavily criticized, partly on the grounds that the case-control approach is supposedly an inherently inferior design. This negative view has been superseded by advances in case-control methodology. The rarity of asthma death, even in severe asthmatics, makes cohort studies and clinical trials impractical in most instances because of the huge numbers of study subjects required. Thus, carefully designed case-control studies are not only a valid option but are usually the only realistic option for studying the role of individual beta agonists in asthma mortality. However, experimental studies are preferable for the investigation of class effects of beta agonists.

ACKNOWLEDGMENT

Neil Pearce and Julian Crane are funded by Senior Research Fellowships from the Health Research Council of New Zealand, and the Wellington Asthma Research Group is funded by a Programme Grant from the Health Research Council of New Zealand.

REFERENCES

1. **Inman, W. H. W. and Adelstein, A. M.,** Rise and fall of asthma mortality in England and Wales in relation to use of pressurized aerosols, *Lancet,* 2, 279, 1969.
2. **Stolley, P. D.,** Asthma mortality: why the United States was spared an epidemic of deaths due to asthma, *Am. Rev. Respir. Dis.,* 105, 883, 1972.
3. **Stolley, P. D. and Schinnar, R.,** Association between asthma mortality and isoproterenol aerosols: a review, *Prev. Med.,* 7, 519, 1978.
4. **Hendeles, L. and Weinberger, M.,** Nonprescription sale of inhaled metaproterenol: deja vu, *N. Engl. J. Med.,* 310, 207, 1984.
5. **Lanes, S. F. and Walker, A. M.,** Do pressurized bronchodilator aerosols cause death among asthmatics?, *Am. J. Epidemiol.,* 125, 755, 1987.
6. **Esdaile, J. M., Feinstein, A. R., and Horwitz, R. I.,** A reappraisal of the United Kingdom epidemic of fatal asthma. Can general mortality data implicate a therapeutic agent?, *Arch. Intern. Med.,* 147, 543, 1987.
7. **Jackson, R. T., Beaglehole, R., Rea, H. H., and Sutherland, D. C.,** Mortality from asthma: a new epidemic in New Zealand, *Br. Med. J.,* 285, 771, 1982.
8. **Crane, J., Pearce, N. E., Flatt, A., Burgess, C., Jackson, R., Kwong, T., Ball, M., and Beasley, R.,** Prescribed fenoterol and death from asthma in New Zealand, 1981–1983: a case-control study, *Lancet,* 1, 917, 1989.
9. **Pearce, N. E., Grainger, J., Atkinson, M., Crane, J., Burgess, C., Culling, C., Windom, H., and Beasley R.,** Case-control study of prescribed fenoterol and death from asthma in New Zealand, 1977–1981, *Thorax,* 45, 170, 1990.
10. **Grainger, J., Woodman, K., Pearce, N. E., Crane, J., Burgess, C., Keane, A., and Beasley, R.,** Prescribed fenoterol and death from asthma in New Zealand, 1981–1987: a further case-control study, *Thorax,* 46, 105, 1991.
11. **Buist, A. S., Burney, P. G. J., Feinstein, A. R., Horwitz, R. I., Lanes, S. F., Rebuck, A. S., and Spitzer, W. O.,** Fenoterol and fatal asthma (letter), *Lancet,* 1, 1071, 1989.
12. **Cole, P.,** The evolving case-control study, *J. Chronic Dis.,* 32, 15, 1979.
13. **Lane-Claypon, J. E.,** A further report on cancer of the breast, in *Reports on Public Health and Medical Subjects,* HMSO, London, 1926, 32.
14. **Strunk, R. C., Mrazek, D. A., Wolfson Fuhrmann, G. S., and LaBrecque, J. F.,** Physiologic and psychological characteristics associated with deaths due to asthma in childhood, *J.A.M.A.,* 254, 1193, 1985.
15. **Elwood, J. M.,** The case-control study, *N.Z. Med. J.,* 103, 7, 1990.
16. **Doll, R. and Hill, A. B.,** Smoking and carcinoma of the lung, *Br. Med. J.,* 2, 739, 1950.
17. **Wynder, E. L. and Graham, E. A.,** Tobacco smoking as a possible etiologic factor in bronchiogenic carcinoma, *J. Am. Statist. Assoc.,* 143, 329, 1950.
18. **Doll, R. and Hill, A. B.,** Mortality in relation to smoking: ten years' observations of British doctors, *Br. Med. J.,* 1, 1399, 1964.
19. **Doll, R. and Peto, R.,** Mortality in relation to smoking: 20 years' observations on male British doctors, *Br. Med. J.,* 2, 1525, 1976.
20. **Savitz, D. A., Greenland, S., Stolley, P. D., and Kelsey, J. L.,** Scientific standards of criticism: a reaction to ''Scientific standards in epidemiologic studies of the menace of daily life,'' by A. R. Feinstein, *Epidemiology,* 1, 78, 1990.
21. **Feinstein, A. R.,** *Clinical Epidemiology: The Architecture of Clinical Research,* W. B. Saunders, Philadelphia, 1985.
22. **Rothman, K. J.,** *Modern Epidemiology,* Little, Brown, Boston, 1986.
23. **Miettinen, O. S.,** *Theoretical Epidemiology,* John Wiley & Sons, New York, 1985.
24. **Checkoway, H. A., Pearce, N. E., and Crawford-Brown, D. J.,** *Research Methods in Occupational Epidemiology,* Oxford University Press, New York, 1989.

25. **Kupper, L. L., McMichael, A. J., and Spirtas, R.,** A hybrid epidemiologic study design useful in estimating relative risk, *J. Am. Statist. Assoc.,* 70, 524, 1975.
26. **Pearce, N. E., Crane, J., Burgess, C., and Beasley, R.,** Study designs for examining death from asthma: the case-control approach, in *Asthma Mortality: Proc. 2nd Natl. Asthma Mortality Workshop,* Ruffin, R. E., Ed., *Excerpta Medica,* Sydney, 1990, 23.
27. **Elwood, J. M. and Skegg, D. C. G.,** *Review of Studies Relating Prescribed Fenoterol to Deaths from Asthma in New Zealand,* Department of Health, Wellington, New Zealand, 1989.
28. **Sears, M. R., Taylor, D. R., Print, C. G., Lake, D. C., Li, Q., Flannery, E. M., Yates, D. M., Lucas, M. K., and Herbison, G. P.,** Regular inhaled beta agonist treatment in bronchial asthma, *Lancet,* 336, 1391, 1990.
29. **Rea, H. H.,** Study designs for examining death from asthma: cohort design, in *Asthma Mortality: Proc. 2nd Natl. Asthma Mortality Workshop,* Ruffin, R. E., Ed., Excerpta Medica, Sydney, 1990, 22.
30. **Pearce, N. E., Beasley, R., Burgess, C., Grainger, J., and Crane, J.,** Confounding by severity does not explain the association between fenoterol and asthma death, Med. J. Aust. N.Z., 20 (Suppl. 1) (Abstr.), 515, 1990.
31. **Burgess, C., Beasley, R., Pearce, N. E., and Crane, J.,** Prescribing of fenoterol and severity of asthma (letter), *N.Z. Med. J.,* 103, 22, 1990.
32. **Pearce, N. E., Crane, J., Burgess, C., Jackson, R., and Beasley, R.,** Beta agonists and asthma mortality: deja vu, *Clin. Exp. Allergy,* 21, 401, 1991.
33. **Beasley, R., Pearce, N. E., Crane, J., Windom, H., and Burgess, C.,** Asthma mortality and inhaled beta agonist therapy, *Aust. N.Z. J. Med.,* 21, 753, 1991.
34. **Spitzer, W. O., Suissa, S., Ernst, P., Horwitz, R. I., Habbick, B., Cockcroft, D., Boivin, J. F., McNutt, M., Buist, A. S., and Rebuck, A. S.,** Beta agonists and the risk of asthma death and near fatal asthma, *N. Engl. J. Med.,* 326, 501, 1992.

Chapter 5

THE NEW ZEALAND CASE-CONTROL STUDIES OF ASTHMA DEATHS AND FENOTEROL: INTERPRETATION AND CLINICAL AND DRUG REGULATORY IMPLICATIONS

J. Mark Elwood

TABLE OF CONTENTS

0-8493-6761-1/93/$0.00 + $.50

I. INTRODUCTION

This chapter consists of a critical review of the two New Zealand case-control studies published in 1989 and 1990, respectively,[1,2] which showed an association between asthma deaths and the prescription of fenoterol, and draws on published comments on these studies and on relevant other literature that was available up to mid 1990. It is primarily a summary of two independent reports prepared in April and November 1989, for the Department of Health in New Zealand.[3,4] After reviewing these reports and much other material,

TABLE 1
Features of the Two Case-Control Studies

	Cases	Controls
First study	Asthma deaths Age 5–45 yr All New Zealand 1981–1983 n = 118 Drug data from GP[a] records	Admissions for asthma Matched aged, ethnicity, hospital, time 1981–1983 4 per case; n = 472 Drug data from hospital records
Second study	Asthma deaths Age 5–45 yr Several areas 1977–1981 n = 58 Drug data from previous discharge	Admissions for asthma Matched age, hospital, time 1977–1981 4 per case; n = 227 Drug data from previous discharge

[a] General practitioner.

the drug regulatory authorities in New Zealand acted to restrict the use of fenoterol. Similar action was subsequently taken in Australia.

Much has since been published containing further information, methodological discussions, and viewpoints, but this chapter summarizes the evidence and opinions available to those first charged with the responsibility for making clinical and public health decisions in light of the new findings from the case-control studies. The last section deals in rather less detail with new information since that time, particularly the third case control study from the Wellington group, an important clinical trial assessing the effects of the regular use of beta agonists, and the case-control study in Canada. To this the reader may add material presented elsewhere in this volume and in other sources to gain a current viewpoint on the issue.

The basic features of the two studies are shown in Table 1. The first study compared all asthma deaths at ages 5–45 in New Zealand in 1981–1983, with patients admitted for asthma during the same period. The second study also compared deaths with admissions, in an earlier time period 1977–1981, with the major modification that both deceased cases and admitted controls had a previous hospital admission for asthma in the preceding 12 months. In the first study, information on drug exposures was based on general practitioner (GP) records for the cases and on hospital records for the controls; in the second study, the drug data for both cases and controls were based on the previous hospital discharge.

A. RESULTS OF BOTH STUDIES FOR BETA AGONISTS

The results of the two studies are shown in Table 2. In comparing them, the second study relates to an earlier time period (1977–1981), compared with 1981–1983 in the first study, but for both cases and controls was restricted

TABLE 2
Comparison of Two Studies: Beta Agonists

	Second Study: Pearce et al.[2] (% use)			First study: Crane et al.[1] (% use)			First study,[1] subjects with previous admission (% use)		
	Cases	Controls	OR[b]	Cases	Controls	OR	Cases	Controls	OR
Oral beta agonist	41.4	37.4	1.18	23.9	22.6	1.07	—	—	0.86
Oral salbutamol	34.5	33.9	1.03	20.5	20.5	1.00	—	—	0.86
Any MDI[a] drug	86.2	83.3	1.26	91.5	87.8	1.48	—	—	—
MDI fenoterol	51.7	35.7	1.93[c]	51.3	40.4	1.55[c]	65.4	46.6	2.16[c]
MDI salbutamol	37.9	46.3	0.71	36.8	45.1	0.71	—	—	0.89
Any nebulizer drug	3.4	4.8	0.70	20.5	8.8	2.69[c]	—	—	1.94
Nebulizer fenoterol	1.7	0.9	1.97	12.0	4.1	3.21[c]	—	—	2.42
Nebulizer salbutamol	1.7	4.0	0.42	8.5	4.5	1.99	—	—	1.34
Any inhaled beta agonist	89.7	86.8	1.32	—	—	—	—	—	—
Inhaled fenoterol	53.4	36.7	1.99[c]	—	—	—	—	—	—
Inhaled salbutamol	39.7	49.8	0.66	—	—	—	—	—	—

[a] Metered dose inhaler.
[b] Odds ratio.
[c] Statistically significant: lower 95% confidence limit >1.00.

to subjects with a prior hospital admission for asthma, which means that they are likely to have had in general more severe asthma.

The results of the two studies are generally consistent. In each, the proportions of cases and controls using oral beta agonists (almost always salbutamol) were virtually identical. Most subjects were prescribed a beta agonist by metered dose inhaler (MDI), and the risk of death was higher in those than in the small number of subjects who did not receive an MDI drug (odds ratio [OR] 1.26 in the second study, 1.48 in the first). In the second study, fenoterol by MDI was prescribed for 52% of cases compared with 36% of controls, giving a relative risk of 1.93; in the first study, the proportions were 51% in cases and 40% in controls, giving an OR of 1.55. A more direct comparison is with subjects in the first study who also had a previous hospital admission; here the proportions using MDI fenoterol were 65% in cases and 47% in controls, with an OR of 2.16. Thus, in the first study (later time period), for a similar selection of cases and controls, the usage of MDI fenoterol was greater than in the earlier time period study, which is in keeping with the increased general use of fenoterol. In both studies the use of MDI salbutamol, which is really a surrogate for the lack of use of MDI fenoterol, was associated with an OR of 0.71. The use of nebulizer drugs was uncommon in the second study; the OR for fenoterol by nebulizer was 1.97, similar to that for MDI fenoterol. The result for nebulizer fenoterol in each study is consistent with that for MDI fenoterol, but the numbers are inadequate for these results to be considered on their own.

Thus, the main association between beta agonist use and death was consistent in the two studies, both showing a positive association between death and the use of MDI fenoterol. It is also relevant to compare the results with those of Rea et al.[5] In this study, 47 patients resident in Auckland up to 60 years of age who died of asthma in 1981–1982 were compared with two sets of controls: (1) patients who had been admitted with acute asthma and (2) the other patients known to have had asthma who consulted their GPs over a 4-week period (community controls). As presented by Crane et al.,[1] reanalysis for the 32 cases and 27 hospital controls who were 4–45 years of age gives an OR for fenoterol of 1.61 (95% limits 0.57–4.54), consistent with the larger studies.

B. MARKERS OF SEVERITY OF ASTHMA: EFFECT MODIFICATION

A central issue in interpretation of these studies concerns the results within subgroups of patients defined by three measures, which were chosen as markers of the severity of the underlying asthma. These were the use of three or more classes of asthma drugs, a previous admission for asthma within a 12-month period (in the second study, this meant an additional admission preceding the admission used to provide the drug exposure data), and the prescription of oral steroids. The validity of these indices as risk markers will be discussed subsequently.

TABLE 3
Modification of Associations by Markers of Asthma Severity

Drug	Odds ratio overall	3+ drugs	Previous admission	Oral steroids	Admission + steroids	Ref.
Fenoterol	1.99[b]	2.98[b]	3.91[b]	5.83[b]	9.82[b]	2
Fenoterol MDI[a]	1.55[b]	2.21[b]	2.16[b]	6.45[b]	13.29[b]	1
Fenoterol	1.61	2.20	3.00	14.1	—	5
Theophylline	1.10	1.19	1.06	5.21	4.14	2
Theophylline	1.44	0.88	1.65	1.50	1.19	1
Oral steroids	2.30	8.24[b]	1.90	1.59	3.42	2
Oral steroids	1.38	1.07	1.33	Infinity	Infinity	1
Inhaled steroids	0.68	0.49	0.54	0.66	0.35	2
Inhaled steroids	1.34	0.95	1.44	1.19	1.34	1

[a] Metered dose inhaler.
[b] Statistically significant: lower 95% confidence limit >1.00.

In the first study, although the overall association with MDI fenoterol had an OR of 1.55, the association was stronger in subjects who had been prescribed three or more categories of asthma drugs (2.21), had an admission in the previous year (2.16), or who had been prescribed oral corticosteroids (OR 6.45, Table 3). The second study had already restricted cases and controls to those who had had an admission in the previous year, and the overall association with MDI fenoterol use was 1.93 similar to the association of 2.16 in those with a previous admission in the first study. In the second study, the same three indicators were used as measures of the severity of underlying asthma; the OR was 2.98 in subjects with three or more categories of asthma drugs, 3.91 in those with a hospital admission prior to the reference admission, and 5.83 in those with prescription of oral corticosteroids at the reference admission (Table 3). All these associations are statistically significant, whereas none of the associations between fenoterol use and death in subjects without each of these three indicators considered separately is statistically significant. Joint tabulation of pairs of these three indicators shows further increases in risk, particularly in the group with oral corticosteroids on admission and a hospital admission in the previous 12 months, where the OR was 13.29 in the first study and 9.82 in the second. The effect modification was similar in each study; the consistency of these results is important. The results within subgroups are also similar to those of the study of Rea et al.,[5] as reanalyzed by Crane et al.[1] (Table 3).

II. GENERAL ISSUES IN INTERPRETATION

Before moving to consider the features of these studies in detail, there are some general issues of interpretation requiring discussion.

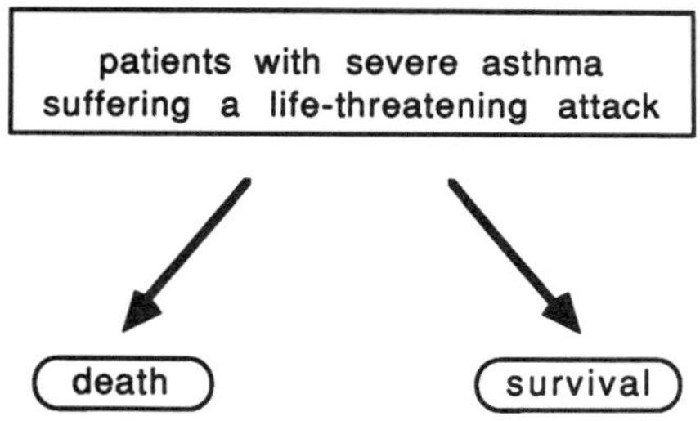

FIGURE 1. Context of study if the central issue is the management of a life-threatening attack.

A. WHAT IS THE MAJOR HYPOTHESIS UNDER TEST?

A major issue is whether the objective of these studies is to look at differences between fatal and nonfatal cases of asthma in terms of drugs prescribed or used in a life-threatening attack or in terms of drugs prescribed or used in a longer period leading up to the final outcome. These two concepts require different approaches.

B. EMPHASIS ON THE OUTCOME OF A LIFE-THREATENING ATTACK

If the main hypothesis relates to the events during a life-threatening asthma attack, the key events are as indicated in Figure 1. Those who approach this subject from an explanatory viewpoint and whose main interest is the physiological mechanism by which death has been precipitated or prevented will emphasize the key question as relating to the drugs actually used in the relevant attack. If this is the key hypothesis, in a case-control design certain principles follow:

1. The relevant exposure comprises the types and amounts of drugs prescribed or taken during the last attack; the onset of the attack needs to be defined. Medication prescribed or taken prior to that attack should not be considered an exposure variable, although it is relevant as an indicator of the severity of the underlying disease.
2. The crucial issue of comparability between cases and controls depends on comparability in regard to the severity of this last attack. The ideal comparison, if any can be considered ideal, would be perhaps between patients who died of acute asthma and subjects who had extremely severe acute asthma and did not die.

Although it is relatively easy to stipulate the theoretical criteria for such a study, it is difficult to see how any study could be designed to adequately explore this question. A possible comparison group would be patients admitted with acute asthma to an intensive care unit, fulfilling certain criteria of severity. Whatever the criteria used, it will be difficult to obtain a comparison group whose asthma attacks were as severe as that of the cases. Because the great majority of asthma deaths occur outside hospital without medical supervision, comparable information for the cases on such measures as blood gases would be unlikely to be available. For the same reason, information on the use of drugs during the last attack would be difficult to obtain and likely be incomplete and inaccurate. The method used in the New Zealand National Asthma Mortality Survey,[6] obtaining a history from friends, relatives, and so on, is probably the best available, although it is clearly difficult to apply objectively, but the national study of asthma deaths did not involve any comparison subjects. The difficulties of a design to test this hypothesis are illustrated by the comments of Lanes and Walker[7] who suggested a study design that would apply only to the seven in-hospital deaths, that is, the study they proposed would be irrelevant to the major issue of studying death in asthmatics. This suggestion is omitted from their later comments.[8] Nor are these difficulties a feature only of the case-control design. Consideration of a prospective cohort study or a randomized trial of this hypothesis, related to medication in the final acute attack, raises the same difficulties and shows what a difficult methodological problem it is. Subjects cannot be randomly allocated to alternative therapies for a life-threatening asthma attack because the management of such attacks is usually carried out by the subjects themselves, without medical supervision until the later stages.

C. EMPHASIS ON THE MANAGEMENT OF SEVERE CHRONIC ASTHMA

The previous argument leads to a consideration of whether a hypothesis emphasizing the acute attack is the most relevant one. Most fatalities occur in an unsupervised out-of-hospital situation, and medication that is taken is self-administered by a subject who is in great difficulty. The only control the physician has over the patients in an acute attack is in terms of what medications the patients have been prescribed in the past, what medication they have available, and what education they have received about dealing with acute attacks. On this basis, the relevant hypothesis relates to differences in the medication prescribed to patients who subsequently die of asthma and patients who subsequently do not, given that both have a severe disease to start with (Figure 2).

Indeed, if a randomized trial of the management of severe asthmatics were planned, the easiest way it could be done would be to randomize the patients to alternative prescribed regimens of regular drugs; the end point would be fatality or survival, irrespective of what drugs were actually used or further prescribed in any acute attack. Studies that evaluate this hypothesis could be called "pragmatic", or "management" studies, given that they assess the impact of the clinical management decisions over which the physician does have control. Consideration of this hypothesis might suggest that it is not the drugs prescribed, but the education given to the patient, and even actions to ensure that patients do not have access to drugs that were not prescribed, which could be important factors. Studies designed to test this

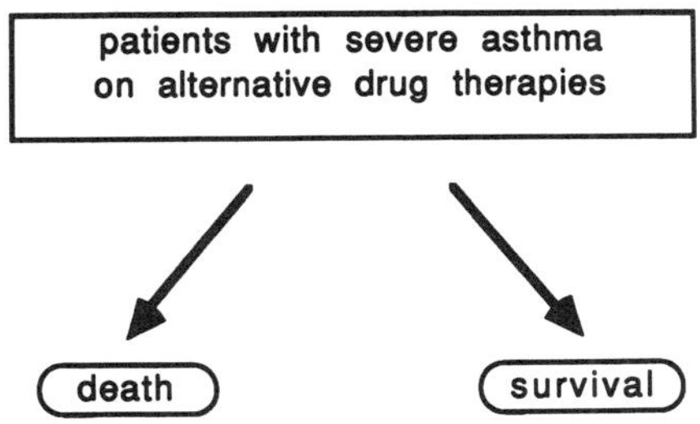

FIGURE 2. Context of study if the central issue is the management of severe asthma.

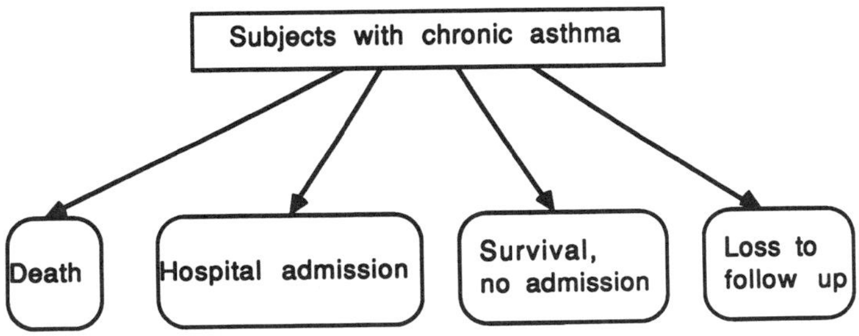

FIGURE 3. The general context of a study of the outcome of severe chronic asthma.

hypothesis are not as useful in relating to the physiological hypotheses of the mechanism causing or preventing death but are directly relevant to the practical issues of how severe asthma can be controlled. A case-control study designed with this as the key issue requires that:

1. The exposure data to be collected refer to drugs regularly prescribed over some specifically defined time period preceding either death or the nonfatal comparison event. For this hypothesis the drugs given in the final phase are not relevant.
2. The important comparative features between fatal cases and nonfatal comparison subjects can be expressed in terms of comparability in the severity of the asthma at the time when the regular prescriptions of drugs were made, and this might be ascertained by various criteria, including clinical and laboratory measurements. The control group should be representative of patients with severe underlying asthma who survive. The use of only a hospital control group may lead to bias if among the survivors, drug use influences the frequency of hospitalization.

D. APPLICATION TO THESE STUDIES

These two hypotheses therefore require different approaches. In the first study, it was not clear which was being assessed, and the authors appeared to mix them. In the second study, perhaps as a result of these arguments, the second (management) hypothesis is clearly the one used.

E. THE DESIGN OF THE STUDIES: CHOICE OF CONTROLS

The architecture of these two studies can be considered as in Figure 3. Consider a source population of patients with a hospital admission for asthma, and their subsequent course in relationship to their drug therapy on discharge after that episode. There are four possible outcomes: death from asthma, a further hospital admission for asthma, survival without a hospital admission, and other events, such as death from other causes, emigration, and so on. In a prospective study one would attempt to compare patients with different discharge medications, controlling for measures of severity of the underlying asthma in terms of their outcome, probably simplified to death compared with survival over a fixed time period after that discharge. The ideal method of achieving comparability in terms of the severity of the underlying asthma, and of other factors, would be to randomize eligible patients between fenoterol and alternative drugs.

To achieve a case-control design that would be comparable in architecture to such a prospective study, one could sample all deaths in this source population as the case events, and take as controls a random sample of subjects in the source population who had not died by the end of an appropriate period. Because it is likely that there would be great differences in underlying severity between all subjects who die and a random sample of those who do not, such a study would have to rely totally on the use of recorded information on measures of severity to control confounding by severity.

The design used in the New Zealand studies was, rather than take a random sample of survivors as the controls, to use subjects who had had another hospital admission for asthma. Although the controls were not a representative sample of the source population, these designs were likely to give a greater degree of comparability with the cases in terms of severity of asthma. It is reasonable to assume that the severity of the underlying asthma in those with another hospital admission for asthma would be greater than in those with no such admission, and therefore, would be more similar to the severity in those subjects who suffered death.

This design is valid on the assumption that within the nondeceased subjects, fenoterol prescription itself did not influence hospital admission (that is, as distinct from any relationship with fenoterol mediated by an effect of differences in underlying severity of disease). If fenoterol had ill effects, or was an ineffective drug so that asthmatics treated by it would tend to get worse, it would be expected not only to increase the risk of death but also to increase the risk of hospital admission; thus, the case-control comparison made would underestimate the true ill effect of fenoterol, by comparing a group with a severe ill effect of fenoterol (death) with a group with a less severe ill effect (hospital admission). In contrast, if among patients who do not die, the prescription of fenoterol were associated with a lower rate of hospital admission, which could occur if it were an effective drug that would allow asthmatic patients to be managed outside hospital, the comparison would exaggerate any true effect of fenoterol, by comparing a group disadvantaged by fenoterol (deaths), with a group whose usage of fenoterol would be relatively low, because fenoterol use tended to prevent hospital admission.

F. DEFINITION OF THE RELEVANT PERIOD OF DRUG USE

Because no particular mechanism for any effect of fenoterol could be assumed, the critical exposure period during which fenoterol would have had to be prescribed to produce an effect on mortality could not be defined *a priori*. In the second study, there were two alternatives: to use the drug history at the time of the reference admission or at the time of the discharge after that hospital admission. The authors chose the latter on the basis presumably that it is closer in time to the outcome event. However, it is unlikely that all drugs prescribed on discharge would be continued because some (e.g., oral steroids) are often given for a short time. If many drugs given to patients on discharge are intended only for short-term use, then the better indicator of likely drug exposure prior to the outcome event (the fatal attack or hospital admission in the controls) may be the drugs prescribed at the time of the previous reference hospital admission. A major effect seen in regard to drugs on discharge should also be seen in regard to drugs prescribed at the time of the reference admission. In the second study, results are given for inhaled fenoterol as assessed at the reference admission, giving an OR of 1.72, increasing to 3.57, 3.10, 16.59, and 14.00 in the four subgroups defined by severity markers shown in Table 3. The results for fenoterol are this similar to those given in Table 3. The differences are considerable for oral steroids. Cases were much more frequently started on oral steroids at the referent hospitalization; this suggests that the severity of asthma at that time was higher for the cases. More of the cases may have been on a short course of oral steroids, which are usually given in decreasing doses; this may be relevant to the mechanisms of the association.

Another method of analysis that might be helpful is to assess the relationships between the outcome event and drug histories in relation to the time interval between the outcome event and the reference admission, which has a range up to 12 months. If a result of the study were biased by incorrect classification, in that a drug used at the time of the reference admission was not used prior to the outcome event, one would expect the association to be weaker if the time interval between outcome event and the reference admission were greater. Consistency of effect, or an effect being seen as stronger when the interval between outcome event and reference admission was short, would argue against such a bias.

III. INTERPRETATION OF THE ASSOCIATION BETWEEN FENOTEROL PRESCRIPTION AND ASTHMA DEATHS

These two studies showed an association between the prescription of fenoterol and death of asthma. The challenge presented in 1989 was to come to a reasonable judgment as to the most likely explanations for these results.

Following general principles,[9] the results obtained must be due to one or more of four general processes:

1. *Bias in the observations,* by which the differences observed between the cases and controls in the recorded data on drug histories could be an overestimate or an underestimate of the true differences;
2. *Confounding,* that is, a true association or difference in drug histories between the cases and controls, due not to a direct association between the drugs prescribed and the risk of death from asthma, but to an association with some other factor or combination of factors;
3. *Chance variation,* meaning that the differences between cases and controls could have arisen purely through chance variation;
4. Or, if these mechanisms can be reasonably excluded, a *cause-and-effect relationship* between the exposure (drug therapy) and the outcome (death or survival).

A. CONSIDERATION OF POSSIBLE OBSERVATION BIAS

1. First Study

The major problem with the first study is the differences in the methods used to collect information from the cases and from the controls. Data for the cases came from questionnaires to the GP usually within 3 months of the patient's death, and described "regular prescribed medication together with medication newly prescribed during the final attack."[1] For the controls, information on "prescribed drug therapy for self-administration at the time of admission" was recorded from "the most complete record in the hospital admission notes."[1] It is difficult to predict what would be the likely differences. The GP questionnaires could be fairly accurate for regularly prescribed medication but might miss medication newly prescribed during the final attack and medication prescribed by other doctors, including hospital specialists. Hospital admission notes might be most complete for medications used by the subject at the time of admission but might omit other medications prescribed. Information provided by the Asthma Task Force giving details on 19 fatal cases in 5–44 year olds[10] shows there were a large number of drugs used or available and considerable differences between the therapy recalled by the family and that prescribed by the GP.

To support the relevance of the drug information used, Crane et al.[1] noted that 91% of cases and 88% of controls used beta agonists by MDI, supporting both the validity of the control group as being true asthma sufferers, and an overall similarity in the frequency of recorded drugs. The frequency of use of oral beta agonists was also similar (24% in cases, 23% in controls). However, for other classes of drugs, beta agonists by nebulizer, oral theophylline, cromoglycate, and inhaled and oral steroids, use was more frequently reported for the cases, which could be interpreted either as showing more severe disease or more complete ascertainment for the cases. The key result is the relative excess of fenoterol compared with salbutamol within the group of subjects prescribed beta agonists by MDI. Differentials in completeness or accuracy of recording would be unlikely to apply to one and not the other of these drugs.

Thus, although the differences in methods of data collection between the cases and controls in this study urge great caution in the interpretation of the results, it is more difficult to see why such differences should have produced a specific effect for MDI fenoterol to be preferentially recorded for the cases and MDI salbutamol for the controls. Our conclusion in regard to bias in the first study[3] was that information bias could be severe. We saw this as the major problem with the study.

2. Second Study

In the second study, the prescribed drug therapy at the time of the prior "reference" hospital episode used data at both admission and discharge. The data on medication were abstracted from case notes, accident and emergency department notes, the GP's letter, and the discharge notes, discharge letter, and discharge prescription; the "data extractors" were instructed to record all drug information and to use the record with the most complete drug information where there was more than one record available. This abstraction process was not carried out in a blind fashion. The assessment of these abstracted data was then made by two of the authors, from copies of the data forms in which information on case or control status was deleted; this was therefore done blind.

Patients at the time of a further acute attack could have had access to other drugs, prescribed earlier or later than the reference admission. Thus, for both cases and controls, the information available on drugs is likely to be incomplete, and there could be important differences between the drug information used in this study and what was actually available to or used by the patient. However, the drug information for both cases and controls was obtained in an identical manner and, therefore, should be free of bias.

Thus, although the drug information may be incomplete, a difference in drugs recorded between cases and controls is likely to represent a true difference in drugs prescribed at the time of discharge from the prior hospital admission. The Boehringer Ingelheim consensus group commented on the limitations of the drug data,[11] using a one-sided argument: "Our main concern here is that fenoterol may have been added after hospital discharge to subjects who subsequently survived and are included as controls. If this is so, then fenoterol use may have been misclassified and underestimated in the control group, resulting in an overestimate of the odds ratio for the fenoterol/asthma death association." They did not mention the possibility that fenoterol may have been added after discharge to the cases, resulting in an underestimate of the association. The usual assumption in these situations, in the absence of any evidence, is that the changes in medication apply to both groups, producing nondifferential misclassification of exposure, which will tend to make the association seem conservative, that is, to underestimate any true difference.

More difficult to assess are the contradictions in the information on the use of drugs for some of the deceased cases as assessed by O'Donnell et al.,[12] Holst,[13] and Rea[14] compared with the data in the first study, and the rejoinder by the authors.[15] A critical issue is that the methods of assessment must be applied similarly to cases and to controls; this indeed was the major weakness of the first study and the major improvement of the second. The reassessments of drugs used have been made only for cases, and unless similar reviews are made for controls, the dangers of information bias are increased by these further post hoc assessments. Members of the Asthma Task Force worked with Pearce et al. in the review of drugs prescribed;[15] there seems reasonable consistency on this but great difficulty in obtaining good data on drugs actually used. The inconsistencies in the records of drugs shown by Rea[14] show that the quality of medical records is low, and the integration of hospital and GP care is poor; the information given to the consensus group on "the high quality of hospital records in New Zealand"[11] is ill-founded.

3. Summary

The major advantage of the second study is that it avoids the serious question of observation bias, which was present in the first study. Those criticisms of the first study, which emphasized this likelihood of observation bias, can therefore be dismissed, given the great similarity of results between the second and first studies. It is reasonable to conclude not only that the results of this second study, but also the results of the first study, were not seriously affected by observation bias.

B. CONFOUNDING

1. Confounding by Selected Markers of Asthma Severity

The main interpretations of the results are that they are due either to a causal relationship or to confounding by the severity of the underlying asthma, that is, patients receiving fenoterol had more severe underlying asthma and for that reason had a higher risk of death. Confounding is dealt with in a case-control study by comparing cases to comparison subjects who have chronic asthma of similar severity. The measures of severity used in both studies are the use of three or more types of drug, the prescription of oral corticosteroids, and a hospital admission for asthma in the year prior to the reference admission.

Are these markers of severity confounders in the association between fenoterol and asthma death? To act as such they need to be associated independently with fenoterol use and with asthma death. The association between the risk indicators and fenoterol use is best assessed in the controls. In the first study, there was a moderate increase in the proportion of the controls prescribed fenoterol when comparing those with three or more drugs with those without (45% to 37%), and those with a hospital admission in a previous year to those without (47% to 37%), although the difference was slightly in the other direction for the prescription of oral steroids (37% compared with 41%). In the first study, the crude OR for the association of fenoterol prescription with death is 1.55; the OR after adjusting (by the Mantel-Haenszel method) for 3+ drugs is 1.45, for a previous admission 1.49, and for oral steroids 1.61. Simultaneous adjustment for the two former factors gives an adjusted risk ratio of 1.41. This suggests that a small proportion of the overall association seen in the first study can be explained by confounding by the measures of severity used, corresponding to the change in OR from 1.55 to 1.41.

In the second study, the proportion of controls prescribed fenoterol was higher in those with three or more categories of asthma drugs (42% compared with 32%), and in those with oral steroid use on admission (41% compared with 35%), but was lower in those with a prior admission (34% compared with 40%). The association between risk indicators and fenoterol was therefore mixed, positive for two of the three indicators. The association between risk indicators and death is best assessed by comparing cases and controls among subjects without exposure to fenoterol, and in the second study shows a surprising pattern in that each of the risk indicators is negatively associated with asthma death. In cases without fenoterol, the percentages on three or more drugs, with a prior admission, and on steroids are 26%, 41%, and 11%, respectively; the corresponding proportions for controls not using fenoterol are 44%, 60%, and 24%, respectively. Thus, the OR for asthma death in subjects not using fenoterol associated with each of the three measures of severity are 0.4, 0.5, and 0.4, respectively. The result of this in terms of confounding is a strong negative association between these risk indicators and death, which taken with the mixed association with fenoterol use, suggests that these risk indicators are likely to have a mild or moderate negative confounding effect. This is confirmed by comparison of the crude OR for fenoterol prescription, 1.99, with the Mantel-Haenszel ORs adjusted for the use of three or more drugs (2.1), for prior admission (2.0), and for oral steroid use (2.0). There is therefore a small negative confounding effect of these measures in the second study.

2. Validity of These Markers as Measures of Asthma Severity

Were the measures of severity used reasonable indicators? There is no independent information that substantiates or refutes the claim that these indicators are adequate measures of the severity of underlying asthma. They have been used in other studies.[1,5] Rea's study,[5] from which these indicators are partially derived, suggested that they are indicators of severity: other indicators suggested were a previous life-threatening attack, an accident and emergency admission, and a previous respiratory arrest. The Boehringer Ingelheim consensus group suggested that information on symptoms, such as nighttime wheezing and cough, time lost from school or work, and measures of lung function and blood gases could be used to develop a clinically relevant index of severity.[11] Work to develop and validate such measures is important for future studies. Some limited data have been provided by Pearce et al.:[16] of 141 asthma admissions at Wellington Hospital in 1977–1987, arterial $PaCO_2$ levels were similar in 17 patients prescribed fenoterol (42.9 ±

10.0 mmHg, mean ± SD) as in 28 other patients (40.2 ± 18.0 mmHg, mean ± SD).

The consensus report[11] stated that "members of the New Zealand Task Force found further evidence to support the conclusion that the data are best explained by fenoterol being prescribed to patients with the more severe asthma." This was the conclusion given by members of the Task Force,[10,12] but data to support that conclusion have not been presented. Nor have data been presented to back up the arguments that alternative measures of severity exist and, if used, would show major differences between fenoterol-treated patients and others.

A general association between the use of fenoterol and more severe asthma outside the context of these studies was supported by comments of experienced physicians,[12,17] by the drug company's marketing approach in advertising Berotec® as "opening the airways for longer",[18] and by data on co-prescribing in a Boehringer Ingelheim report.[18] In general in New Zealand since 1983, prescriptions for fenoterol more commonly represented a change in therapy than did prescriptions for salbutamol, and oral steroids were more frequently co-prescribed with fenoterol than they were with salbutamol. The conclusion that these data present "unequivocal" evidence,[18] that fenoterol was used in more severe patients must however be disputed. It merely provides a general case that fenoterol may have been used in more severe asthmatics than salbutamol. Data presented from The Netherlands provide a similar viewpoint for that country.[18] The relevance of this to the interpretation of the major case-control studies is limited, however, because the crucial issue is whether *within these studies* there are strong relationships between severity, fenoterol prescribing, and asthma death.

3. Associations Seen with These Markers of Severity

In the second study, the factors taken as markers of asthma severity were actually more common in the hospital admission group than the asthma death group for the subjects who were not given fenoterol. As discussed, the measure of outcome in these studies is the ratio of the risk of death to the risk of hospital admission, where both refer to events in an undefined inception cohort of patients with asthma. Patients who suffer neither death nor admission were not sampled. If a factor increases the rate of hospital admission more than it increases the risk of death, a comparison between deaths and admissions will show an apparently aberrant result. The best example is from the Rea et al. case-control study,[5] which used samples of deaths, admissions, and also asthma patients in the community. The risk factor of "previous hospital admission for asthma" showed a relative risk of 16 in comparing deaths with community controls, but comparing deaths with hospital admissions gave a relative risk of 0.8 (a protective effect). This means that for patients with asthma in general, this factor was associated with an increase in the risk of a subsequent hospital admission (about 20 times increased) and a smaller increase in the risk of death (about 16 times). Given this example, the observation that in subjects not prescribed fenoterol, the three chosen risk factors (previous admission, prescription of oral steroids, or of three or more types of asthma drug) were as common or more common in subjects who had a further admission for asthma than in those who died is not totally surprising. It suggests that for asthma patients, in general, these indicators of severity (or of therapy) give greater increases in admissions than in deaths. It is still reasonable to refer to these factors as risk factors in the context of the wider population of asthma patients.

Such data do not invalidate the studies, as has been implied,[19] although they show their complexity. The positive association seen with fenoterol could be due to fenoterol not increasing the risk of death but decreasing the risk of hospital admission. This possibility has to be considered, but there is little direct evidence to support it.[20] The Boehringer Ingelheim consensus group[11] considered this issue and put considerable emphasis on the ''non-representativeness'' of the controls, but took little account of the difficulties introduced by using a wider control group in terms of greater differences in severity of disease.

4. Random Misclassification of a Confounder

The ability of the analyses to deal with confounding effects depends on whether the measures used for confounders are accurate and appropriate. It has been shown[21] that if the measure used for a confounder is simply inaccurate, that is, if there is random misclassification, not only is the ability to control confounding limited, but apparent heterogeneity of effect can be produced. This raises the question of whether the lack of reduction in the OR when the results are stratified by the confounders, and also the strengthening of effect when the analysis is restricted to patients within certain subgroups, could be due to the measures used for confounding having a high degree of random misclassification. However, the issue of random misclassification has been modeled, and it has been shown that the results in these studies could not have been produced by this mechanism.[22] Thus, the demonstration of the increasing OR in subgroups of patients defined by the given severity markers remains the strongest evidence against the association being produced by confounding by severity.

5. Other Confounding Factors

There are several other potential confounding factors. In the previous Auckland case-control study,[5] although numbers were small, positive associations with asthma mortality were seen with a ''below average medical care score'' (OR 1.9), patient's noncompliance with treatment (OR 1.4), and psychosocial problems (OR 3.5). High ORs were also seen with one or more previous respiratory arrests (OR 5.0) and one or more previous life-threatening asthma attacks (OR 3.8), suggesting that these are also relevant measures of severity. The importance of such factors was supported by the comments by the Asthma Task Force.[12] It is relevant in that in regard to the choice of controls, these studies are based partially on the previous Auckland study. In the second major study,[2] the authors referred to the Auckland study,[5] which noted that patients dying of asthma and patients admitted to hospital come from a similar portion of the asthmatic population, using this to support their use of the hospital comparison group. However, the next sentence in the Auckland paper[5] stated that "there is however a suggestion of some dissimilarities between those who die and the hospital controls. Those who die may have had more severe disease (previous life threatening attacks), received poorer medical care, had more discontinuous general practice care, and had more psycho-social problems. The importance of some of these factors was, however, hard to judge." Although these factors are indeed difficult to assess and measure, their influence again raises the possibility of uncontrolled confounding.

Another potential confounder is that of regional or local geographical variation. Large variations occurred in both fenoterol prescribing and in asthma mortality in New Zealand. Cases and controls were matched on area or hospital, but the matching was not used in the analysis, so confounding could still remain. Also, if such variations in prescribing are due to large variations between practices or individual GPs, area matching may be insufficient; matching by GP practice or individual doctor may be needed.

On the basis of these arguments, it seems that despite the authors' appropriate attempts to measure and adjust for confounding factors, there could still be some residual confounding primarily by the severity of underlying disease, and also by other social, psychosocial, and medical care factors. Because the primary association in these studies is not strong, it is conceivable that this association could be produced largely by uncontrolled confounding. It must be pointed out, however, that a study design that would avoid such confounding is by no means simple. It is more difficult to see how the strong associations within those subjects who had one or more of the indicators of severity could be produced by such confounding.

6. Conclusion

Within both of these studies, the severity of asthma appears generally similar in subjects prescribed fenoterol and in those prescribed other drugs. In both studies, the fact that the OR relating fenoterol use to asthma death was greater for subjects with one or more of these measures of severity argues strongly against the association being due to confounding by asthma severity. The overall association in this study could be produced by confounding. However, we did not agree with the Asthma Task Force's conclusion[10,12] that the association "is fully explained" by confounding; the data do not show this, and in fact the data from the two studies are in general not consistent with an explanation of confounding.

C. CHANCE VARIATION

The overall association between death and inhaled fenoterol in each study was statistically significant, although the lower 95% confidence limits were not much above the null value. Within subgroups categorized by one or more of the "indicators of severity", the ORs, and the lower 95% limits were substantially higher, despite the reduced numbers of subjects. The results of the two studies, given the differences in design, were generally consistent both in terms of the magnitude of the ORs and their significance. Chance variation is therefore an unlikely explanation of the results.

IV. INTERPRETATION OF THE JOINT ASSOCIATION WITH FENOTEROL AND ORAL STEROIDS

As noted (Table 3), the association with fenoterol was stronger in subjects with one or more of the measures of severity in both studies. Joint tabulation of pairs of these three indicators showed further increases in risk, particularly in the group with oral corticosteroids on admission and a hospital admission in the previous 12 months, where the OR was 13.29 in the first study and 9.82 in the second.

The assessment of the interaction with steroids is made more difficult because of the lack of detail on oral steroids: the drugs prescribed, dosages, and duration of therapy are unknown. It is possible to look at the interaction between fenoterol on discharge (from the reference hospital episode) and oral steroids on admission, which has been taken as an indicator of disease severity, and may be a good indicator of the likelihood of continued steroid use a considerable time after the reference episode (Table 4).

The data (second study) show a significant excess risk of fenoterol overall, both crude (OR = 1.99) and after adjustment for steroids (OR = 2.02). Although the effect of fenoterol is considerably larger in those subjects also on steroids (fenoterol OR = 5.83 with steroids, 1.46 without), the contrast, as assessed by the test for homogeneity, is not significant. In the first study, the situation is similar except that the difference in the association between steroid users (OR = 6.45) and nonusers (OR = 0.96) is statistically significant. The consistency of the two studies is striking, although the data on steroids are not defined identically.

The results for risk in association with oral steroids are more complex (Table 4). In the second study, steroids on admission at the reference hospital episode showed no association with asthma death (OR = 0.99); this is 0.91 when adjusted for fenoterol use. However, the risk associated with oral steroids is reduced in subjects without fenoterol (OR = 0.39) and increased in those with fenoterol (OR = 1.55). The results of the first study are similar to these. The combined analysis of the two studies shows a significant interaction between oral steroids and fenoterol; the increased risk applies to subjects treated with both; fenoterol alone gives no significant increase in risk, and steroids alone are associated with a decrease in risk.

The observed results could be explained by confounding only if the confounding effects are greater in the high-risk subgroup than in the study as a whole. The Asthma Task Force[12] suggested that in the first study, for the fatal cases the data from the GP questionnaire would pick out subjects on long-term steroid dosage, indicating chronic severe asthma, while from the hospital records controls categorized as being on steroids would include a

TABLE 4
Combined Analysis of Two Studies: Fenoterol and Oral Steroids

	Crane et al.[1]		Pearce et al.[2]		Combined data		Test of homogeneity between studies	
Drugs	**OR[a]**	**CI[b]**	**OR**	**CI**	**OR**	**CI**	**Chi-Square**	**(1 *df*)**
Fenoterol								
Overall	1.55	1.04–2.33	1.99	1.12–3.55	—	—	—	—
With oral steroids	6.45	2.27–15.33	5.83	1.62–20.96	6.24	2.90–13.45	0.04	NS
Without oral steroids	0.96	0.59–1.56	1.46	0.74–2.89	1.10	0.74–1.64	0.99	NS
Adjusted for steroids	1.53	0.98–2.38	2.02	1.09–3.74	1.67	1.16–2.40	—	—
Oral Steroids								
Overall	1.38	0.87–2.17	0.99	0.51–1.92	—	—	—	—
With fenoterol	3.04	1.65–5.58	1.55	0.65–3.69	2.39	1.43–4.00	1.53	NS
Without fenoterol	0.45	0.20–1.03	0.39	0.11–1.33	0.43	0.21–0.87	0.01	NS
Adjusted for fenoterol	1.35	0.75–2.43	0.91	0.41–2.02	1.18	0.74–1.90	—	—
Homogeneity test between drugs (chi-square, 1 *df*)	12.53	$p < 0.001$	2.88	NS[c]	—	—	—	—

Note: All results for combined data are adjusted for study. The homogeneity statistics test variation between the strata used; thus, there is no evidence of variation between the studies, but there is statistically significant interaction between the drugs. In the Pearce et al. study,[2] oral steroid data apply to the admission at the reference hospital episode.

[a] Odds ratio.
[b] 95% confidence interval test-based.
[c] Not significant.

higher proportion given steroids only in the acute phase, which might not mean that they had long-term severe asthma. In the first study, of cases classified as being given steroids, 24 of 33 (73%) had "continuous" steroids, compared with 52% (54 of 104) of the controls. Rea[14] and Taylor[23] also suggested that the subgroup of oral steroid users will select cases with long-term use, i.e., severe asthma, but controls with short-term use. However, the risk is also apparent within the subgroup of those defined as being on "continuous" steroids, with an OR of 4.75 (95% confidence limits 1.61, 14.0),[1] which is a strong argument against the aforementioned concept, although it depends on the accuracy of the classification of steroid use being reasonable.

As the authors emphasized,[2,16,24] few of the commentators on the study adequately emphasized this strong result in patients who had also been given oral steroids, although the first Boehringer Ingelheim submission stressed the corresponding fact that no association with fenoterol was found in the majority of asthma patients, as 72% of cases and 78% of controls had not been prescribed oral steroids.[25] The Boehringer Ingelheim group interpreted the findings as showing that "addition of steroids to therapy increases the mortality risk for fenoterol treated patients."[25] The association seen suggested that patients treated with both drugs have a higher risk of death, without any implications for the time relationship of the two therapies. Moreover, the data do not allow a firm distinction between a direct effect from the two drugs, or a confounding effect by oral steroid prescription being an indicator of severity of disease.

The observed high risk of asthma death in subjects on both oral steroids and fenoterol could be explained by several mechanisms.

1. These patients could have the most severe or unstable asthma. A comparison of patients on steroids and fenoterol, one only of these, and none, in terms of other drugs prescribed, age, sex, ethnic origin, and other characteristics of their disease would be useful. Data sets from several studies could be combined for such analyses.
2. Such patients may have an undue concentration of other risk factors, such as poor compliance and difficult social circumstances.[5] Further data from the studies or from new reviews could be helpful.
3. There could be a pharmacological interaction between oral steroids and fenoterol. Here the difficulty in distinguishing short- from long-term steroids is important. Those subjects who were not prescribed oral steroids at the reference admission but were at discharge, that is, who were newly prescribed oral steroids, are worth examining specifically. A possibility worth considering is if the use of a short-term, decreasing dose, oral steroid regimen in severe asthma could produce at some point a period of bronchial hyperresponsiveness or in other ways lead to hypersensitivity to an asthma attack or to aberrant effects of beta agonist therapy. Alternatively, perhaps the use of fenoterol could block the beneficial effects of steroids.

V. MODIFICATION OF THE EFFECT OF FENOTEROL BY SEX, AGE, AND ETHNIC ORIGIN

In the second study, the association with fenoterol was greater in males than in females, although the difference is not significant. In the first study, a slight difference in the other direction was found. In the second study, the association with fenoterol was much stronger in non-Europeans (5.20) than in Europeans (1.20), and this difference was statistically significant; however, in the first study, a slight difference in the other direction was found. In both studies, the association with fenoterol was stronger in subjects under the age of 20; in the second study the ORs were 4.02 and 1.33 in those under and over 20, respectively, and in the first study they were 2.08 and 1.34, respectively. However, it is more important to know if the major effect, the high risk with fenoterol in subjects with other risk markers, such as oral steroid use, shows these modifications by age and ethnic origin. Such data have not been published, and would be limited by small numbers.

VI. SUMMARY OF THE INTERPRETATION OF THE STUDIES: OTHER CRITERIA FOR CAUSALITY

The main results of the two studies are consistent. The second case-control study has the major advantage that the problem of observation bias can be dismissed. On the basis of the substantially raised and statistically significant increased risk, particularly in high-risk subgroups and the consistency of the three available studies, chance variation can be dismissed.

The remaining possibilities are as follows: (1) the results of these studies demonstrate an empiric causal relationship between the prescription of fenoterol and an increased risk of death from asthma or (2) the relationship is due to confounding, most likely by the severity of underlying asthma. The main evidence against the confounding hypothesis is the strengthening of the association between fenoterol and risk of death when the analysis is confined to subjects with indicators of greater severity of underlying asthma, and also the fact that there is no strong association between fenoterol prescription and the risk indicators in either of the main studies. Confounding by severity of underlying asthma can be confidently dismissed if one can assume that the measures of severity used in the two case-control studies adequately represent the severity of underlying asthma. However, this may not be so and further measures of severity are desirable.

A. TIME RELATIONSHIP

There are few data on the time aspects of the relationship, and there is no information that would distinguish long-term effects related to the use of medication over a reasonable period leading up to death, from acute effects due to drugs available and presumably used during the severe premorbid attack.

B. STRENGTH

The strength of the overall relationship is not so high as to make unrecognized bias or confounding unlikely, but it is the much higher risk ratios in the apparently more severe subgroups which are particularly important.

C. DOSE-RESPONSE

There is little useful evidence available on dose-response because there is not adequate heterogeneity of dose within subjects in the studies.

D. CONSISTENCY AND SPECIFICITY

By 1989 there were three case-control studies performed in New Zealand that showed consistent results in terms of the overall association of deaths with fenoterol prescription and the association within apparent high-risk subgroups. Both the major studies showed a concentration of the effect in younger subjects, aged under 20, and this consistency suggests that this modification of effect may be real, which raises several questions relating to the possible mechanism. The differences between the sexes and the differences between European and non-European subjects were not consistent between the two studies.

E. PLAUSIBILITY: THE MECHANISM OF THE ASSOCIATION

The possibilities of mechanisms were reviewed in the 1989 reports,[3,4] and the following summarizes the considerations at that time:

1. Pharmacological Effects

1. A pharmacological mechanism could involve acute toxicity. There is evidence that fenoterol has greater potential to produce cardiac arrhythmias, hypokalemia, bronchial hyperresponsiveness, and down-regulation of beta receptors than have some other drugs, such as salbutamol,[1,2,26,27] although others dispute this.[16] There are no direct observational data on the metabolic state of subjects who die of asthma, understandably so because the great majority die out of hospital without observation. The dosages given by self-administration by asthma patients in a severe, frightening attack are understandably much greater than those recommended or those on which most assessments of side effects have been made.[27] This raises the question of the safety of self-administration of powerful drugs and the need for evidence on the side effects of such drugs when used in high dosages and in the presence of conditions such as hypoxia. Buist[30] stated that Adverse Reaction Reports "provide no evidence" for a causal role of fenoterol in asthma deaths. These reports, lacking any systematic method of assessment or any comparison group, are of limited value, although they do argue against a sudden short-term or hypersensitivity type effect.

2. The long-term use of fenoterol could have an ill effect, perhaps mediated by a change in bronchial sensitivity to beta agonists or to other metabolic or cardiac effects.
3. The concentration of the effect in subjects with apparently more severe asthma has to be explained. The possibilities are that the use of fenoterol is associated with risk, particularly in subjects with particularly severe asthma or specifically in those using oral steroids. It would be important to determine whether the effects of fenoterol on hypokalemia and cardiac responsiveness are increased in subjects on oral steroids, but no clear evidence exists.[18]

2. Nonpharmacological Effects

1. Fenoterol or the fenoterol-steroid combination may be misapplied, giving subjective relief in an acute attack but leading to a delay in seeking more effective medical help.[3] It has been suggested that,[28] "it is possible, even likely, that the fenoterol MDI provided temporary relief in individuals with a steadily deteriorating condition, giving the patients an inappropriate and inaccurate sense of improvement and security." The concentration of the effect in younger subjects may be explicable on this basis. The specificity of the risk of death with fenoterol rather than salbutamol would therefore suggest that fenoterol when used in maximum or excessive dosages in an acute attack gives more symptomatic relief than does salbutamol used under the same circumstances. If so, in the management of asthma, pharmacologically effective drugs are not necessarily those that are most clinically effective. There does not seem to be any direct evidence that can support or refute this hypothesis. This suggests that if fenoterol were not used in these subjects and another powerful bronchodilating drug were used instead, this same effect might apply (although the data still suggest salbutamol would be safer); however, it also suggests possible means of controlling such an effect through patient education in the management of acute attacks, modifying the drug delivery apparatus to prevent overuse, or using regular medications to reduce reliance on acute relief.
2. Fenoterol may be prescribed as part of an unsuitable therapy regimen, in which more effective drugs or combinations of drugs are needed by virtue of severity of the underlying disease. This could happen if physicians had an exaggerated opinion of the effectiveness of fenoterol in severe asthma.[3,29,30] This mechanism could explain the particular association between fenoterol use and death in subjects with other indicators of severe asthma. Given that the data on oral steroid use in both the major studies are clearly incomplete and in particular do not distinguish between acute or long-term use, a particular suggestion emerges that the patients on fenoterol who are also prescribed oral steroids have had a short course of oral steroids in relation to previous acute attacks.

There is evidence for this in the second case-control study, as reviewed. If these patients have severe asthma that is unstable, but they are not on long-term steroids, they may be being undertreated. This is supported by the review by Buist[30] of case reports of patients who died of asthma, wherein she suggested that undertreatment and particularly the lack of adequate long-term steroid treatment may be important: "the consistent theme is one of severe disease which was inadequately treated."[28] To explain the association of these conditions with fenoterol use rather than salbutamol use implies that perhaps the real effectiveness of these two drugs is not greatly different, but fenoterol has been marketed and has been regarded by physicians as the more powerful drug and therefore suitable for use in patients with more severe asthma, removing the need to prescribe other medications, such as steroids. This seems a reasonable hypothesis. The differences in severity would need to be subtle, not adequately described by the risk indicators used in the main studies. There does not seem to be any direct evidence that can clarify this idea further.

3. Prescribed fenoterol could be linked to a high risk of death not because of the overuse of the drug in the acute attack, but because of underuse if there were any reason why effective therapy would not be used in subjects with fenoterol. This would imply that self-administration of fenoterol would, in contradistinction to the aforementioned hypotheses, not produce adequate airway response and relief of acute symptoms compared with the use of salbutamol in the acute attack, or that some factor, perhaps the occurrence of side effects, would prevent patients from using it adequately in an acute attack. There seems to be no evidence that can be used in relation to this hypothesis.

F. IS THE ASSOCIATION SPECIFIC TO FENOTEROL OR IS IT A DOSE EFFECT?

One important general question is whether the observed association, and any of the discussed mechanisms, whether pharmacological or other, are specific to fenoterol, or whether they are merely characteristic of a potent high-dosage bronchodilator drug. Fenoterol (Berotec®) has been marketed at twice the effective dose per puff than its main alternative, salbutamol (Ventolin®), and the marketing strategy of offering it as a more powerful drug is a characteristic of the dose as well as the pharmacological preparation. The studies therefore in principle could have been written as a comparison of "inhaled beta agonists at 200 μg per puff compared to inhaled beta agonists at 100 μg per puff." The similarities between fenoterol and newer, and future, beta agonist drugs need to be considered.

G. COHERENCE: THE RELATIONSHIP TO TIME TRENDS AND INTERNATIONAL VARIATION IN ASTHMA MORTALITY

The analysis of time and geographical differences is a much less precise scientific method than that of an analytical study, such as a case-control study.

The ability to control for other factors is extremely limited. The comparability of mortality data for asthma between countries is questionable, although comparability within a country across fairly short time intervals should be reasonable. Death statistics are age-specific, whereas the information on drug use is expressed either as sales of the drugs in puffs per total (all age) population, or as a market share of a drug compared with all drugs of a comparable type.

Drug use will be related to the frequency and intensity with which asthma is treated. Data presented by Boehringer Ingelheim[18] showed a weak but generally positive association between death rates and the use expressed as puffs per person per year of fenoterol, beclomethasone, and salbutamol between countries. Of the countries noted, New Zealand had the highest mortality rate from asthma and the highest utilization rates for fenoterol and beclomethasone. This gives rise to a statistical problem; if there is a cluster of points with one outlier in terms of both the axes, a fitted regression line will readily give a high and often statistically significant correlation coefficient, which is dependent on the one outlying observation. The Boehringer Ingelheim submission shows that the relationship between mortality and most of these drugs is weak or nonexistent if the New Zealand outlier is ignored. It is clearly arbitrary and inaccurate to ignore one point, but at the same time the finding of a high correlation coefficient is indicating only that New Zealand has high asthma mortality and high drug utilization, rather than any general trend over all the countries surveyed.

H. TIME TRENDS IN NEW ZEALAND

Variations in diagnostic and certification practices over a relatively short time period should not be major. The death rate from asthma in young adults in New Zealand rose between 1976 and 1980 in parallel with the increasing market share of beta agonists held by fenoterol, although thereafter the mortality rate dropped, whereas the market share stayed the same. Crane et al.[1] suggested that this initial consistency and later discrepancy could be due to the early use of the drug in severe asthmatics, followed by its diffusion to the less severely affected asthmatic population. There is no evidence to support this, and it can explain only a leveling off of the trend; the decrease must be due to other factors, such as, perhaps, improvements in the management of asthma following the attention given to the topic in recent years. Substantial increases in asthma mortality between 1975 and 1985 were seen for Austria, Belgium, West Germany, the United Kingdom, and Australia, with 1985 market shares of fenoterol of 34%, 46%, 50%, 2%, and 5%, respectively. No major trend was seen for Canada, The Netherlands, or Sweden with market shares of 7%, 23%, and 7%, respectively.[18] These data are open to many difficulties of interpretation, and in total seem neither to support nor refute the association of asthma deaths with fenoterol seen in the case-control studies. Again, there is the difficulty of comparing age-specific mortality data with drug data, which are based on total units sold or on total population. Boehringer Ingelheim presented a graph[18] of asthma mortality in New Zealand from 1970 to 1986 divided into ages 5–20 and ages 20–45. This is appropriate because the two major case-control studies have shown a concentration of the association in subjects younger than 20 years; however, the data should be presented on a logarithmic scale to give directly the proportional change in the two mortality rates. The comparison of rates around the early 1980s with rates in the pre-fenoterol period shows an approximate doubling of rates in each age group, and the decrease from the peak in the early 1980s is about 50% in each age group. This does not fit with the results of the case-control studies showing the concentration of effect in the under 20s. However, the drug data are not age-specific, and the effect on the mortality rate in a particular age group, if the case-control study results are correct, depends both on the relative risk associated with fenoterol use and on the exposure to fenoterol in that age group.

The results of the case-control studies show a concentration of effect in subjects with risk markers of severe asthma; therefore, a more appropriate comparison could be with the extent of use of fenoterol in such subjects. Co-prescription data could be relevant; these show a considerable decrease in the co-prescription of Berotec® and oral steroids from 1983 (the earliest data given) to 1985.[18] Could this be related to the declining mortality rate during the same period? Thus, to assess trends more carefully, information on the use of fenoterol, the use of other drugs, and the joint use of various combinations of drugs, within age groups of patients over the last 15 years or so, is needed.

These considerations emphasize the weakness of making conclusions based on single factor comparisons of drug sales and asthma mortality. Although these trend data and international data are of interest, they do not add greatly to the arguments for or against a causal relationship in the case-control studies. The data show that fenoterol use is not a complete explanation for either the high death rate from asthma in New Zealand or the mortality trends over the last 10 years.

Crane et al.[31] compared fenoterol sales in New Zealand up to 1990 with asthma deaths at ages 5–34 up to 1989. Fenoterol sales, given by market share of inhaled doses of beta agonists, remained fairly steady until the first half of 1989, but fell in late 1989 and in 1990, when the market share was around 12% compared with around 28% in previous years. A general decline in asthma mortality has been seen from 1979 through the 1980s, with a lot of irregularity, but the 1989 mortality rates show a particular decrease being lower than any rates since 1975. Further data on 1990 and beyond will be needed. Crane et al.[31] commented that this pattern is consistent with an effect of fenoterol but is inconsistent with a more general hypothesis relating risk to beta agonist use in general, as this has not fallen.

VII. SUMMARY OF FINDINGS IN 1989

The evidence implicating fenoterol with an increased risk of death from asthma from the two case-control studies, although it did not constitute scientific certainty, was strong enough to support clinical and public policy decisions, and there were no strong counterbalancing arguments for the benefits of this particular drug. The review of the first study[3] concluded that the association between fenoterol and asthma death could be causal, but also could be produced by "a combination of information basis, confounding, and chance." With the second study, it was possible to dismiss information bias and chance variation as likely. The main options[4] were as follows:

1. That the association was causal, meaning that the prescription of fenoterol rather than alternatives did result by some mechanism as yet not understood, in a higher risk of death in subjects who had severe underlying asthma. A causal interpretation includes the possibilities both of pharmacological effects and of nonpharmacological effects related to the method of use of the drug by patients and doctors. The implications of a causal relationship depend on the mechanism and whether it is specific to fenoterol or is shared by other drugs.
2. That the association between fenoterol and asthma deaths was due to confounding, in that patients who are prescribed fenoterol had a disease that was more severe or more unstable, and for that reason had a higher risk of death.

The main evidence consistent with a causal interpretation was summarized as follows:[4]

1. An association between the prescription of fenoterol and death from asthma in subjects aged 5–45 in New Zealand had been shown in two reasonably large case-control studies and an earlier small study.
2. The results of these two major studies were consistent.
3. The association was statistically significant.
4. In the second study, data were collected in an identical manner for all subjects.
5. The association became stronger when the comparisons were restricted to subjects who had characteristics that were likely to be markers of more severe asthma.
6. There was an association in time between the introduction of fenoterol in New Zealand and an abrupt, rapid increase in the death rate from asthma.

The evidence in favor of the causal hypothesis was therefore empiric and from within the studies, rather than subjective and from general considerations. The evidence against confounding was based on the analysis of data on factors that were taken as indicators of severity of underlying asthma: previous hospital admissions, multidrug treatment, and prescription of oral steroids. Using these indicators, within the two major studies, there was no strong association between these risk indicators and the prescription of fenoterol, and controlling for these indicators made no major difference to the overall association between fenoterol prescription and death. Stratification for these measures showed that the association became much stronger in the subjects who had one or more of these markers of severity, showing that confounding by these measures of severity did not explain the observed association between fenoterol and asthma death. Random misclassification of the confounding effect, which would occur if these measures of severity were an unbiased but inaccurate guide to the underlying severity of asthma, did not explain the observed results.

The main evidence in favor of the confounding hypothesis was summarized as follows:[4]

1. The difficulty in finding a mechanism for the observed relationship between fenoterol prescription and death from asthma.
2. The opinion of experienced physicians that fenoterol had tended to be used in patients with more severe asthma.
3. The data on prescribing of fenoterol, suggesting that it had been used more often as a second-line therapy and in conjunction with oral steroids, than alternative drugs.
4. The lack of concordance between recent decreases in asthma mortality and the continued high usage of fenoterol.
5. Consideration of case histories, suggesting that patients who die of asthma often have complex medical and social situations, and suggesting various alternative hypotheses, for example, that fenoterol has been used in patients with severe unstable asthma when it is not an adequately powerful drug to deal with their condition.

The evidence in favor of the confounding hypothesis was indirect, circumstantial, and considerably subjective; support of the hypothesis depended on the limitations of the studies done. Ideally, the main studies would have been sufficiently detailed to allow a full description of all drug therapy prescribed to (and better, used by) the subjects in a defined period preceding death or the equivalent event in the controls, and would have extensive data on the severity of their asthma. The confounding hypothesis depended on this lack of detail. If the confounding hypothesis held, it should have been possible to demonstrate within the context of patients with severe asthma treated in New Zealand, that subjects treated with fenoterol had more severe underlying disease than those treated with alternatives, such as salbutamol, using appropriate indices of severity of chronic asthma. There was insufficient information on the ideal measures of severity of asthma as predictors of death.

The conclusion reached therefore was that the balance of the available information was in favor of the causal rather than the confounding hypothesis. However, there were several unresolved issues identified:

1. All the relevant data related to drugs prescribed to patients over a variable time period; the relationships to drugs actually used, and to how and when they were used, were unknown.
2. The association could be due to either a pharmacological or a medical care mediated mechanism; thus, the relevance of the relationship to other, and to new and future drugs was unknown.
3. A particularly high risk in subjects who had been prescribed both oral steroids and fenoterol was shown and had not been explained.
4. The association appeared stronger in young subjects, under the age of 20, for unknown reasons; it was not, however, restricted to such subjects.

In regard to implications for clinical practice and public policy, there were therefore two main possible interpretations of the data in scientific terms: (1) the association was causal or (2) the association was due to confounding factors. Two subtly different questions could be posed:

1. *Do these results demonstrate an increased mortality risk due to fenoterol?*

   The implication of this question is that the burden of proof is on the study to demonstrate an effect. This is the question that had been addressed by the panel convened by Boehringer Ingelheim,[11] who emphasized their findings in terms of whether the evidence provided could be interpreted unequivocally as demonstrating a cause-and-effect relationship between fenoterol use and asthma death. (For example, the consensus report, page 11: ''The alternative hypotheses of confounding by disease severity and bias in control selection require adequate testing before concluding that chronic fenoterol use increases the risk of asthma death.'' The corresponding proposition, which would read ''The alternative hypotheses of confounding by disease severity and bias in control selection require adequate testing before concluding that the association between fenoterol and asthma death can be explained by these hypotheses,'' was not mentioned). This question is relevant in the context of general scientific knowledge, for which an extremely high level of confidence is demanded before concluding that a cause-and-effect relationship exists, restricting it to situations in which all reasonable noncausal explanations have been tested and shown not to apply. The answer to the question as set in this way was ''no'', there remained a number of possibilities of noncausal explanations, which had not been adequately tested and therefore could not be confidently dismissed.

2. *Do these results show that the relationship between fenoterol and asthma death is due to confounding factors?*

In this question the burden of proof is put on the critics of the study to demonstrate that alternative mechanisms are responsible for the results produced. To answer this question in the affirmative requires empiric data rather than merely hypotheses, and such data were not available. Indeed, the data that were available and relevant to the assessment of the confounding hypothesis within these two studies showed that confounding did not explain the results seen; the answer to this question was also "no." The clinical and public policy question was whether fenoterol should be used where an acceptable alternative existed, and in this context it is this second question, which was the more relevant; the principle of *primum non nocere* applied.

The relevant studies, the independent reports, and submissions from the manufacturers were discussed in December 1989 by the two committees responsible for drug regulations in New Zealand and, as a result, fenoterol was removed from the drug tariff from August 1990, which provides subsidies for listed drugs. The drug is still available in New Zealand for patients for whom the physician makes a special case to the Department of Health that they should use it. Action to restrict the drug to use in only mild or moderate asthma sufferers has been taken in Australia.[32]

VIII. THE IMPORTANCE OF THE USE OF CASE-CONTROL METHODOLOGY

The New Zealand case-control studies led to an increase in interest in empiric, clinically based, epidemiological studies with appropriate controls and the sophisticated methodology required to deal with confounding and effect modification. In the management of asthma where relatively few large-scale and long-term randomized trials have been carried out, such studies have the potential to contribute greatly to progress. Such studies are difficult and complex to perform, and few similar studies relevant to asthma deaths and drug therapy have been published. This is a limitation; the fuller understanding of the effects of drugs in asthma will be aided by a range of study designs by different investigators in areas that have differing environmental situations and medical care practices. In the future there should be more such studies, including multicenter international studies. The development of such studies should also increase awareness of the limitations of studies that are small, short-term, use end points chosen for their ease of measurement rather than for the ultimate relevance, and relate to highly selected groups of individuals; such studies should lead to a higher standard of critical appraisal of the evidence.

A. THE THIRD NEW ZEALAND CASE-CONTROL STUDY

A third case-control study from the Wellington group[33] was designed primarily to deal with some of the limitations of the control selection mechanisms used in the earlier studies, by using two control groups. The cases and a first control group, control group A, were selected in the same way as in the second case control study described earlier. The cases were subjects 5–45 years of age who died of asthma in New Zealand between 1981 and 1987, and who had been admitted to one of 32 major hospitals studied during the 12 months before death, with a discharge diagnosis of asthma. The study eligibility period of 1981–1987 overlapped with the study period 1981–1983 used in the first case control study; therefore, some asthma deaths were included in both studies. The control group A were subjects who had an admission for asthma in the same year as the death in the cases and who had had an admission within the previous 12 months to one of the 32 hospitals, with a discharge diagnosis of asthma.

Control group B was selected from all patients with an admission and a discharge diagnosis of asthma in the hospitals surveyed in the study period, and matched for age and hospital. The purpose of control group B was to be representative of all subjects who had a previous admission for asthma to the hospitals chosen, irrespective of their later outcome; indeed, their later outcome was presumably unknown because follow up of the control group B subjects was not done. This corresponds with the ideal of the control group being a representative sample of the original incidence cohort of discharged patients, as shown in Figure 3. However, because control group B subjects were chosen irrespective of their subsequent progress, subjects who subsequently died or were subsequently readmitted and would therefore be eligible as cases or as members of control group A could also be represented in control group B. It is not clear if this overlap was allowed, which would bring in a small dilution effect in the comparison of cases with control group B. The difference is not likely to be important in practice.

The drug treatment data for all subjects were that recorded at the time of discharge after this previous index admission. The measures of severity and of other therapy used were the same as in the first two studies, including the use of data on drug therapy at the time of admission in these index admissions; in addition, markers of acute asthma severity at the time of the index admission were collected where available. These included arterial carbon dioxide tension ($PaCO_2$), plasma potassium concentration, forced expiratory volume in 1 s (FEV_1) and peak expiratory flow (PEF). On the basis of the arguments presented earlier, it would be expected that the results comparing deaths with control group A would be similar to the results of the second case-control study, and the results comparing the deaths with control group B would show stronger associations, as the subjects in control group B would have generally less severe asthma than those in control group A. The residual association after confounding control should ideally be similar whichever control group were used, although the amount of confounding being controlled would be

TABLE 5
Main Results of Third New Zealand Case-Control Study

	% use			Odds ratio	
	Cases	Controls (Group A)	Controls (Group B)	Group A	Group B
Oral beta agonist	25.0	22.2	13.8	1.16	2.08[b]
Oral salbutamol	24.1	20.8	13.4	1.21	2.05[b]
Any MDI[a] drug	90.2	92.5	92.4	0.74	0.75
MDI fenoterol	59.8	45.9	40.0	1.75[b]	2.24[b]
MDI salbutamol	33.0	46.8	51.3	0.56[b]	0.47[b]
Any nebulizer drug	16.1	7.7	4.9	2.29[b]	3.71[b]
Nebulizer fenoterol	10.7	3.5	2.2	3.30[b]	5.26[b]
Nebulizer salbutamol	6.3	4.2	2.7	1.51	2.42
Any inhaled beta agonist	95.5	94.4	94.9	1.27	1.16
Inhaled fenoterol	65.2	47.1	41.3	2.10[b]	2.66[b]
Inhaled salbutamol	37.5	48.7	52.7	0.63[b]	0.54[b]

[a] Metered dose inhaler.
[b] Statistically significant: 95% confidence limits exclude 1.00.

expected to be greater with control group B. The OR for death in association with inhaled fenoterol was 2.10 using control group A and 2.66 using control group B; the ORs for inhaled salbutamol were equivalently 0.63 and 0.54, respectively (Table 5). The ORs for fenoterol MDI were 1.75 and 2.24, respectively; for nebulizer fenoterol they were higher, 3.30 and 5.26, respectively. Thus, for all these comparisons the ORs in comparison with control group B are higher than those with control group A, as predicted. Stratification for measures of severity, as used in the previous studies, showed a much less impressive specificity of effect. Combining categories of severity markers did not show the particular concentration in apparently high-risk patients, as were shown earlier.

The three quantities suggested *a priori* as markers of chronic asthma severity showed significant associations with asthma death only when compared with control group B. However, for the comparison between cases and control group A, the ORs were only slightly and nonsignificantly elevated. In the more relevant comparison excluding subjects prescribed fenoterol, the ORs comparing cases with control group B for the three markers of asthma severity were 1.69, 3.54, and 1.25; comparing with control group A gave ratios of 0.90, 1.18, and 0.67. Thus, selecting controls with a previous hospital admission for asthma (group A) gives subjects with fairly severe asthma, therefore, the residual difference between them and the cases in terms of markers of chronic severe asthma is fairly small. Using a more representative series of asthma patients (group B) produces a greater distinction in severity between these subjects and the cases, which is shown by larger ORs for these markers of chronic severity. This evidence provides justification that these measures of severity used in all the Wellington studies have reasonable validity, and also that the selection of controls with a previous asthma admission has some advantages over the concept of selecting controls as a representative sample of all asthma patients.

Similar arguments should be applicable to the use of the respiratory function and blood gas measurements collected in this study, but the authors do not present a comparison of these values for the cases compared with the controls. They do present a comparison of group A with group B controls, which shows few differences between them and also demonstrates that there are only small differences between controls in either group prescribed fenoterol and controls in the same group not prescribed fenoterol. Another useful result is that the prescription of psychotropic drugs, which might be a marker for psychosocial problems which have previously been shown to be related to asthma death,[5] was related to asthma death but was not associated with the prescription of fenoterol and therefore was not a confounding factor.

The results of this study are therefore consistent with the results of the first two major New Zealand studies in regard to the primary association with fenoterol. They differ in that the concentration of the risk with fenoterol in subjects apparently with more severe asthma is much less obvious in the earlier studies, and also in the relationship between this excess risk and other characteristics of the patients. In this third study, the relative risks in association with fenoterol were similar in males and females, as had been found earlier. The risk was higher in Europeans than in non-Europeans, the opposite of what had been found earlier. Strikingly, the relative risk was lower in younger subjects than in subjects over the age of 20, the opposite of the situation found in both previous studies. This third study covers a long time period, and the ORs for fenoterol were higher for the comparisons relating to deaths in 1981–1983 (2.92 and 3.07 for control groups A and B) than for 1983–1987 (ratios 1.70 and 2.41). During the period of the whole study, the efforts of the National Asthma Task Force and the publicity given to the asthma problem in New Zealand are likely to have caused many changes in the management of asthma by physicians and by the subjects themselves. It is impossible to obtain any consistent documentation of such effects, or indeed any details about how a drug, such as fenoterol, was described and used, and this makes it difficult to do other than speculate on the reasons for the changes in the modifying factors in the fenoterol-asthma death relationship in this study compared with earlier studies. The authors pointed out that the changes in the relative risk seem consistent with the course of the epidemic of fatal asthma, which in the early years was particularly severe in younger people and in Maori patients, but this specificity disappeared later. If these modifications are meaningful, they would seem more easily explained by a non-pharmacological mechanism, such as over use in an acute attack, or delay in other therapy, than by a pharmacological effect at recommended dosages.

B. STUDIES OF THE EFFECTS OF BETA AGONIST THERAPY

This chapter is concerned with epidemiological studies and cannot usefully comment on the many studies of shorter-term clinical and laboratory effects of beta agonists. However, studies of reasonably typical patients, looking at major clinical end points and at longer-term therapy are relevant, and there are few of these. Sears et al.[34] presented a study, although still small and short-term by general standards (89 subjects entered and 64 completed the 1-year study), is one of the largest and most relevant studies of beta agonist use in asthma. In these patients with generally mild asthma, this randomized double-blind crossover trial compared therapy with regular fenoterol 400 mg four times daily to a placebo, the patients continuing to use their other therapies, including corticosteroids, cromoglycate, and aerosol bronchodilators, including fenoterol, salbutamol, and terbutaline. Outcomes were assessed blind and included a hierarchy of clinical end points. While on regular fenoterol the patients showed worse outcomes in measures, including morning peak expiratory flow rate, bronchial responsiveness, and several symptom descriptions. Particularly relevant, although numbers are small, may be that while on regular fenoterol there were five severe exacerbations compared with one while on placebo. The authors concluded that regular beta agonist use produces clinical deterioration. It is not unreasonable to take this result along with the associations with asthma death to suggest that the regular use of potent beta agonists may lead to an increase in the risk of a severe and even a life-threatening or fatal asthma attack.

Thus, the evidence that regular use, or overuse, of beta agonists may be contributing to the high death rate, and perhaps to the high prevalence of severe disease, is growing. Whether these results are specific to one drug, or to a high-dose regimen, or apply to all such drugs, is an important question that is still unresolved. It is disturbing that the clinical management of large numbers of patients seems to depend on a limited amount of reliable evidence from evaluative studies. The detailed discussion of the case-control studies in this chapter has shown that an essential issue is to distinguish conclusions based on documented evidence from those based only on opinion and uncontrolled observations. This issue will clearly be at the center of discussions on asthma therapy for a long time yet.

C. OTHER STUDIES OF BETA AGONISTS AND ASTHMA DEATH

The several studies that consistently relate fenoterol with asthma death have been carried out in New Zealand. The other countries where fenoterol is used most extensively are Germany and Holland, countries that unfortunately do not have a strong tradition of analytical epidemiology. A study using case-control methods in those countries was proposed by Spitzer et al. and referred to in early discussions of the fenoterol issue, but was not completed.

D. SASKATCHEWAN CASE-CONTROL STUDY

Saskatchewan has the particular advantage that drugs dispensed to eligible residents are recorded on a computer file. A cohort of 68,813 Saskatchewan residents aged 5–54 years between 1980 and 1987 who had had at least one prescription of medication for commonly used asthma drugs was identified, and from this subset the 12,301 patients who had had at least ten prescriptions for one or more of the asthma drugs dispensed between 1978 and 1987 were selected.[35] The cohort was further defined by dates of entry and exit.

The study then compared deaths from asthma, ''near-deaths'', and controls. One hundred eighty deaths were identified, and available documents were found for 165 of these and reviewed blindly by consultants, resulting in classification of 44 deaths as probably due to asthma. Near-death from asthma was identified as a hospital event related to asthma in which hypercarbia or nonelective intubation occurred. Again, the data were reviewed blindly by consultants. Eighty-five subjects with such episodes were identified. Controls were matched to each case in respect to region of residence, receipt of social assistance, age at entry and date of entry into the cohort, and hospitalization at least once in the 2 years before the event. Controls were required to have been at risk for the outcome at the time of the event of the case patient. The analysis was based on the comparison of 44 deaths with 233 matched controls and on the comparison of 129 deaths or near-deaths with 655 matched controls; the two sets of analyses are not independent. Adjustment variables used included the number of hospitalizations for asthma, the number of visits to a physician, in the 2 years before the index event, and the use of drugs other than those to treat asthma, divided into several categories.

Comparing the deaths with controls showed a significant increased risk with the use of fenoterol MDI (OR 9.1) and also with the use of theophylline (OR 3.3); nonsignificant elevated risks were seen with the use of albuterol (salbutamol) by nebulizer, oral beta agonists, oral corticosteroids, and inhaled corticosteroids. An analysis that combined deaths with near-deaths with therefore considerably increased statistical power, showed significantly elevated ORs in association with fenoterol MDI (6.1), albuterol MDI (4.1), albuterol by nebulizer (2.5), other inhaled beta agonists (2.6), theophylline (2.4), and oral corticosteroids (2.5). The risks increased with the total dose of inhaled beta agonists, measured as the number of inhalers dispensed during the 12-month period before the index date, for both fenoterol and albuterol. For deaths and near-deaths combined, the results were similar, with ORs of 21 to 24 in the highest exposure category. For the analysis of deaths only, the ORs reached were higher for fenoterol, 113 in the highest dose group, compared with albuterol with an OR of 29, although the precision of the estimates was poor. Estimates of the crude overall death rate from asthma could be made, which was 9.2 per 10,000 person-years. For those taking neither of the two major beta agonists, the rate was 1.8 per 10,000; for those taking albuterol, it was 8.6 per 10,000, and for fenoterol the rate was 34.6 per 10,000.

The overall conclusion was that the use of beta agonists by MDI was associated with an increased risk of death from asthma and of combined death or near-death from asthma. For deaths the use of fenoterol gave an OR of 5.4 per dose compared with 2.4 per dose for albuterol. Because the single dose of fenoterol was 200 μg compared with 100 μg for albuterol, the risks are thus similar on an equivalent weight basis.

Information available to classify subjects by severity of asthma was weaker in this study than in the New Zealand studies. The main variable used was prior hospitalization for asthma. ORs are given for those without this indicator of high risk, giving ORs of 2.4 for albuterol and 2.1 for fenoterol; results are not given for the higher risk group. The overall results are therefore generally consistent with the New Zealand studies in regard to fenoterol, although they also raise the question of whether other drugs carry similar risks. The ability to distinguish an effect from a confounding effect by severity of asthma seems to be weaker in this study than in the New Zealand studies.

Burrows and Lebowitz[36] noted this difficulty and that no medication appeared to prevent deaths or near-deaths. They pointed to the need for controlled trials of beta agonists in high-risk patients. They concluded, "there is enough doubt about the safety of fenoterol to avoid it altogether and to be suspicious of other new very long-acting beta-agonists." On the basis of this and the study of Sears et al.,[34] they did not recommend prescribing beta agonists on a regular schedule, and noted that a patient's increasing need for beta agonists should be considered a sign of worsening disease. In a comment on the Spitzer et al. study,[35] Pearce et al.[37] noted that the findings in regard to fenoterol are similar to the New Zealand findings. They commented that the argument presented by Spitzer et al.[35] for a general beta agonist effect depends on comparison of a large group of patients who received either fenoterol or albuterol with a small group of patients who received neither drug. The latter group would be expected to have much less severe asthma both on general considerations, and by their demonstrated low mortality rate. The same issue of confounding by severity would apply to the dose-response estimates.

IX. CONCLUSIONS

There is still much unknown about the effect of fenoterol and of beta agonists in general on the natural history of asthma and their role in the etiology of death from asthma. This chapter has described the process of consideration of the new findings that came to light in New Zealand in 1989, which raised important clinical and public policy issues. The debates on the specific issue of fenoterol were to a considerable extent covering a wider concern about the appropriate ways to study the effects of therapy for asthma, and the requirements in terms of quality of evidence to justify clinical actions. It has become clear that many major clinical decisions and often the "normal" management plans for asthma were supported by only poor and limited evidence for their benefits. The methods used in the new work on the asthma deaths problem will be of great value in the future, as similar issues will need to be faced.

REFERENCES

1. **Crane, J., Pearce, N. E., Flatt, A., Burgess, C., Jackson, R., Kwong, T., Ball, M., and Beasley, R.,** Prescribed fenoterol and death from asthma in New Zealand, 1981-3: case-control study, *Lancet,* 1, 917, 1989.
2. **Pearce, N. E., Grainger, J., Atkinson, M., Crane, J., Burgess, C., Culling, C., Windom, H., and Beasley, R.,** Prescribed fenoterol and death from asthma in New Zealand 1977–81: a further case-control study, *Thorax,* 45, 170, 1990.
3. **Elwood, J. M. and Skegg, D. C. G.,** *Review of studies relating prescribed fenoterol to deaths from asthma in New Zealand,* Report to the New Zealand Department of Health, 1989.
4. **Elwood, J. M.,** *Prescribed fenoterol and deaths from asthma in New Zealand: second report,* Report to the New Zealand Department of Health, 1989.
5. **Rea, H. H., Scragg, R., Jackson, R., Beaglehole, R., Fenwick, J., and Sutherland, D. C.,** A case-control study of deaths from asthma, *Thorax,* 41, 833, 1986.
6. **Sears, M. R., Rea, H. H., Beaglehole, R., Gillies, A. J. D., O'Donnell, T. V., Rothwell, R. P. G., and Sutherland, D. C.,** Asthma mortality in New Zealand; a two year national study, *N. Z. Med. J.,* 98, 271, 1985.
7. **Lanes, S. F. and Walker, A. M.,** *Draft review,* 15 Feb 1989, in New Zealand Department of Health Document File, 1989, 160.
8. **Lanes, S. F. and Walker, A. M.,** *Review: prescribed fenoterol and death from asthma in New Zealand, 1981–1983: A case-control study,* 10 Mar 1989, in New Zealand Department of Health Document File, 1989, 112.
9. **Elwood, J. M.,** *Causal Relationships in Medicine,* Oxford University Press, Oxford, 1988.
10. **O'Donnell, T. V., Rea, H. H., Holst, P. E., and Sears, M. R. (on behalf of Asthma Task Force),** *Prescribed fenoterol and death from asthma in New Zealand, 1981–1983: a case-control study,* in New Zealand Department of Health Document File, 1989, 141.
11. **Spitzer, W. O., Buist, S., Burney, P., Ernst, P., Horwitz, R., Leeder, S., Poole, C., Rebuck, A. S., and Seale, J. P.,** *Consensus report: an appraisal of a manuscript by N. Pearce et al.,* unpublished manuscript, 30 August 1989.
12. **O'Donnell, T. V., Rea, H. H., Holst, P. E., and Sears, M. R.,** Fenoterol and fatal asthma, *Lancet,* 1, 1070, 1989.
13. **Holst, P. E.,** Fenoterol and severe asthma mortality, *N. Z. Med. J.,* 102, 296, 1989.
14. **Rea, H. H.,** Fenoterol and asthma death, *N. Z. Med. J.,* 102, 356, 1989.
15. **Pearce, N., Crane, J., Burgess, C., Beasley, R., and Jackson, R.,** Fenoterol and asthma mortality, *Lancet,* 1, 1196, 1989.
16. **Pearce, N., Grainger, J., Beasley, R., Crane, J., and Burgess, C.,** Fenoterol: confounding again, *N. Z. Med. J.,* 101, 619, 1989.
17. **Grant, I. W. B.,** Fenoterol and asthma deaths in New Zealand, *N. Z. Med. J.,* 103, 160, 1990.
18. **Boehringer Ingelheim (NZ) Ltd.,** *Submission summary from Boehringer Ingelheim concerning fenoterol,* 2 Oct 1989, New Zealand Department of Health, 1989.
19. **Poole, C., Lanes, S. F., and Walker, A. M.,** Fenoterol and fatal asthma, *Lancet,* 1, 920, 1990.
20. **Elwood, J. M.,** Fenoterol and fatal asthma, *Lancet,* 1, 436, 1990.
21. **Greenland, S.,** The effect of misclassification in the presence of covariates, *Am. J. Epidemiol.,* 112, 564, 1980.
22. **Cox, B. and Elwood, J. M.,** The effect on the stratum-specific odds ratios of nondifferential misclassification of a confounder measured at 2 levels, *Am. J. Epidemiol.,* 133, 202, 1991.
23. **Taylor, R.,** *Letter to chairman, Medical Adverse Reactions Committee,* 20 Feb 1989, in New Zealand Department of Health Document File, 1989, 112.

24. **Beasley, R., Burgess, C., Crane, J., Jackson, R., and Pearce, N.,** *A response to the submissions to the Medicine Adverse Reactions Committee by Boehringer-Ingelheim and the MRC Asthma Task Force,* in New Zealand Department of Health Document File, 1989, 234.
25. Boehringer Ingelheim Ltd., *Submission to Medicine Adverse Reactions Committee,* 13 Mar 1989, in New Zealand Department of Health Document File, 1989, 247.
26. **Pearce, N., Crane, J., Burgess, C., Grainger, J., and Beasley, R.,** Fenoterol and asthma mortality in New Zealand, *N. Z. Med. J.,* 103, 73, 1990.
27. **Windom, H. H., Burgess, C. D., Crane, J., Pearce, N., Kwong, T., and Beasley, R.,** The self-administration of inhaled beta agonist drugs during severe asthma, *N. Z. Med. J.,* 103, 205, 1990.
28. **Sackett, D. L., Browman, G., and Marrett, L.,** *Manuscript review,* 3 Mar 1989, in New Zealand Department of Health Document File, 1989, 434.
29. **Sackett, D. L., Shannon, H. S., and Browman, G. W.,** Fenoterol and fatal asthma, *Lancet,* 1, 45, 1990.
30. **Buist, A. S.,** *Expert report on Boehringer Ingelheim records of asthma deaths in patients receiving fenoterol MDI,* 29 Aug 1989, Department of Health Document File, 1989, 157.
31. **Crane, J., Pearce, N., Burgess, C., Beasley, R., and Jackson, R.,** Asthma deaths in New Zealand, *Br. Med. J.,* 304, 1307, 1992.
32. Australian Adverse Drug Reactions Bulletin, *Revised Indications for Fenoterol,* Australian Government Publishing Service, Canberra, 1990.
33. **Grainger, J., Woodman, K., Pearce, N., Crane, J., Burgess, C., Keane, A., and Beasley, R.,** Prescribed fenoterol and death from asthma in New Zealand, 1981-7: a further case-control study, *Thorax,* 46, 105, 1991.
34. **Sears, M. R., Taylor, D. G., Print, C. G., Lake, D. C., Li, Q., Flannery, E. M., Yates, D. M., Lucas, M. K., and Herbison, G. P.,** Regular inhaled beta-agonist treatment in bronchial asthma, *Lancet,* 1, 1391, 1990.
35. **Spitzer, W. O., Suissa, S., Ernst, P., Horwitz, R. I., Habbick, B., Cockcroft, D., Boivin, J.-F., McNutt, M., Buist, A. S., and Rebuck, A. S.,** The use of beta-agonists and the risk of death and near death from asthma, *N. Engl. J. Med.,* 326, 501, 1992.
36. **Burrows, B. and Lebowitz, M. D.,** The beta-agonist dilemma, *N. Engl. J. Med.,* 326, 560, 1992.
37. **Pearce, N., Crane, J., Burgess, C., Beasley, R., and Jackson, R.,** Fenoterol, beta agonists, and asthma deaths, *N. Engl. J. Med.,* 326, 1992.

Section 4

The Pharmacological Effects of Beta Receptor Agonist Drugs

Chapter 6

AN OVERVIEW OF EXPERIMENTAL METHODS

Carl D. Burgess

TABLE OF CONTENTS

0-8493-6761-1/93/$0.00 + $.50

I. INTRODUCTION

At a time when Lands et al.[1] were publishing data extending the classification of beta receptors into two populations subserving different functions (Table 1), others[2] were reporting the occurrence of an epidemic of asthma deaths in young individuals. The most likely cause was excessive use of high-dose isoprenaline,[3] and because the deaths were sudden and unexpected, the putative mechanism was thought to be cardiovascular through the occurrence of ventricular arrhythmias. The new proposed classification[1] seemed to offer a ready-made solution for new drug development of bronchodilators in that it proposed that the rate and force of cardiac contraction were due to $beta_1$ receptor stimulation, whereas bronchodilatation was due to stimulation of $beta_2$ receptors. It therefore seemed possible that the development of agonists that selectively stimulated $beta_2$ receptors would be free of cardiovascular toxicity and therefore safer than isoprenaline.

As reviewed in Chapter 1, a number of agonists were developed during the 1960s and 1970s (Figure 1), the most commonly used being salbutamol, terbutaline, orciprenaline, and fenoterol. Together, these agents have become the most popular form of treatment for patients with asthma. However, doubt about their safety has once again surfaced since the recent publication of three case-control studies from New Zealand[4-6] that positively associated the prescription of fenoterol with the epidemic of asthma deaths, which occurred from the late 1970s in that country. If the cause(s) for this latter epidemic is/are similar to those that occurred with high-dose isoprenaline, the question arises of whether potential problems with fenoterol could have been predicted during the experimental stages of its development. Because of these concerns, a number of questions relating to assessment of beta receptor selectivity arise, including the following:

1. Are selectivity studies in *in vitro* tissues applicable to the *in vivo* state?
2. Can one extrapolate results from one species to another?
3. What models in animals and humans should be used to assess selectivity?
4. Is selectivity dose-related?

In this chapter some of the issues concerning the experimental approach to the assessment of the pharmacodynamic effects of beta agonists are considered, concentrating particularly on assessment of selectivity. The long-term effects of beta agonist therapy are considered in depth in Chapter 9.

II. CLASSIFICATION OF BETA RECEPTORS

The Lands et al.[1] classification that $beta_1$ and $beta_2$ receptors were response-specific and likely to be distributed to specific organs or tissues has

TABLE 1
Classification of Beta Adrenoceptors

Beta$_1$ receptor responses	Beta$_2$ receptor responses
Increase in heart rate	Smooth muscle relaxation in bronchi, vascular muscle, uterus
Increase in cardiac contractility	Decrease in twitch tension in skeletal muscle
Lipolytic activity	Glycolysis
	Glycogenolysis

Adapted from Lands, A. M., Arnold, A., McAuliffe, J. P., Luduena, F. P., and Brown, T. G., *Nature,* 214, 597, 1967.

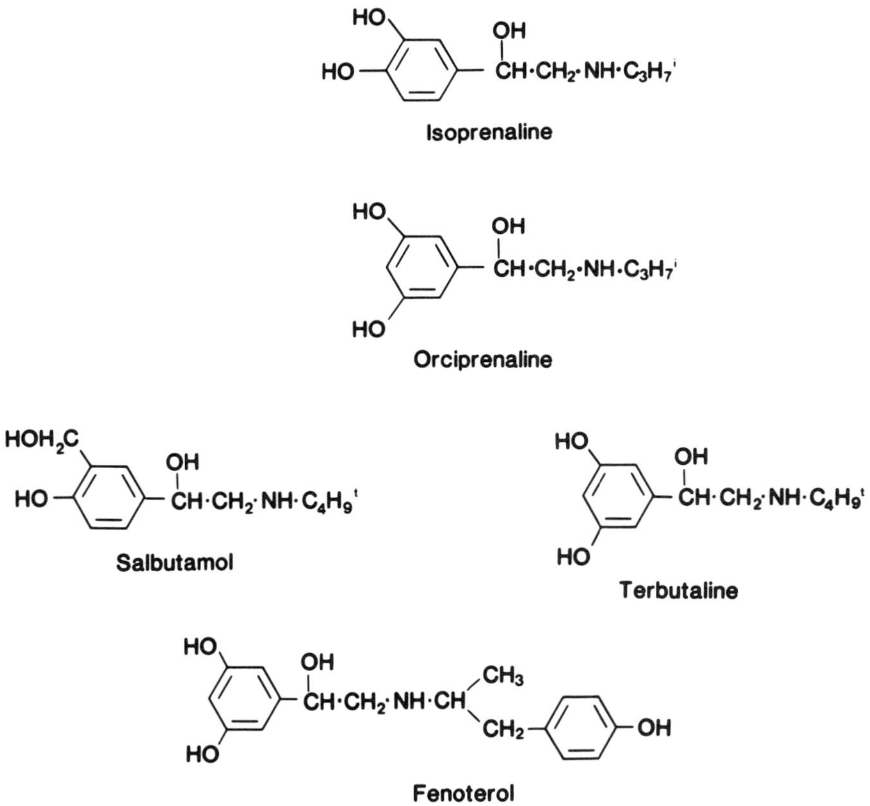

FIGURE 1. Structural formulas for the commonly used beta agonists.

been proven incorrect. Initially, stimulation of $beta_1$ receptors alone was thought to be responsible for both positive chronotropic (heart rate increase) and inotropic (increase in contractility) effects. There is now ample evidence that both $beta_1$ and $beta_2$ receptors are present and functional,[7] in atrial and ventricular myocardium in all species including humans, but with different numbers of the two types of receptors across the species.[7-10] In general, in myocardium $beta_1$ receptors are present in greater numbers than $beta_2$ receptors.

The role of the two different receptors is still not completely understood, although it is now largely accepted that $beta_2$ receptors are involved in positive chronotropic responses following physiological or pharmacological stimuli.[7] However, the type of receptor involved in positive inotropic responses remains controversial. It is also not known whether stimulation of $beta_2$ receptors alone results in the same maximal response as stimulation of $beta_1$ receptors. Studies in humans have suggested that the dominant catecholamine mediating both positive inotropy and chronotropy is noradrenaline.[11] This evokes its responses by stimulating the $beta_1$ receptor. $Beta_2$ receptor stimulation can result in additional increases in contractility and heart rate, which become evident during stress. These responses are mediated by adrenaline.[11] Theoretically, selective $beta_2$ agonists could affect both inotropy and chronotropy.

III. CONCEPTS OF SELECTIVITY/PARTIAL AGONIST ACTIVITY

Selectivity of beta agonists is defined in terms of relativity to the effects of isoprenaline, a nonselective agonist at beta receptors. It has stimulatory activity at both receptor types for any dose. An agonist selective at the $beta_2$ receptor would stimulate that receptor with little or no effect at the $beta_1$ receptor. Selectivity can be dose-related so that at high doses a $beta_2$ receptor agonist could lose its selective profile. Selectivity may also depend on the intrinsic activity of the agonist for a particular receptor.

Partial agonist activity (PAA) implies that for any given occupancy of a receptor the response with a partial agonist is always less than that obtained with a full agonist (Figure 2). A drug with PAA will obviously have a lower intrinsic activity at the receptor than a full agonist. The property of PAA should not be confused with drugs having both agonist and competitive antagonist activity at the same receptor. Antagonist activity can be present even though a maximal response is attained when the drug acts purely as an agonist. What occurs is that the dose-response curve is shifted to the right, but the same maximal effect could theoretically occur. Whether this latter property is of importance clinically is unknown, but theoretically it could become important if high doses are used. The properties of selectivity and PAA have been extensively investigated in animal studies.

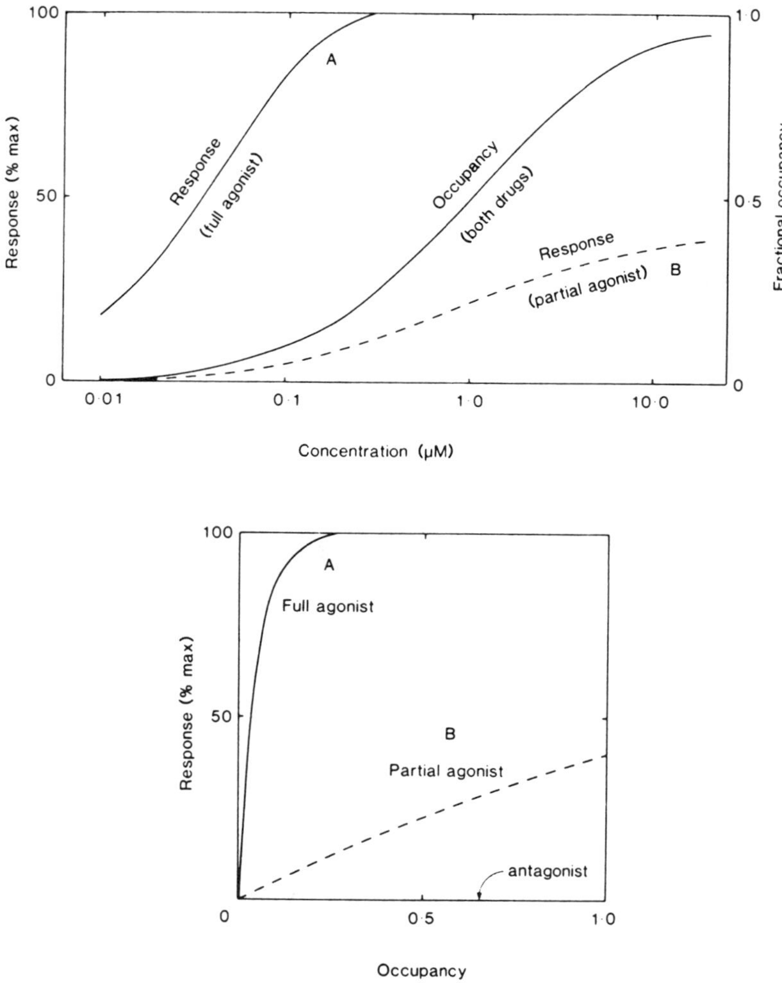

FIGURE 2. Theoretical occupancy and response curves for full and partial agonists. (Top) Occupancy curve for both drugs. (Bottom) Relationship between response and occupancy for full and partial agonists corresponding to curves in top graph. (From Rang, H. P., Dale, M. M., *Pharmacology,* Churchill Livingstone, New York, 1987. With permission.)

IV. PHARMACOLOGICAL EFFECTS IN ANIMALS

Much of the original work investigating the pharmacological effects of beta agonists were performed before ligand-binding studies to $beta_1$ and $beta_2$ receptors were established; thus, definitions of selectivity may have been inaccurate. *In vitro* studies were receptor directed in that they used tracheal relaxation as an indicator of $beta_2$ receptor activation, whereas increase in

TABLE 2
Potency of Intravenous Beta Receptor Agonists in the Anesthetized Guinea Pig

Beta stimulant	50% decrease in intratracheal pressure	50% decrease in skeletal muscle tension during submaximal tetanus	25% increase in heart rate
Isoprenaline	1	1	1
Fenoterol	4.3	3.2	83
Orciprenaline	56	63	226
Salbutamol	5.2	5.2	245
Terbutaline	15	18.5	266

Note: Values are mean beta stimulant potency relative to isoprenaline = 1.

From Brittain, R. T., Dean, C. M., and Jack, D., *Pharmacol. Ther.*, 2, 423, 1976. With permission.

heart rate and contractility were thought to represent $beta_1$ receptor stimulation. More recent binding studies have shown that agents, such as salbutamol, fenoterol, and terbutaline, act as nonselective beta agonists *in vitro,* although they act as selective agents *in vivo.*[12,13] It is thought that these drugs may antagonize $beta_1$ receptors rather than stimulate them, as binding studies do not describe functional effects.[12]

In vivo studies were performed in anesthetized animals, with the effects on heart, lung (bronchodilatation), arteriolar smooth muscle relaxation, and skeletal muscle tremor being monitored. Selectivity for the $beta_2$ receptor can be inferred by comparing equivalent bronchodilatory doses with the effects on the heart. One of the confusing elements with *in vivo* studies is that potent vasodilatation may result in reflex tachycardia, which could confuse attempts at estimating selectivity.

A. BRONCHODILATOR RESPONSES

Both *in vitro* and *in vivo* studies[14-19] have shown that all beta agonists are full agonists at the $beta_2$ receptor, with the exception of one study that showed that with severe bronchoconstriction salbutamol acts as a partial agonist compared with fenoterol.[20] Whether this effect would be relevant in clinical practice is unknown. Although all are accepted as being full agonists, these drugs differ in their potency, with isoprenaline being the most potent followed by fenoterol, salbutamol, terbutaline, and orciprenaline on a weight basis (Table 2). This is reflected in the doses used clinically with the exception of fenoterol, which although being approximately twice as potent as salbutamol as a bronchodilator,[20] is prescribed in double the dose per puff in a metered dose inhaler (MDI). Although it could be argued that studies on guinea pigs should not be extrapolated to other animals or humans, there is remarkable uniformity in the bronchodilating effect of the different bronchodilators in animal studies.[21] There is no reason to suppose humans would differ in this response.

Orciprenaline, terbutaline, and salbutamol can act as $beta_2$ receptor antagonists,[18] whereas fenoterol does not.[20] The relevance of this property is unknown, but theoretically it could partially explain deterioration in respiratory function observed with isoprenaline and fenoterol,[22,23] as they would be more likely to cause down-regulation of $beta_2$ receptors.

B. CARDIAC, VASCULAR, AND SKELETAL MUSCLE EFFECTS

In vitro and *in vivo* studies in the guinea pig have shown that salbutamol and terbutaline have PAA on atrial myocardium,[14,17,18] whereas fenoterol, isoprenaline, and orciprenaline are full agonists on this tissue.[16,18] In isolated animal tissues, fenoterol, salbutamol, and terbutaline are highly selective for the $beta_2$ receptor compared with isoprenaline.[24] However, when examined in the *in vivo* cat, the degree of selectivity was markedly decreased. Furthermore, in this preparation, all the drugs acted as full agonists on the cardiovascular system.[24] Studies in dogs have shown that salbutamol is more selective for the $beta_2$ receptor than either orciprenaline or isoprenaline and causes little increase in myocardial oxygen consumption compared with the other two agents.[19,25] All these drugs cause peripheral vasodilatation, which in turn can increase heart rate through baroreceptor reflex mechanisms. Efforts to try and separate either the peripheral vascular or skeletal muscle effect of $beta_2$ agonists from their bronchodilating activity have failed.[15]

The differences in response between different animal species probably relate to differences in functional $beta_1$ and $beta_2$ receptors in atria and ventricles. This emphasizes the difficulty in extrapolating data from animals to humans. However, animal studies have shown that there are pharmacological differences between the newer beta agonists. These could relate to differences in potency, efficacy, or selectivity. Therefore, the potential for different pharmacodynamic effects with the newer $beta_2$ agonists in humans could have been predicted.

V. HUMAN STUDIES

The effects of beta receptor stimulation in humans are shown in Table 3. Note the differences in response to stimulation of the receptors between those proposed by Lands et al.[1] (Table 1) and those of today. Both rate and contractile responses in the myocardium are subserved by $beta_1$ and $beta_2$ receptors.[11] Pure $beta_2$ receptor effects relate not only to bronchodilatation but also to arteriolar vasodilatation, and to the movement of potassium from the extracellular to the intracellular compartment.[26] Beta receptor stimulation activates adenyl cyclase with production of cyclic adenosine monophosphate (cAMP).[27] cAMP acts as a second messenger modulating responses to beta receptor stimulation.[28]

There is controversy regarding the role of cAMP due to $beta_1$ receptor stimulation. Some authors have noted that only $beta_2$ receptor stimulation resulted in activation of adenyl cyclase (and increase in cAMP)[29] and that plasma cAMP levels do not change in response to exogenously administered

TABLE 3
Effect of Beta Receptor Stimulation on Different Organs and Tissues in Humans

	$Beta_1$ receptor	**$Beta_2$ receptor**
Bronchial smooth muscle	0[a]	Relaxation
Heart rate	Increase[b]	Increase
Cardiac contractility	Increase[b]	Increase
Vascular smooth muscle	0[a]	Relaxation
Plasma potassium	0[a]	Decrease
Blood glucose	0[a]	Increase
Cyclic AMP[c] (plasma)	Increase	Increase[b]
Skeletal muscle	0[a]	Tremor

[a] No effect.
[b] Dominant control.
[c] Adenosine monophosphate.

noradrenaline while they increase following administration of isoprenaline and adrenaline, suggesting that there may be non-cAMP mechanisms for $beta_1$ receptor inotropic responses.[30,31] Others, however, have demonstrated that adenyl cyclase is coupled to $beta_1$ receptors.[32,33] It is difficult to understand the disparity in the results between different investigators, but it may relate to the different preparations used and the fact that $beta_1$ receptors outnumber $beta_2$ receptors in myocardium, although $beta_2$ receptors are more effectively coupled to adenyl cyclase than $beta_1$ receptors. It has also been shown that the magnitude of contractility for $beta_2$ receptor stimulation in the atrium is different from that in the ventricle, with the latter only amounting to 50% of that produced by $beta_1$ receptor stimulation.[33]

Other actions of $beta_2$ agonists that may result in cardiovascular changes include activation of presynaptic $beta_2$ receptors, which result in enhanced release of noradrenaline, which in turn can stimulate $beta_1$ receptors.[34] At present, there is little evidence to support the theory that there may be vagal withdrawal following vasodilatation due to $beta_2$ receptor stimulation.[7]

These factors have made it more difficult to design clinical studies to assess comparative selectivity between $beta_2$ agonists. Study designs investigating selectivity should also consider the way patients use their drugs during an attack. In a recent study overuse of beta agonists was common in a group of 101 patients who were admitted to hospital with severe asthma. Of those patients whose attack had lasted longer than 24 h, 52% had taken more than 30 puffs of their inhaler in the 24 h prior to admission, whereas of those using a home nebulizer 76% had self-administered this device more than four times during the 24-h period prior to admission. In addition, the patients using a home nebulizer had also taken a median of 24 doses of their inhaler during this same period.[35] Furthermore, the British Thoracic Society's recent guidelines recommended that doses of between 20 and 50 puffs of a beta agonist be administered by an MDI during acute severe asthma.[36] Therefore, it is important that an assessment is made of the pharmacological effects of beta agonists after frequent use.

A. STUDIES IN NONASTHMATIC INDIVIDUALS

1. *In Vitro*

Because of the potential problems in demonstrating selectivity in the intact individual, some studies have been performed using *in vitro* methodology. A recent comparative study investigating the effects of fenoterol and salbutamol on contractility using human ventricular strips has shown that fenoterol has much greater intrinsic activity than salbutamol (maximum increase in force of contraction 130% with fenoterol versus 11% with salbutamol).[37] Furthermore, salbutamol caused its effects entirely through $beta_2$ receptor stimulation, whereas fenoterol stimulated both $beta_1$ and $beta_2$ receptors. Under the same study conditions, isoprenaline was shown to exert its positive inotropic effects almost entirely through $beta_1$ receptor stimulation. Another study, using human atrial myocardium, confirmed that salbutamol exerted its positive inotropic effect entirely through $beta_2$ receptor stimulation.[38] When compared with isoprenaline, it acted as a partial agonist.

These studies support the view that there are discernible differences in selectivity, potency, and intrinsic activity between beta agonists, which may prove relevant in clinical practice. One criticism that could be leveled against the *in vitro* studies is that the tissues were taken from patients undergoing operations for various cardiovascular disease states. $Beta_1$ receptor responsiveness alters with varying degrees of cardiac failure (down-regulation), and beta-blocking agents (taken by some patients) can also alter both $beta_1$ and $beta_2$ receptor responsiveness. Even so, there is no doubt that beta receptor stimulation can increase contractility and that less selective drugs seem to cause greater responses.

2. *In Vivo*

Early studies of agents, such as fenoterol, salbutamol, and terbutaline, concentrated on the cardiovascular responses to intravenous doses.[39-41] They demonstrated that fenoterol was two to three times more potent than salbutamol in its effect on heart rate and contractility on a weight basis, but maximal responses were not defined. Terbutaline was shown to be more selective than orciprenaline.[41] Since the reports of increased asthma mortality in New Zealand,[42] attention has once again focused on the pharmacology of the $beta_2$ agonists, and more particularly on any differences between fenoterol and other agents.

In a number of studies, our group has shown that fenoterol had significantly greater positive chronotropic and inotropic effects than salbutamol and terbutaline. It also had greater hypokalemic effects than salbutamol but not terbutaline.[43-45] The inotropic and chronotropic effects of fenoterol following multiple inhalations were not different from those demonstrated after equivalent doses of isoprenaline.[43] The greater cardiovascular effects of fenoterol (compared with salbutamol or terbutaline) could relate to the drug being less selective for $beta_2$ receptors. Alternatively, the differences seen may be simply due to greater potency. The evidence for the latter is that it causes a greater degree of hypokalemia than salbutamol; thus, the argument would be that in equihypokalemic doses it would have had similar cardiovascular effects. However, there is evidence that for an equihypokalemic effect of terbutaline, fenoterol causes significantly greater inotropic and chronotropic effects,[44,45] suggesting that it (fenoterol) has greater intrinsic myocardial effects than terbutaline.

Some authors[46] have suggested that the differences in the systemic effects between fenoterol and salbutamol may also be due to fenoterol being more lipid-soluble (and thus better absorbed) than salbutamol. This is unlikely to be correct because it ignores the intravenous studies referred to and also ignores the potential difference of salbutamol acting as a partial agonist.

Estimation of selectivity and PAA could be studied by giving incremental doses of the drug to be tested and assessing heart rate and contractility as $beta_1$ and $beta_2$ receptor functions (contractility is mainly a $beta_1$ receptor response) and plasma potassium as a $beta_2$ receptor function. Because the drugs are thought to be full agonists at the latter receptor, the maximal effect of the agonist can be assessed. One would assume that $beta_2$ receptors in myocardium would be maximally stimulated at such doses; thus, any differences in either inotropy or chronotropy would be due to differing stimulation of the $beta_1$ receptor. In this way we recently showed that after frequent dosing, fenoterol and formoterol (a long-acting $beta_2$ agonist) had similar maximum hypokalemic effects but that the inotropic and chronotropic effects were approximately 40% less with formoterol (Table 4), indicating that the latter is more selective for the $beta_2$ receptor.

Another method that has been used to assess the selectivity of the beta agonists is to assess their cardiovascular activity with and without treatment with selective ($beta_1$) and nonselective ($beta_1$ and $beta_2$) beta receptor blocking agents. Wellstein et al.[47] investigated the chronotropic and inotropic effects of isoprenaline infusions before and after administration of bisoprolol ($beta_1$ receptor blocking agent) and propranolol (nonselective beta blocker). They showed that the chronotropic response was equally mediated by both receptors, whereas the inotropic response (shortening of electromechanical systole) of isoprenaline was mainly mediated by stimulation of $beta_1$ receptors.

In other studies,[48,49] it was shown that at low doses terbutaline exerts its chronotropic and inotropic effects through stimulation of $beta_2$ receptors in the myocardium, whereas at higher doses $beta_1$ receptor stimulation plays a significant role. Whether this is due to a direct effect or presynaptic $beta_2$ receptor stimulation is not known. In a study investigating the functional role of $beta_2$ receptors in the human heart, Hall et al.[49] injected the same dose of

TABLE 4
Maximum Cardiovascular and Metabolic Effects of Fenoterol, Formoterol, and Salbutamol in 12 Healthy Volunteers

	Fenoterol	Formoterol	Salbutamol	Placebo
Heart rate (beats/min)	29.8 ± 3.9	16.7 ± 2.7	12.8 ± 3.3	−2.7 ± 1.6
QS_2I[a] (ms)	−53.8 ± 4.0	−35.5 ± 3.9	−31.5 ± 2.6	−7.6 ± 2.4
QTc (ms)	61.4 ± 7.6	40.2 ± 8.4	32.5 ± 5.2	7.1 ± 3.0
Systolic blood pressure	12.3 ± 2.7	9.2 ± 1.9	3.0 ± 2.2	−0.2 ± 2.2
Plasma potassium (m*M*)	−1.13 ± 0.07	−0.96 ± 0.09	−0.55 ± 0.06	−0.08 ± 0.07

Note: Values are mean ± SEM in this double-blind crossover study. The doses administered were as follows: 2000 μg fenoterol, 2000 μg salbutamol, and 120 μg formoterol. These represent cumulative doses over 120 min. Although the hypokalemia of fenoterol equals formoterol, the effect on heart rate and QS_2I is significantly greater with the former agent.

[a] QS_2I = total electromechanical systole, a measure of inotropy (the greater the negative result, the greater the degree of positive inotropy[43]).

salbutamol into the right coronary artery and into the root of the aorta in patients undergoing cardiac catheterization. They showed that intracoronary injection resulted in sinus tachycardia, although such a dose caused no effect when the drug was given into the aorta. Therefore, salbutamol caused its effect by direct action on the heart. In a subsequent study in similar patients,[50] the authors showed that pretreatment with propranolol increased the mean dose of salbutamol from 2.6 μg to 64 μg, necessary for an increase in heart rate of 30 beats/minute, whereas pretreatment with practolol (a selective $beta_1$ receptor blocker) did not increase the dose of salbutamol for the same response, demonstrating that $beta_2$ receptor stimulation is responsible for the chronotropic effect of salbutamol.

To assess PAA in more detail, one could extend studies until there was no further increase in inotropy, or decrease in plasma potassium, and thus compare maximal responses. Our group[50] compared the maximal responses to fenoterol and salbutamol in eight healthy males. Doses of 400 μg of either drug were administered double-blind through a spacing device, at 10-min intervals until there was a plateau in the response measured or the subject had inhaled a total of 48 puffs (9600 μg). All subjects reached a plateau for both a decrease in plasma potassium ($beta_2$ receptor response) and decrease in total electromechanical systole (QS_2I, mainly $beta_1$ receptor response). The results of the study are of interest and are shown in Figures 3 to 6. The maximum response (E_{max}) for fenoterol was significantly greater than salbutamol for plasma potassium, QS_2I, and cAMP (Table 5), and the dose of salbutamol required to produce 50% of the maximum response to fenoterol (ED_{50F}) was significantly greater with potency ratios of 1.75, 1.61, and 2.26 for plasma potassium, QS_2I, and cAMP, respectively (Table 5). These results show that salbutamol acts as a partial agonist at both $beta_1$ and $beta_2$ receptors

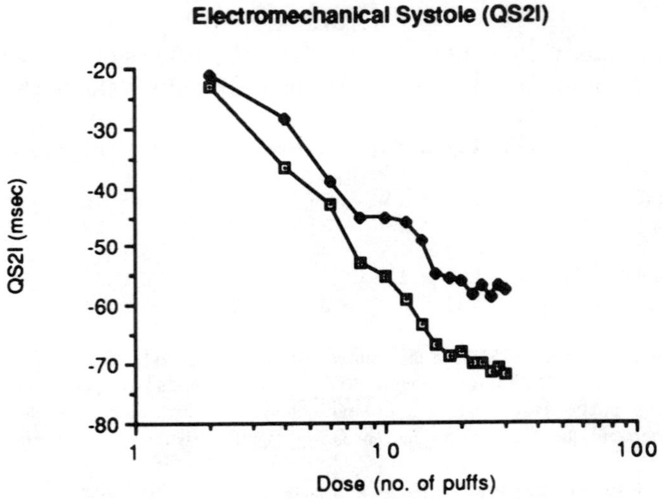

FIGURE 3. Cumulative log-dose response curve for QS_2I following fenoterol (□) and salbutamol (♦).

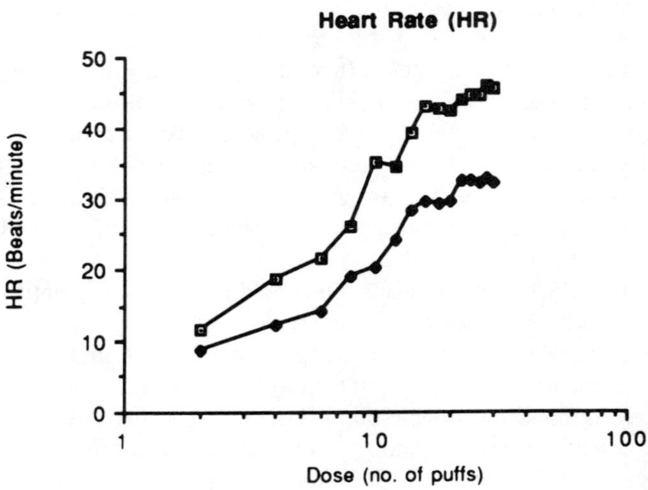

FIGURE 4. Cumulative log-dose response curve for heart rate following fenoterol (□) and salbutamol (♦).

compared with fenoterol. Because the doses we used are within those recommended by the British Thoracic Society[36] for treatment in severe asthma, it is likely that salbutamol would be safer than fenoterol under such circumstances. This study highlights the importance of examining the effects of beta agonists in the doses in which they are recommended.

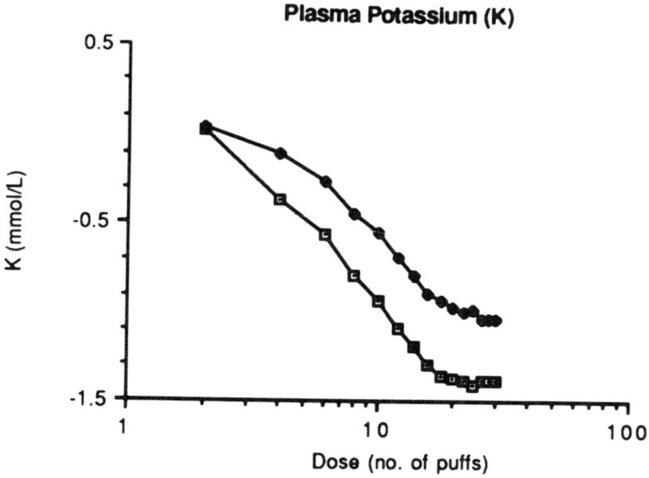

FIGURE 5. Cumulative log-dose response curve for plasma potassium following fenoterol (□) and salbutamol (♦).

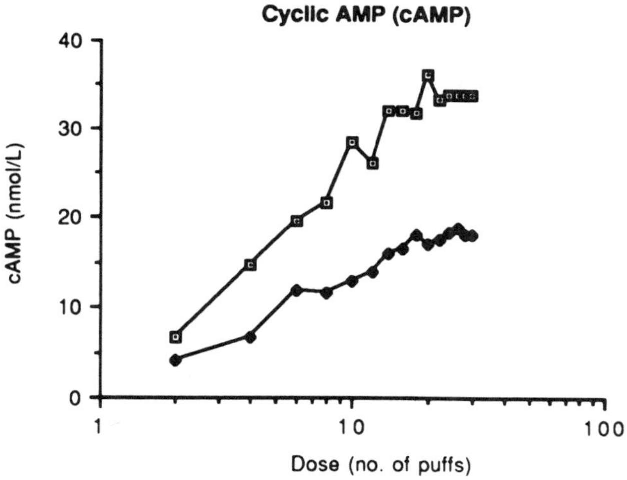

FIGURE 6. Cumulative log-dose response curve for plasma cAMP following fenoterol (□) and salbutamol (♦).

Volunteer studies have definitely shown that when therapeutically equivalent doses are used, terbutaline and salbutamol have lesser cardiovascular effects than fenoterol and orciprenaline. The underlying mechanisms are not fully understood, but in high doses direct effects on myocardial beta receptors seem a more plausible explanation than either vagal withdrawal through baroreceptor stimulation (there is evidence that beta agonist stimulation may cause

TABLE 5
The Maximum (E_{max}) Responses and Dose Required to Reach ED_{50F} of Fenoterol and Salbutamol in Eight Normal Volunteers

	E_{max}		ED_{50F}[a] (μg)	
	Fenoterol	Salbutamol	Fenoterol	Salbutamol
QS_2I (ms)	−71.8	−57.5	767	1234
	(−42.8 to −94.5)	(−30.4 to −97.7)	(300 to 2100)	(800 to 2950)
Plasma potassium (m*M*)	−1.40	−1.03	1348	2365
	(−0.9 to −1.72)	(−0.47 to −1.50)	(550 to 2600)	(1400 to 3250)
cAMP (n*M*)	33.8	18.1	1085	2454
	(18.0 to 59.7)	(14.2 to 21.4)	(420 to 2160)	(900 to 4800)
Heart rate (beats/min)	44.9	32.5	1170	2312
	(14.7 to 70.3)	(10.1 to 52.0)	(370 to 2350)	(1600 to 4800)

Note: Values are means, with ranges given in parentheses.

[a] The mean dose (range) of salbutamol and fenoterol (μg) required to reach 50% of the maximum fenoterol effect.

vagal stimulation rather than withdrawal[48]) or reflex mechanisms through stimulation of presynaptic $beta_2$ receptors.

B. STUDIES IN ASTHMATIC SUBJECTS

Studies should be able to be performed when the patient's condition is stable or when the asthma is severe. There have been no comparative pharmacological studies of beta agonists under conditions of severe asthma. The studies that have been performed have compared intravenous salbutamol with aminophylline[51] and aminophylline with adrenaline.[52] A number of repeated-dose studies have been performed when the patient's asthma has been stable. These have compared the pharmacodynamic effects of terbutaline, salbutamol, fenoterol, orciprenaline, and isoprenaline (Table 6).[53-58] In general, where the drugs have been administered in equibronchodilator doses, salbutamol and terbutaline have been found to be more bronchoselective (less cardiovascular activity) in their action than fenoterol and orciprenaline (Table 5). In one study neither fenoterol nor orciprenaline showed any benefit over isoprenaline;[57] however, the study was of relatively short duration. The mechanisms for the relative bronchoselectivity of salbutamol and terbutaline in patients with asthma are not known but suggest less intrinsic activity on the heart, although this has yet to be unconditionally proven.

It could be argued that the extrapulmonary responses of beta agonists are diminished by regular usage;[59] therefore, most of the studies examining these effects are clinically irrelevant. However, most patients on regular long-term beta agonist therapy take steroids either by inhalation or by oral administration. Steroids up-regulate beta receptors,[60] which may overcome tolerance and return responses to pretolerance levels. This has yet to be formally assessed in clinical trials.

TABLE 6
Respiratory and Cardiac Effects Following Multiple Inhaled Doses of Beta Receptor Agonists in Asthmatic Patients

Drug and dose (total)	Respiratory effects	Cardiac effects	Ref.
F 400 μg/800 μg O 1500 μg/3000 μg	F > 0	F > 0, heart rate	54
F 1500 μg T 3750 μg	F = T	F > T, heart rate and palpitations	53
I 1600 μg F 1600 μg S 1600 μg	F = I = S	F and I > S, inotropic activity	55
A 2800 μg F 2000 μg I 1000 μg O 7500 μg	F = I = O > A	F = O > A and I, heart rate, QTc interval and inotropic activity I > A, heart rate and inotropic activity	57
F 5200 μg S 2600 μg T 6500 μg	F = S = T	F > S = T, heart rate and QTc interval	58

Note: A = adrenaline; F = fenoterol; I = isoprenaline; O = orciprenaline; S = salbutamol; T = terbutaline.

VI. FACTORS ALTERING RESPONSES TO BETA RECEPTOR AGONISTS

Asthma deaths may be associated with excessive use of beta agonists. The majority of deaths occur outside hospital where patients are likely to be hypoxemic and perhaps hypercapnic. As reviewed in Chapter 7, studies in animals have shown that hypoxemia influences the cardiovascular response to isoprenaline. Lockett[61] showed in the cat heart-lung preparation that isoprenaline or orciprenaline could cause heart failure and death when given in the presence of a high work load, but under normal loading conditions the same dose of drug was not harmful.

Alterations in blood gases are known to affect the cardiovascular system, and it is important to determine whether such alterations alter the cardiovascular effects of beta agonists. Hypoxemia can increase heart rate and cardiac output and decrease the peripheral vascular resistance.[62,63] With more severe degrees of hypoxemia (PaO_2 = 40 mmHg) stroke volume can increase. If hypoxemia becomes worse, bradycardia and cardiac standstill can occur. Hypercapnia, with or without hypoxemia, is also associated with tachycardia, increase in blood pressure, peripheral vascular resistance, and increase in cardiac contractility.[64] Leitch et al.[65] showed that the positive chronotropic effect of salbutamol was potentiated by both hypoxemia and hypercapnia.

Our group has investigated the cardiovascular effects of fenoterol in nonasthmatics who breathed room air or a gas mixture, which resulted in an arterial oxygen saturation of 90% (all subjects were studied under both conditions; the subjects were blind to the gas mixture inhaled).[66] The dose of fenoterol inhaled was 800 μg (four puffs; one or two puffs is a therapeutic dose). Hypoxemia increased heart rate and the electrocardiographic QTc interval. Fenoterol under conditions of normoxia increased cardiac contractility, heart rate, and the QTc interval. When given under conditions of hypoxia, the effects on heart rate and QTc interval with fenoterol were additive. Prolongation of the QTc interval has been associated with an increased risk of ventricular arrhythmias,[67] and increases in heart rate will result in increase in myocardial oxygen demand. Therefore, these changes could suggest one mechanism by which fenoterol could increase the risk of death in patients with severe asthma.

In another (unpublished) study, we examined the effect of hypercapnia alone, hypercapnia and hypoxia ($PaCO_2$ 50 mmHg, PaO_2 60 mmHg), and room air on the cardiovascular responses to isoprenaline (400 μg by inhalation) in a randomized crossover study in nine subjects. Compared with room air, the hypercapnia-hypoxic gas mixture increased heart rate, systolic and diastolic blood pressure, inotropic indices (of the echocardiogram), and the QTc interval (Table 7). The changes in heart rate, systolic blood pressure, QTc interval, and the contractile indices were all additive with isoprenaline, demonstrating that abnormal arterial gases in patients could potentiate the cardiovascular changes from a beta agonist alone. No studies have been performed comparing the extrapulmonary effects of different beta agonists under conditions of hypoxia and/or hypercapnia.

VII. LONG-TERM EFFECTS

All of the aforementioned studies have involved acute effects of beta agonists. More recently, some studies have reported deterioration in lung function with long-term use of regular beta agonists.[68] The underlying cause for such occurrences is not known, although they may relate to increases in bronchial hyperresponsiveness. However, not all studies with regular beta agonist use have been able to demonstrate deterioration in lung function,[23,69] and it may relate to certain beta agonists, such as isoprenaline and fenoterol.[22,23,68] Study designs to assess the underlying mechanism and incidence of potential deterioration in respiratory function are difficult to define. At present, such basic questions as what dosage constitutes regular use sufficient to downregulate beta receptors and duration of treatment, remain elusive. Studies with enantiomers instead of racemic mixtures may also be relevant in assessing this problem.[70] Plainly it is of major importance with the introduction of new long-acting beta agonists, such as salmeterol and formoterol.

TABLE 7
Cardiovascular Effects of Isoprenaline (I) (400 μg) When Subjects Breathed Room Air (RA) or Gas Mixtures to Produce Hypercapnia (HC) or HC and Hypoxia (HYP)

	RA	RA + I	HC	HC + I	HC/HYP	HC/HYP + I
Heart rate (beats/min)	−0.6 ± 2.1	3.1 ± 2.8	3.1 ± 3.4	8.4 ± 4.6	16.2 ± 4.3	23.9 ± 4.9
SBP (mmHg)	−4.0 ± 2.4	6.3 ± 1.9	4.2 ± 1.9	12.3 ± 5.1	6.9 ± 3.8	16.0 ± 3.8
DBP (mmHg)	−1.7 ± 1.5	−2.3 ± 2.7	1.9 ± 3.6	−0.3 ± 2.6	7.1 ± 2.1	7.2 ± 2.9
CI (l/min/m^2)	0.06 ± 0.12	0.51 ± 0.17	0.26 ± 0.26	0.7 ± 0.27	1.0 ± 0.24	1.57 ± 0.24
EF (%)	0.9 ± 0.8	6.0 ± 1.6	6.7 ± 2.2	10.6 ± 2.8	7.4 ± 1.7	14.2 ± 2.3
FS (%)	0.8 ± 0.7	4.9 ± 1.3	5.2 ± 1.7	8.9 ± 2.1	6.2 ± 1.5	12.9 ± 2.2
QTc (ms)	2.7 ± 4.5	14.1 ± 4.9	12.2 ± 5.7	23.9 ± 6.4	25.4 ± 6.2	37.0 ± 5.5

Note: Values are change from control (mean ± SEM). SBP = systolic blood pressure; DBP = diastolic blood pressure; CI = cardiac index; EF = ejection fraction; FS = fractional shortening.

TABLE 8
Suggested Design for Testing Selectivity of $Beta_2$ Receptor Agonists

Animal studies
- *In vitro*
  - Ligand binding studies
  - Guinea pig, trachea, atrial myocardium
  - Assessments of partial agonist activity versus isoprenaline
  - Beta receptor blockade studies
- *In vivo*
  - Cat/guinea pig versus isoprenaline

Human
- *In vitro*
  - Ligand binding studies
  - Myocardial strips, including beta receptor blockade studies
- *In vivo*
  - Volunteer
    - Multiple dose
    - Measurements: heart rate, contractile indices (echocardiogram or systolic time intervals), plasma potassium, tremor
    - Comparisons including salbutamol, isoprenaline, and fenoterol
    - Under conditions of hypoxemia, hypercapnia
    - Co-administer with $beta_1$ and $beta_2$ receptor blockade
  - Patients
    - Doses used in severe asthma
    - Measurements: cardiovascular/FEV_1/PEFR
    - Comparisons including salbutamol, isoprenaline, and fenoterol
    - Comparisons, in acute asthma, ECG tape recordings

VIII. CONCLUSIONS

In vitro studies can predict *in vivo* pharmacodynamic responses in the same animal, but there are differences between species. Ligand-binding studies can aid the investigator to identify the type of receptors present in the tissue to be studied. Selectivity is a relative term and is dose-dependent. PAA has now been demonstrated to be important in assessing the actions of any new beta agonist. A proposed scheme for studying selectivity to any new agent is shown in Table 8. Long-term studies assessing effects on lung function should also be added. Studies should include the effect of inhaled steroids on these measures because patients on regular beta agonists should be using prophylactic drugs.

REFERENCES

1. **Lands, A. M., Arnold, A., McAuliffe, J. P., Luduena, F. P., and Brown, T. G.,** Differentiation of receptor systems activated by sympathomimetic amines, *Nature,* 214, 597, 1967.
2. **Speizer, F. E., Doll, R., and Heaf, P.,** Observations on recent increase in mortality from asthma, *Br. Med. J.,* 1, 335, 1968.
3. **Speizer, F. E., Doll, R., Heaf, P., and Strang, L. B.,** Investigation into use of drugs preceding death from asthma, *Br. Med. J.,* 1, 339, 1968.
4. **Crane, J., Pearce, N., Flatt, A., Burgess, C., Jackson, R., Kwong, T., Ball, M., and Beasley, R.,** Prescribed fenoterol and death from asthma in New Zealand, 1981–83: case-control study, *Lancet,* 1, 917, 1989.
5. **Pearce, N., Grainger, J., Atkinson, M., Crane, J., Burgess, C., Culling, C., Windom, H., and Beasley, R.,** Case-control study of prescribed fenoterol and death from asthma in New Zealand, 1977–81, *Thorax,* 45, 170, 1990.
6. **Grainger, J., Woodman, K., Pearce, N., Crane, J., Burgess, C., Keane, A., and Beasley, R.,** Prescribed fenoterol and death from asthma in New Zealand, 1981-7: a further case-control study, *Thorax,* 46, 105, 1991.
7. **Brodde, O.-E.,** β1 and β2-adrenoceptors in the human heart: properties, function and alterations in chronic heart failure, *Pharmacol. Rev.,* 43, 203, 1991.
8. **Carlsson, E., Ablad, B., Brändstrom, A., and Carlsson, B.,** Differentiated blockade of the chronotropic effects of various adrenergic stimuli in the cat heart, *Life Sci.,* 11, 953, 1972.
9. **Spiker, B. A., McKeon, W. B., and Arnold, A.,** Guinea pig atrial and pulmonary beta adrenoceptors, *Arch. Intern. Pharmacodyn. Ther.,* 207, 220, 1974.
10. **Ablad, B., Carlsson, B., Carlsson, E., Dahlöf, C., Ek, L., and Hultberg, E.,** Cardiac effects of beta adrenergic receptor antagonists, *Adv. Cardiol.,* 12, 290, 1974.
11. **Motomura, S., Zerkowski, H. R., Daul, A., and Brodde, O.-E.,** On the physiologic role of β2 adrenoceptors in the human heart: in vitro and in vivo studies, *Am. Heart J.,* 119, 608, 1990.
12. **Minneman, K. P., Hegstrand, L. R., and Molinoff, P. B.,** Simultaneous determination of β1 and β2 adrenergic receptors in rat heart and lung in vitro, *Mol. Pharmacol.,* 16, 21, 1979.
13. **Minneman, K. P., Hedberg, A., and Molinoff, P. B.,** Comparison of beta adrenergic receptor subtypes in mammalian tissues, *J. Pharmacol. Exp. Ther.,* 211, 502, 1979.
14. **Brittain, R. T., Dean, C. M., and Jack, D.,** Sympathomimetic bronchodilator drugs, *Pharmacol. Ther.,* 2, 423, 1976.
15. **Apperley, G. H., Daly, M. J., and Levy, G. P.,** Selectivity of adrenoceptor agonists and antagonists on bronchial, skeletal, vascular and cardiac muscle in the anesthetised cat, *Br. J. Pharmacol.,* 57, 235, 1976.
16. **O'Donnell, S. R.,** An examination of some beta-adrenoreceptor stimulants for selectivity using the isolated trachea and atria of the guinea pig, *Eur. J. Pharmacol.,* 19, 371, 1972.
17. **Raper, C. and Malta, E.,** Salbutamol: agonistic and antagonistic activity at beta adrenoceptor sites, *J. Pharm. Pharmacol.,* 25, 661, 1973.
18. **Malta, E. and Raper, C.,** Non-catechol phenylethanolamines: agonistic and antagonistic actions on beta adrenoreceptors in isolated tissues from the guinea pig, *Clin. Exp. Pharmacol. Physiol.,* 1, 259, 1974.

19. **Daly, M. J., Farmer, J. B., and Levy, G. P.,** Comparison of the bronchodilator and cardiovascular actions of salbutamol, isoprenaline and orciprenaline in guinea pigs and dogs, *Br. J. Pharmacol.,* 43, 624, 1971.
20. **O'Donnell, S. R. and Wanstall, J. C.,** Evidence that the efficacy (intrinsic activity) of fenoterol is higher than that of salbutamol on beta adrenoceptors in guinea pig trachea, *Eur. J. Pharmacol.,* 47, 333, 1978.
21. **Bowman, W. C. and Raper, C.,** Sympathomimetic bronchodilators and animal models for assessing their potential value in asthma, *J. Pharm. Pharmacol.,* 28, 369, 1976.
22. **Van Metre, T. E.,** Adverse effects of inhalation of excessive amounts of nebulised isoproterenol in status asthmaticus, *J. Allergy,* 43, 101, 1969.
23. **Trembath, P. W., Greenacre, J. K., Anderson, M., Dimmock, S., Mansfield, L., Wadsworth, J., and Green, M.,** Comparison of four weeks' treatment with fenoterol and terbutaline aerosols in adult asthmatics, *J. Allergy Clin. Immunol.,* 63, 395, 1979.
24. **Wagner, J., Reinhardt, D., and Schumann, H. J.,** Comparison of the bronchodilator and cardiovascular action of isoprenaline, TH 1165 A, terbutaline and salbutamol in cats and isolated organ preparations, *Res. Exp. Med.,* 162, 49, 1974.
25. **Nayler, W. G. and McInnes, I.,** Salbutamol and orciprenaline-induced changes in myocardial function, *Cardiovasc. Res.,* 6, 725, 1972.
26. **Struthers, A. D. and Reid, J. L.,** The role of adrenomedullary catecholamines in potassium homeostasis, *Clin. Sci.,* 66, 377, 1984.
27. **Hazeki, O. and Ui, M.,** Beta 1 and beta 2 adrenergic receptors responsible for cyclic AMP accumulation in isolated heart and lung cells, *Mol. Pharmacol.,* 17, 8, 1980.
28. **Katz, A. M.,** Cyclic adenosine monophosphate effects on the myocardium: a man who blows hot and cold with one breath, *J. Am. Coll. Cardiol.,* 2, 143, 1983.
29. **Waelbroeck, M., Taton, G., Delhaye, M., Chatelain, P., Camus, J. C., Pochet, R., Leclerc, J. L., De Smet, J. M., Robberecht, P., and Christophe, J.,** The human heart beta adrenergic receptors. II. Coupling of beta 2 adrenergic receptors with the adenylate cyclase system, *Mol. Pharmacol.,* 4, 174, 1983.
30. **Hjemdahl, P., Akerstedt, T., Pollare, T., and Gillberg, M.,** Influence of beta adrenoreceptor blockade by metoprolol and propranolol on plasma concentrations and effects of noradrenaline and adrenaline during IV infusion, *Acta Physiol. Scand.* [*Suppl.*], 515, 45, 1983.
31. **Fairfax, A. J., Rehahn, M., Jones, D., and O'Malley, B.,** Comparison between the effects of inhaled isoprenaline and fenoterol on plasma cyclic AMP and heart rate in normal subjects, *Br. J. Clin. Pharmacol.,* 17, 165, 1984.
32. **Ikezono, K., Michel, M. C., Zerkowski, H.-R., Beckeringh, J. J., and Brodde, O.-E.,** The role of cyclic AMP in the positive inotropic effect mediated by β1- and β2-adrenoceptors in isolated human right atrium, *Naunyn Schmiedebergs Arch. Pharmacol.,* 335, 561, 1987.
33. **Lemoine, H., Schönell, H., and Kaumann, A. J.,** Contribution of β1 and β2 adrenoceptors of human atrium and ventricle to the effects of noradrenaline and adrenaline as assessed with (-)-atenolol, *Br. J. Pharmacol.,* 95, 55, 1988.
34. **Langer, S. Z.,** Pre-synaptic regulation of the release of catecholamines, *Pharmacol. Rev.,* 32, 337, 1980.
35. **Windom, H. H., Burgess, C. D., Crane, J., Pearce, N., Kwong, T., and Beasley, R.,** The self-administration of inhaled beta agonist drugs during severe asthma, *N.Z. Med. J.,* 103, 205, 1990.
36. British Thoracic Society, Guidelines for management of asthma in adults II-acute severe asthma, *Br. Med. J.,* 301, 797, 1990.
37. **Mügge, A., Posselt, D., Reimer, U., Schmitz, W., and Scholz, H.,** Effects of the beta 2 adrenoceptor agonists fenoterol and salbutamol on force of contraction in isolated human ventricular myocardium, *Klin. Wochenschr.,* 63, 26, 1985.

38. **Hall, J. A., Kaumann, A. J., and Brown, M. J.,** Selective β1-adrenoceptor blockade enhances positive inotropic responses to endogenous catecholamines mediated through β2-adrenoceptors in human atrial myocardium, *Circ. Res.*, 66, 1610, 1990.
39. **Coleman, A. J., Leary, W. P., and Asmal, A. C.,** Cardiovascular effects of fenoterol, *S. Afr. Med. J.*, 47, 618, 1973.
40. **Coleman, A. J. and Leary, W. P.,** Cardiovascular effects of hexoprenaline sulphate and salbutamol in man, *S. Afr. Med. J.*, 47, 621, 1973.
41. **Arner, B., Bertler, A., Karlefors, D., and Westling, H.,** Circulatory effects of orciprenaline, adrenaline and a new sympathomimetic beta receptor stimulating agent, terbutaline, in normal subjects, *Acta Med. Scand.* [*Suppl.*], 512, 25, 1970.
42. **Jackson, R. T., Beaglehole, R., Rea, H. H., and Sutherland, D. C.,** Mortality from asthma: a new epidemic in New Zealand, *Br. Med. J.*, 285, 771, 1982.
43. **Crane, J., Burgess, C., and Beasley, R.,** Cardiovascular and hypokalaemic effects of inhaled salbutamol, fenoterol and isoprenaline, *Thorax*, 44, 136, 1989.
44. **Flatt, A., Crane, J., Purdie, G., Kwong, T., Beasley, R., and Burgess, C.,** The cardiovascular effects of beta adrenergic agonist drugs administered by nebulisation, *Postgrad. Med. J.*, 66, 98, 1990.
45. **Burgess, C. D., Flatt, A., Siebers, R., Crane, J., Beasley, R., and Purdie, G.,** A comparison of the extent and duration of hypokalaemia following three nebulised β2 adrenoceptor agonists, *Eur. J. Clin. Pharmacol.*, 36, 415, 1989.
46. **Lipworth, B. J. and McDevitt, D. G.,** Inhaled β2-adrenoceptor agonists in asthma: help or hindrance, *Br. J. Clin. Pharmacol.*, 33, 129, 1992.
47. **Wellstein, A., Belz, G. G., and Palm, D.,** Beta adrenoceptor subtype binding activity in plasma and beta blockade by propranolol and beta 1 selective bisoprolol in humans: evaluations with Schild-Plots, *J. Pharmacol. Exp. Ther.*, 246, 328, 1988.
48. **Levine, M. H. and Leenen, F. H. H.,** Role of β1-receptors and vagal tone in cardiac inotropic and chronotropic responses to a β2 agonist in humans, *Circulation*, 79, 107, 1989.
49. **Hall, J. A., Petch, M. C., and Brown, M. J.,** Intracoronary injections of salbutamol demonstrate the presence of functional β_2 adrenoceptors in the human heart, *Circ. Res.*, 65, 546, 1989.
50. **Burgess, C., Bremner, P., Beasley, R., Siebers, R., Crane, J., D'Souza, W., and Pearce, N.,** A comparison of the maximum cardiovascular and metabolic effects of salbutamol and fenoterol, *Am. Rev. Respir. Dis.*, 145(4) A67, 1992.
51. **Evans, W. V., Monie, R. D. H., Crimmins, J., and Seaton A.,** Aminophylline, salbutamol and combined intravenous infusion in acute severe asthma, *Br. J. Dis. Chest.*, 74, 385, 1980.
52. **Josephson, G. W., Kennedy, H. L., MacKenzie, R. J., and Gibson, G.,** Cardiac dysrhythmias during the treatment of acute asthma, *Chest*, 78, 429, 1980.
53. **Gray, B. J., Frame, M. H., and Costello, J. F.,** A comparative double-blind study of the bronchodilator effects and side effects of inhaled fenoterol and terbutaline administered in equi-potent doses, *Br. J. Dis. Chest*, 76, 341, 1982.
54. **Beardshaw, J. and Chan-Yeung, M.,** Comparison of the bronchodilator and cardiac effects of hydroxyphenylorciprenaline and orciprenaline, *Chest*, 65, 507, 1974.
55. **Windom, H. H., Burgess, C. D., Siebers, R. W. L., Purdie, G., Pearce, N., Crane, J., and Beasley, R.,** The pulmonary and extrapulmonary effects of inhaled beta agonists in patients with asthma, *Clin. Pharmacol. Ther.*, 48, 296, 1990.
56. **Tandon, M. K.,** Cardiopulmonary effects of fenoterol and salbutamol aerosols, *Chest*, 77, 429, 1980.
57. **Burgess, C. D., Windom, H. H., Pearce, N., Marshall, S., Beasley, R., Siebers, R. W. L., and Crane, J.,** Lack of evidence for β2 receptor selectivity: a study of metaproterenol, fenoterol, isoproterenol and epinephrine in patients with asthma, *Am. Rev. Respir. Dis.*, 143, 444, 1991.

58. **Wong, C. S., Pavord, I. D., Williams, J., Britton, J. R., and Tattersfield, A. E.,** Bronchodilator, cardiovascular and hypokalaemic effects of fenoterol, salbutamol and terbutaline in asthma, *Lancet,* 1, 1396, 1990.
59. **Bengtsson, B. and Fagerstrom, P. O.,** Extrapulmonary effects of terbutaline during prolonged administration, *Clin. Pharmacol. Ther.,* 31, 726, 1982.
60. **Mano, K., Akbarzadeh, A., and Townley, R. G.,** Effect of hydrocortisone on beta adrenergic receptors in lung membranes, *Life Sci.,* 25, 1925, 1979.
61. **Lockett, M. F.,** Dangerous effects of isoprenaline in myocardial failure, *Lancet,* 2, 104, 1965.
62. **Phillips, B. A., McConnell, J. W., and Smith, M. D.,** The effects of hypoxaemia on cardiac output, *Chest,* 93, 471, 1988.
63. **Kontos, H. A., Levasseur, J. E., Richardson, D. W., Macick, H. P. Jr., and Patterson, J. L. Jr.,** Comparative circulatory responses to systemic hypoxia in man and in unanaesthetized dogs, *J. Appl. Physiol.,* 23, 381, 1967.
64. **Downing, S. E., Mitchell, J. H., and Wallace, A. G.,** Cardiovascular responses to ischemia, hypoxia and hypercapnia of the central nervous system, *Am. J. Physiol.,* 204, 881, 1963.
65. **Leitch, A. G., Clancy, L. J., Costello, J. F., and Flenley, D. C.,** Effect of intravenous infusion of salbutamol on ventilatory response to carbon dioxide and hypoxia on heart rate and plasma potassium in normal men, *Br. Med. J.,* 1, 365, 1976.
66. **Bremner, P., Burgess, C. D., Crane, J., McHaffie, D., Galletly, D., Pearce, N., Woodman, K., and Beasley, R.,** The cardiovascular effects of fenoterol under conditions of hypoxaemia, *Thorax,* 47, 814, 1992.
67. **Krikler, D. M. and Curry, P. V. L.,** Torsade de pointes an atypical ventricular tachycardia, *Br. Heart J.,* 38, 117, 1976.
68. **Sears, M. R., Taylor, D. R., Print, C. G., Lake, D. C., Qingquing, Li, Flannery, D. M., Yates, D. M., Lucas, M. K., and Herbison, G. P.,** Regular inhaled β-agonist treatment in bronchial asthma, *Lancet,* 336, 1391, 1990.
69. **Haahtela, T., Jarvinen, M., Kava, T., Kiviranta, K., Koskinen, S., Lehtonen, K., Nikanda, K., Persson, T., Reinikainen, K., Selroos, O., Sovijarvi, A., Stenius-Aarniala, B., Svahn, T., Tammivara, R., and Laitenen, L.,** Comparison of β2 agonist terbutaline with an inhaled corticosteroid, budesonide, in newly detected asthma, *N. Engl. J. Med.,* 325, 388, 1991.
70. **Sanjar, S., Kristersson, A., Mazzoni, L., Morley, J., and Schaeublin, E.,** Increased airway reactivity in the guinea-pig follows exposure to intravenous isoprenaline, *J. Physiol.,* 425, 43, 1990.

Chapter 7

THE ROLE OF HYPOXEMIA IN DETERMINING THE CARDIOVASCULAR RESPONSE TO BETA RECEPTOR AGONIST DRUGS

Robin G. Shanks

TABLE OF CONTENTS

0-8493-6761-1/93/$0.00 + $.50

I. INTRODUCTION

During the past 30 years, beta adrenoceptor agonists have been increasingly used in the treatment of bronchial asthma especially with the introduction of pressurized aerosols delivering a metered dose of drug. The first drug to be extensively prescribed using this type of administration was isoprenaline, but during the past 15 years it has been largely replaced by drugs that selectively stimulate $beta_2$ adrenoceptors, for example, salbutamol and terbutaline. Isoprenaline is an agonist at $beta_1$ and $beta_2$ receptors with stimulation of $beta_1$ receptors in the heart producing positive chronotropic and inotropic effects, although these effects are less marked when the drug is given in therapeutic doses using an aerosol. The increase in deaths from asthma in England and Wales in young people in the early 1960s was attributed to excessive use of aerosols containing isoprenaline and in those delivering a large dose.[1,2] The association between the use of isoprenaline forte and this epidemic of deaths is reviewed in Chapters 2 and 3. It was thought that the increase in deaths with isoprenaline resulted from its cardiac effects and that the introduction of $beta_2$-selective agonists would enable a comparable degree of bronchodilation to be achieved with much less effect on the heart.

Even though $beta_2$-selective agonists had by the 1970s become the bronchodilator drugs of choice for the treatment of asthma, a second epidemic of deaths occurred in New Zealand. This epidemic could not be attributed to isoprenaline or apparently to toxicity from bronchodilators in general, as the increase in deaths began in 1975 and lasted until 1979, but the increase in total sales of bronchodilator drugs did not start to rise until 1979.[3] The epidemic of deaths in New Zealand was temporarily associated with the introduction of and increase in the use of high-dose preparation of the beta agonist fenoterol, and the major epidemiological studies investigating this relationship are reviewed in Chapter 5. Even though there may be doubts about the exact relationship between the use of bronchodilator drugs and the increase in deaths that have occurred twice in some countries in the last 25 years, these drugs are widely used to treat patients, some of whom die of the disease.

The mechanism of death in patients with asthma has not yet been elucidated, but it may well be that beta agonists contribute. The increase in deaths associated with large doses of isoprenaline were attributed to its effects on cardiac $beta_1$ receptors. With the development of more selective $beta_2$ agonists, it was assumed that such drugs would be safer, but if these drugs are given in sufficient doses, there is considerable stimulation of $beta_1$ receptors with an increase in heart rate, which is accompanied by marked effects of stimulation of $beta_2$ receptors, including a reduction of serum potassium.[4]

The actual cause of death in patients with asthma has not been clearly established, and in particular the mechanism of death has not been elucidated.[5] Although some of the increase in deaths may be attributed to an increase in incidence of asthma, it would appear that most deaths arise from inadequate assessment and treatment of the disease or to the adverse effects of treatment. The epidemic of asthma deaths in the United Kingdom and several other countries in the late 1960s was attributed to increased use of concentrated aerosols delivering isoprenaline in a dose of 0.4 mg per puff. Canada and the United States, which had not licensed the stronger aerosols, did not have an increase in asthma deaths.

The increase in sales of bronchodilator aerosols could reflect an increase in the prevalence or severity of asthma, and these may in themselves contribute to the increase in mortality. However, the description of patients dying clutching an aerosol or being surrounded by empty aerosols maintained the view that it was the contents of the aerosol that caused death, although this scenario might have indicated that the patient had a severe attack of asthma or that the disease had been undertreated. If the sympathomimetic agents were responsible for the deaths of patients with asthma, the exact mechanism has not yet been elucidated. Because isoprenaline administered by inhalation is absorbed into the bloodstream and affects the heart,[6,7] it has been suggested that the deaths in the asthmatic patients may result from sympathomimetic-induced cardiac arrhythmias.[8,9] There is little evidence to support this conclusion because electrocardiographic studies have rarely been made in the patients before their death. The intravenous infusion or injection of small doses of isoprenaline in normal people or of larger doses in animals, although increasing heart rate, did not produce cardiac arrhythmias.[10,11] Grant[12] indicated that many patients with asthma who use pressurized aerosols are not normal and suggested that the reduction in the tension of oxygen in arterial blood in patients with asthma may alter the effects of a sympathomimetic agent on the heart and on the bronchi and that this may contribute to their deaths.

II. INITIAL EXPERIMENTS WITH ISOPRENALINE

Because the effects of sympathomimetic agents on the cardiovascular system of animals or humans had not previously been studied during arterial hypoxemia and it seemed to be of importance in the use of these drugs in asthma, observations were made in anesthetized dogs. The details of experimental methods and a more detailed analysis of some aspects of this work have been published.[13] All observations were made in dogs anesthetized by the subcutaneous injection of morphine sulfate (0.5 mg/kg) followed 1 h later by the intravenous injection of pentobarbitone (20 mg/kg) and respired with room air or a mixture of 12% oxygen/88% nitrogen. Drugs were injected intravenously. Heart rate, the electrocardiogram, and arterial pressure were recorded in all experiments. Arterial blood samples were taken at frequent intervals and analyzed for oxygen and carbon dioxide tensions.

The intravenous injection of a series of increasing doses (0.1 to 1000 μg/kg) of isoprenaline in a dog respired with room air increased heart rate

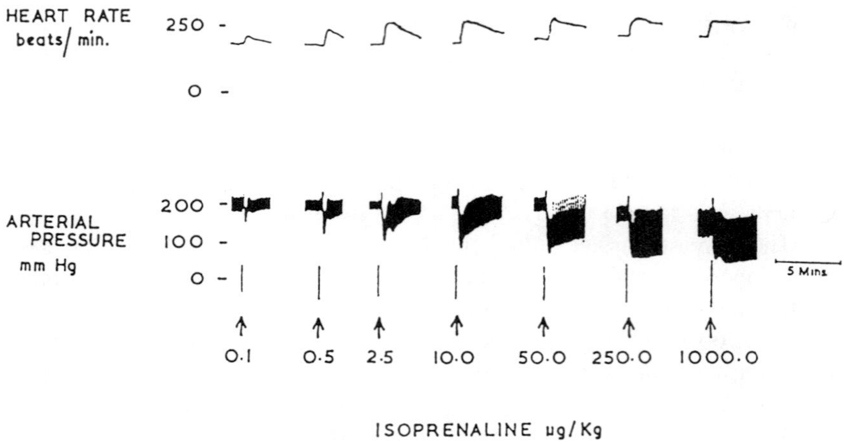

FIGURE 1. Records of heart rate and arterial pressure in an anesthetized dog respired with room air. Responses to the intravenous injection of increasing doses of isoprenaline. (From Shanks, R. G. and Swanton, J. G., *Excerpta Medica International Congress Series,* No. 220, 147, 1971. With permission.)

and reduced arterial pressure (Figure 1). As the dose of isoprenaline was increased, the changes in these two parameters became maximal at 10 μg/kg; larger doses produced more prolonged responses. All survived the largest dose of isoprenaline, 100 or 500 μg/kg. Ventricular ectopic beats were occasionally produced by the administration of isoprenaline; their incidence was not dose-related.

The intravenous injection of a series of doses of isoprenaline during respiration with 12% oxygen/88% nitrogen to reduce the tension of oxygen in arterial blood to 40 mmHg with no change in the tension of carbon dioxide is shown in Figure 2. The administration of 0.1, 0.5, 2.5, and 10 μg/kg isoprenaline produced the normal responses, an increase in heart rate and a decrease in arterial pressure, although the heart rate response to 10.0 μg/kg was reduced. The responses to 50.0 μg/kg isoprenaline were not normal. An initial increase in heart rate was followed by rapid and progressive decreases in heart rate and in systolic, diastolic, and pulse pressures. Sinus rhythm persisted until arterial pressure was less than 50 mmHg when a slow idioventricular rhythm developed, which progressively slowed until cardiac asystole occurred. Ventricular fibrillation did not occur. Observations of this type were made in five dogs. Three died after the administration of isoprenaline 10 μg/kg, one after 25.0 μg/kg, and one after 50.0 μg/kg. In all five death occurred from cardiac asystole. Arrhythmias did not develop until the final stage of the reaction when arterial pressure was less than 50 mmHg.

Further observations were made in another series of experiments in which a single dose of isoprenaline (2.5 μg/kg) was injected on six occasions with 5 min between each injection (Figure 3). During respiration with room air, each dose of isoprenaline increased heart rate and reduced arterial pressure.

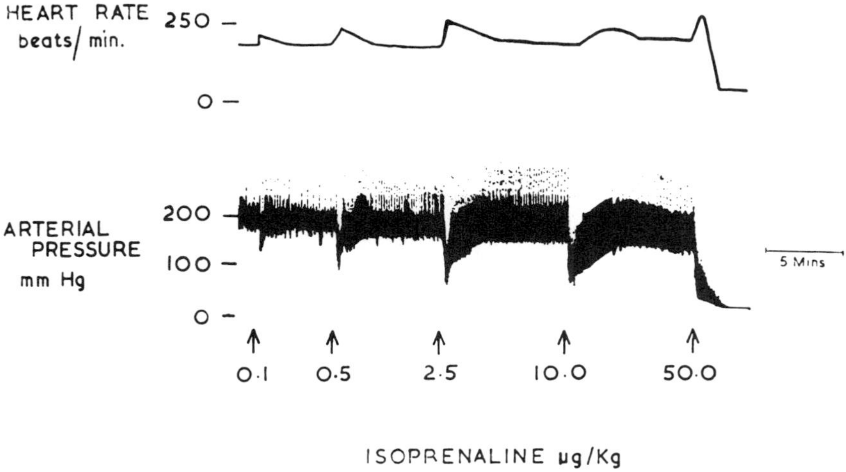

FIGURE 2. Records of heart rate and arterial pressure in an anesthetized dog respired with 12% oxygen, 88% nitrogen. Responses to the intravenous injection of increasing doses of isoprenaline. (From Shanks, R. G. and Swanton, J. G., *Excerpta Medica International Congress Series,* No. 220, 147, 1971. With permission.)

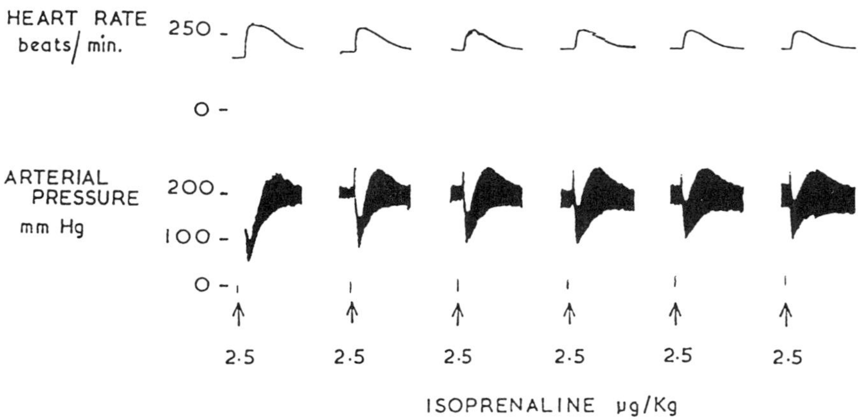

FIGURE 3. Records of heart rate and arterial pressure in an anesthetized dog respired with room air. Responses to the repeated injection of isoprenaline (2.5 µg/kg). (From Shanks, R. G. and Swanton, J. G., *Excerpta Medica International Congress Series,* No. 220, 147, 1971. With permission.)

During respiration with 12% oxygen/88% nitrogen, the responses to the first to fourth dose of a series of doses were as described, but the fifth dose in all experiments produced a transient increase in heart rate and arterial pressure followed by a rapid and progressive decrease in both parameters with death occurring from cardiac asystole (Figure 4).

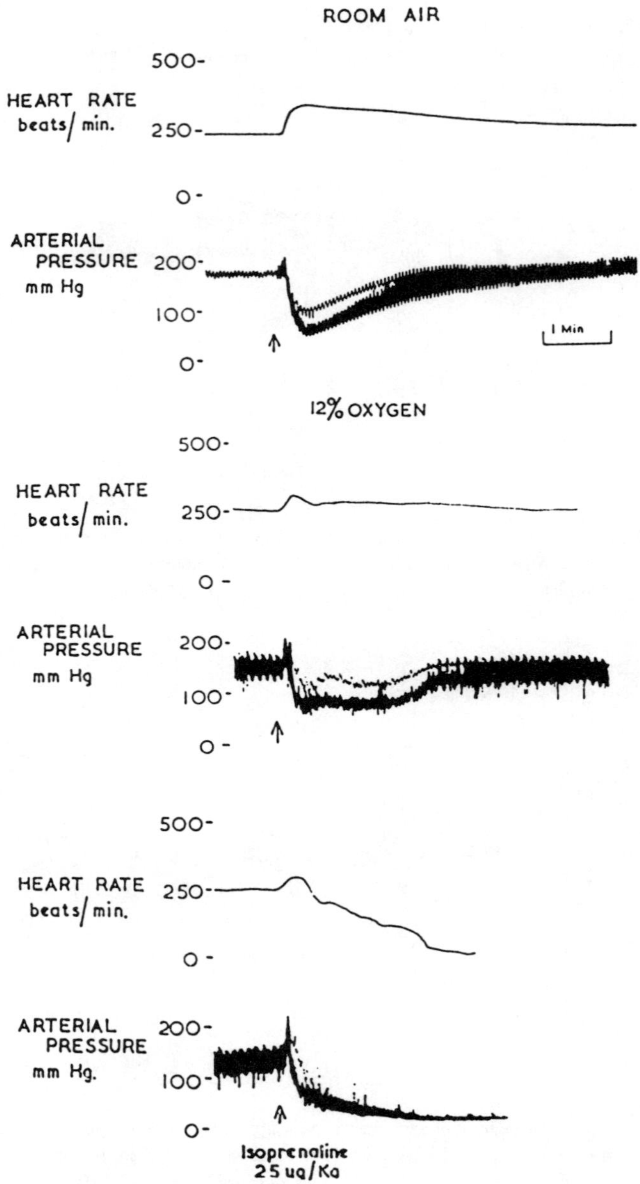

FIGURE 4. Records of heart rate and arterial pressure in an anesthetized dog respired with 12% oxygen, 88% nitrogen. Responses to the intravenous injection of isoprenaline (2.5 μg/kg) during respiration with room air (upper panel) and later with 12% oxygen, 88% nitrogen (lower two panels). The middle and lower sets of records are the responses to the 4th and 5th doses of isoprenaline, respectively. (From Shanks, R. G. and Swanton, J. G., *Excerpta Medica International Congress Series,* No. 220, 147, 1971. With permission.)

Observations were made in three dogs in which a probe for an electromagnetic flowmeter was placed around the ascending aorta to measure stroke volume and the rate of ejection of blood from the left ventricle. The responses to the injection of isoprenaline (2.5 μg/kg) were obtained in each animal during respiration with room air and at 5-min intervals after starting respiration with 12% oxygen/88% nitrogen (Figure 5). During respiration with room air, isoprenaline increased heart rate, stroke volume, and the rate of ejection of blood from the left ventricle; arterial pressure was decreased. During respiration with 12% oxygen/88% nitrogen, normal responses were obtained with the first four of a series of doses (0.2 μg/kg) of isoprenaline. The fifth dose initially produced increases in heart rate and the rate of ejection of blood, but 1 min after the injection of isoprenaline both had fallen to below the preinjection levels, although sinus rhythm was still present. All parameters continued to decline; idioventricular rhythm developed 4 min after injection of isoprenaline and death from asystole occurred after another minute. Similar observations were found in two other experiments.

III. FURTHER EXPERIMENTS WITH DIFFERENT BETA RECEPTOR AGONIST DRUGS

Because several other drugs used for the relief of bronchospasm also act through stimulation of beta adrenoceptor, the effects of some of these drugs were compared in dogs respired with room air and with 12% oxygen/88% nitrogen mixture. The drugs studied were orciprenaline and salbutamol. Orciprenaline stimulates all beta adrenoceptors, and salbutamol has a greater effect on adrenergic $beta_2$ receptors responsible for bronchodilation and vasodilation than on $beta_1$ receptors responsible for cardiac stimulation.[14] Studies in anesthetized dogs have shown that the intravenous administration of all three drugs increased heart rate and that the order of activity was isoprenaline, orciprenaline, and salbutamol. If isoprenaline is given an activity of 1000, the relative activity of the other drugs was orciprenaline 39.8 and salbutamol 4.75. The effect of the intravenous injection of increasing doses (0.1, 1.0, 10.0, and 100.0 μg/kg) of isoprenaline, orciprenaline, and salbutamol was studied in anesthetized dogs respired with room air. Each drug was given to four animals and all survived the largest dose.[15]

Similar observations were made in groups of animals respired with 12% oxygen/88% nitrogen, which reduced the tension of oxygen in arterial blood to 35 to 40 mmHg without altering the tension of carbon dioxide. As the dose of isoprenaline was increased, the characteristic fatal response from cardiac asystole occurred, all with doses less than 200 μg/kg. Increasing doses of orciprenaline were given in nine experiments. The two smallest doses (0.4 and 2.0 μg/kg) produced an increase in heart rate and a decrease in arterial pressure. The previously described fatal reaction to isoprenaline occurred after the administration of orciprenaline (10 μg/kg) in five, after 50 in two, and

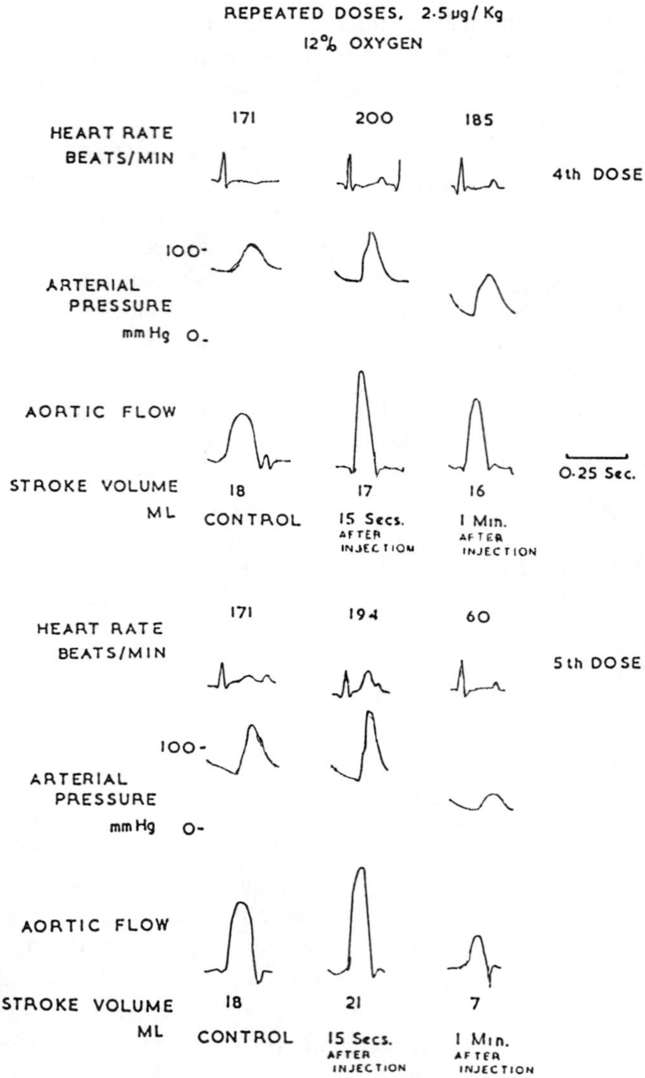

FIGURE 5. Records of the electrocardiogram, arterial pressure and flow through the ascending aorta in an anesthetized dog respired with 12% oxygen, 88% nitrogen. The heart rate (beats/min) and stroke volume (ml) are shown. The responses to the intravenous injection of the 4th and 5th of a series of doses of isoprenaline (2.5 µg/kg) are shown. The time after the injection of isoprenaline at which the records were taken is indicated. (From Shanks, R. G. and Swanton, J. G., *Excerpta Medica International Congress Series,* No. 220, 147, 1971. With permission.)

after 200 in one. The final dose of orciprenaline produced a transient increase in heart rate followed by a progressive decrease, which developed into a progressively slow idioventricular rhythm; arterial pressure decreased rapidly with a marked reduction in pulse pressure.

The effects of salbutamol were studied in four experiments. The administration of 0.1 and 1.0 μg/kg increased heart rate and reduced arterial pressure. One animal died after 10 and two after 100 μg/kg. The final fatal dose of salbutamol produced the characteristic reductions in heart rate and arterial pressure from which the animal did not recover.

These observations suggest that the reversal of the cardiac actions of isoprenaline by hypoxia is due to stimulation of adrenergic beta receptors because it also occurred with orciprenaline and salbutamol, which stimulate beta adrenoceptors. Although these two drugs have less effect on the heart than isoprenaline, reversal of their cardiac effects with death occurred with doses of the same order as those of isoprenaline, which were reversed.

Propranolol was administered in doses that blocked the effects of isoprenaline on heart rate and blood pressure during respiration with room air. Following pretreatment with propranolol, the repeated injection of isoprenaline during respiration with 12% oxygen/88% nitrogen did not produce the abnormal response leading to cardiac asystole and death.

IV. DISCUSSION

The observations summarized in this chapter indicate that in animals respired with room air the intravenous injection of isoprenaline produces the characteristic hemodynamic responses of an increase in heart rate and a decrease in blood pressure and large doses of isoprenaline were tolerated. However, the responses to isoprenaline were reversed during respiration with 12% oxygen/88% nitrogen, so that relatively small doses produced marked cardiovascular depression and death. The cardiac actions of salbutamol and orciprenaline were also reversed by hypoxemia. These effects of the drugs did not occur after pretreatment with propranolol. The cardiovascular collapse produced by these drugs during hypoxemia was attributed to an effect on beta adrenoceptor because it occurred with isoprenaline, orciprenaline, and salbutamol and was prevented by propranolol.

The mechanism responsible for the reversal of the cardiac actions of these drugs is not known. It appears to be related to their cardiac action either through a direct action on cardiac muscle or through changes in coronary blood flow. It does not result from a cardiac arrhythmia, peripheral circulatory failure, or changes in the tension of carbon dioxide in arterial blood. It may be related to the unexplained observations of Lockett[16] who showed in the isolated heart that small doses of isoprenaline produced cardiac asystole in the presence of a high work load. It is not clear if the effects were due to stimulation of $beta_1$ or $beta_2$ receptors. All three drugs affect both sets of receptors, although salbutamol has a greater effect on $beta_2$ receptors. Activation of $beta_1$ or $beta_2$ receptors has not previously been shown to produce cardiac depression. Thus, it is not possible to conclude if the effect resulted from $beta_1$ or $beta_2$ receptors or both. The response was prevented by propranolol, but no studies were completed using drugs to selectively block either $beta_1$ or $beta_2$ receptors. It is still not known if these observations are important in the use of any or all beta agonists in the treatment of asthma.

A number of questions remain unanswered. The reversal of the normal cardiovascular responses to three beta adrenoceptor agonists (isoprenaline, salbutamol, and orciprenaline) has been demonstrated. Newer beta agonists (terbutaline, fenoterol, and salmeterol) have been introduced for the treatment of asthma. The effects of hypoxia and their cardiovascular responses have not been examined. The mechanism of death in patients with asthma and its relationship to the use of bronchodilator drugs is unclear because a precise causal relationship has not been established. The severe impairment of cardiovascular function that takes place during an asthmatic attack may in itself be fatal or, if not, the patient may be tipped into death by drugs that have a well-defined and pronounced cardiovascular effect. The experiments described in this chapter show that the responses in such patients may be different from those in normal subjects.

Although the observations summarized in this chapter were made over 20 years ago, they still appear to be important for a number of reasons, including the following:

1. Asthma is still a common disease and deaths due to asthma have not declined despite the introduction of several new treatments.
2. The mechanism of those deaths is largely unknown in that it is not entirely clear if they occur from undertreatment or overtreatment.
3. The role of sympathomimetic drugs in asthma deaths has still to be clarified.

REFERENCES

1. **Stolley, P. D.,** Asthma mortality: why the United States was spared an epidemic of deaths due to asthma, *Am. Rev. Respir. Dis.*, 105, 883, 1972.
2. **Benatar, S. R.,** Fatal asthma, *N. Engl. J. Med.*, 314, 423, 1986.
3. **Keating, G., Mitchell, E. A., Jackson, R., Beaglehole, R., and Rea, H.,** Trends in sales of drugs for asthma in New Zealand, Australia and the United Kingdom, 1975–81, *Br. Med. J.*, 289, 348, 1984.

4. **Wong, C. S., Pavora, I. D., Williams, J., and Tattersfield, A. E.,** Bronchodilator, cardiovascular and hypokalaemic effects of fenoterol, salbutamol and terbutaline in asthma, *Lancet,* 1, 1396, 1990.
5. **McFadden, E. R.,** Fatal and near-fatal asthma, *N. Engl. J. Med.,* 324, 409, 1991.
6. **Chamberlain, D. A.,** The role of the sympathetic innervation of the heart in man, M. D. thesis, University of Cambridge, 1967.
7. **Paterson, J. W., Connolly, M. E., Davies, D. S., and Dollery, C. T.,** Isoprenaline resistance and the use of pressurised aerosols in asthma, *Lancet,* 2, 426, 1968.
8. **Speizer, F. E., Doll, R., and Heaf, P.,** Observations on recent increase in mortality from asthma, *Br. Med. J.,* 1, 335, 1968.
9. **Speizer, F. E., Doll, R., Heaf, P., and Strange, L. B.,** Investigation into use of drugs preceding death from asthma, *Br. Med. J.,* 1, 339, 1968.
10. **Krasnow, N., Rolett, E. L., Yurchak, P. M., Hood, W. B., and Gorbin, R.,** Isoproterenol and cardiovascular performance, *Am. J. Med.,* 37, 514, 1964.
11. **Shanks, R. G.,** Unpublished observations, 1969.
12. **Grant, I. W. B.,** Deaths from asthma, *Br. Med. J.,* 1, 575, 1968.
13. **Collins, J. M., McDevitt, D. G., Shanks, R. G., and Swanton, J. G.,** The cardiotoxicity of isoprenaline during hypoxia, *Br. J. Pharmacol.,* 36, 35, 1969.
14. **Kofi Ekue, J. M., Shanks, R. G., and Zaidi, S. A.,** Observations on the subdivision of β-adrenoceptors in the circulation of the dog, *Br. J. Pharmacol.,* 39, 184P, 1970.
15. **McDevitt, D. G., Shanks, R. G., and Swanton, J. G.,** Further observations on the cardio-toxicity of isoprenaline during hypoxia, *Br. J. Pharmacol.,* 50, 335, 1974.
16. **Lockett, M. F.,** Dangerous effects of isoprenaline in myocardial failure, *Lancet,* 2, 104, 1965.
17. **Shanks, R. G. and Swanton, J. G.,** Changes in the pharmacological response to isoprenaline under conditions of hypoxia in dogs, *Excerpta Medica International Congress Series,* No. 220, 147, 1971.

Section 5

The Acute and Long-Term Effects of Beta Receptor Agonist Therapy

Chapter 8

THE ACUTE UNWANTED EFFECTS OF $BETA_2$ RECEPTOR AGONIST THERAPY

Martin J. Kendall and Christine A. Haffner

TABLE OF CONTENTS

0-8493-6761-1/93/$0.00 + $.50

I. INTRODUCTION

Adverse effects of drugs are often classified as type A (pharmacologically predictable) and type B (idiosyncratic).[1] The majority of unwanted actions of $beta_2$ agonists belong to the former category and result from stimulation of beta receptors in organs and tissues other than the bronchi. In this review, therefore, the classification of adrenoceptors will be reviewed and $beta_2$ receptor-mediated functions identified.

From the beginning of this century, physiologists have appreciated that the catecholamine response to such stimuli as fear, stress, and exercise produce many different effects in the body.[2,3] Ahlquist[4] divided adrenoceptors into two groups, alpha and beta, according to the effect on them of different pharmacological agents. Lands et al.[5] further characterized beta receptors as $beta_1$ or $beta_2$. Table 1 illustrates the effects of stimulation of these receptors. Initially the picture was oversimplified: alpha receptor stimulation caused vasoconstriction; $beta_1$ receptor stimulation resulted in positive inotropic and chronotropic effects on the heart and lipolysis; $beta_2$ receptors mediated all other adrenoceptor functions. This view led to the concept of *selectivity:* each tissue contained one type of receptor, stimulation of which produced a single characteristic response. Subsequently, however, two facts were established which contested this concept. First, most tissues containing beta receptors were found to possess a mixture of both subtypes[8,9] even if one, for instance, $beta_2$ in bronchi, was functionally more important. Second, beta receptor antagonist drugs were shown to be more selective, binding to one subtype at low concentrations but binding to the other at high concentrations.[10] Thus, true "selectivity" of beta agonist or antagonist drugs is more complex than originally suggested and involves all the factors listed in Table 2. Other factors affecting the actions of $beta_2$ agonists are also shown in this table. It is important to bear these in mind as the acute unwanted effects of various $beta_2$ agonist medications are discussed.

When $beta_2$ agonists are administered for the purpose of bronchodilatation (and increased mucociliary transport, reduced bronchial venous congestion, and inhibition of chemical mediator release), their other sympathomimetic actions could then be described as "unwanted". These comprise the other physiological responses to stress (fight or flight) shown in Table 1 and include (1) metabolic functions, such as glycogenolysis and lipolysis, (2) cardiovascular adaptations, and (3) other effects, such as changes in skeletal muscle function. In this review, acute unwanted effects of $beta_2$ agonists will be considered under these broad headings. Those that are clinically harmful or could prove fatal are highlighted, although it is yet to be established that such effects are responsible for increased asthma mortality and morbidity.

II. BIOCHEMICAL AND METABOLIC EFFECTS

The pharmacological responses to $beta_2$ agonists described in this section can be subdivided into those concerned with energy substrates (glucose, free fatty acids [FFAs], insulin), those influencing cation concentrations (potassium and magnesium), and finally the production of lactic acidosis.

A. GLUCOSE

Catecholamines stimulate glycogenolysis and gluconeogenesis, thus increasing glucose production: this is a vital response to physical stress.[6,13] The importance of $beta_2$ adrenoceptors in these processes has been demonstrated in three ways. First, infusion or inhalation of selective $beta_2$ agonists, such as salbutamol or terbutaline, produces an increase in plasma glucose.[14-18] Second, infusion of selective $beta_1$ agonists, such as prenalterol, does not have this effect.[19] Lastly, nonselective beta blockers, such as propranolol, impair recovery from insulin-induced hypoglycemia more than selective beta blockers, for example, metoprolol or atenolol.[20-22]

The hyperglycemic response to acute administration of $beta_2$ agonists has been described in healthy volunteers, women in premature labor, asthmatic subjects, and diabetic patients. Rolf Smith et al.[15] and Kendall et al.[18] described a marked dose-dependent increase in plasma glucose (from mean 4.4 to mean 8 m*M*) within 20 min of infusing terbutaline into healthy subjects, reaching a maximum after 60 min. They also showed a similar plasma glucose increase after nebulized salbutamol. This occurs with all $beta_2$ agonists: comparison of equimolar doses of intravenous (IV) salbutamol (long half-life) and rimiterol (shorter half-life) showed a similar time course for the plasma glucose response, but rimiterol caused a less marked increase at all doses (maximum 3.0 versus 5.0 m*M*).[23] Different modes of administration alter the glucose response. In asthmatics significant increases in plasma glucose occurred after IV boluses of salbutamol (4 μg/kg), but there was only a small, short-lived increase in plasma glucose after aerosol inhalation of salbutamol (200 μg dose).[16] However, the response is also dose-related: with higher doses of inhaled salbutamol (up to 4 mg) in asthmatic patients, producing greater increases in plasma glucose (maximum 1.46 m*M*).[17] Mouth rinsing or gargling, although removing around 24% of inhaled salbutamol dose, did not alter the effect on plasma glucose in eight asthmatic patients.[24] $Beta_2$ agonists may have less effect on plasma glucose of asthmatics, especially if they are acutely ill, than of healthy volunteers,[25,26] possibly due to regular use. Tolerance to the plasma glucose response develops much more quickly than to bronchodilatation,[27,28] although this has been disputed.[29,30]

This increase in plasma glucose in response to $beta_2$ agonist treatment should be remembered when managing diabetic asthmatics or pregnant women.

TABLE 1
Adrenoceptor Function

Adrenoceptor	Function
$Alpha_1$	Smooth muscle contraction
	Blood vessels
	Genitourinary tract
	Mydriasis
	Bronchoconstriction
	Stimulation of
	Release from mast cells
	Gluconeogenesis
	Glycogenolysis (liver)
$Alpha_2$	Smooth muscle relaxation
	Gastrointestinal tract
	Platelet aggregation
	Inhibition of
	Lipolysis
	Renin release
	Insulin release
	Noradrenaline release
	Promotion of
	K^+ and water secretion by salivary glands
$Beta_1$	Cardiac
	Automaticity, force of contraction, conduction velocity
	Coronary vasodilation
	Glycogenolysis
	Lipolysis
	Reduced mast cell release
$Beta_2$	Smooth muscle relaxation
	Bronchi
	Blood vessels
	Genitourinary tract
	Gastrointestinal tract
	Promotion of
	Noradrenaline release
	Glycogenolysis and gluconeogenesis (liver)
	Glycogenolysis (muscle)
	Insulin and glucagon secretion
	Renin release

Data taken from Lees, G. M., *Br. Med. J.*, 283, 173, 1981. Also, from Strosberg, A. E., *Am. J. Cardiol.*, 59, 3F, 1987.

Comparison of salbutamol infusion in normal and diabetic subjects revealed greater hepatic glucose production and resultant increase in plasma glucose as well as ketone body production in diabetic patients.[31] Reports of ketoacidosis induced by $beta_2$ agonist therapy in diabetic women in premature labor[32,33] emphasized the need for vigilance. Diabetics produce less $beta_2$ stimulated insulin release and so cannot limit hyperglycemia. There has also been a

TABLE 2
Factors Affecting Severity and Frequency of Unwanted Effects of $Beta_2$ Receptor Agonists

Selectivity of Drug
- Affinity for $beta_1$ and $beta_2$ receptors
- Proportion of $beta_1$:$beta_2$ receptors subserving function
- Pharmacokinetic factors

Efficacy of Drug
- Capacity of drug to stimulate receptor to produce response

Sensitivity of receptors
- Tolerance
- Asthmatic versus normal individual (Are $beta_2$ receptors in asthmatics different?)

Risks in patient
- Disease state: acutely ill and hypoxic
  - chronic poor control — tolerance
  - difference between young asthmatic and older chronic bronchitic[12]
- Interaction of effects: low K^+ predisposes to cardiac rhythm disturbances

report of $beta_2$ agonist therapy of premature labor inducing ketoacidosis in a woman not known to have diabetes mellitus.[34] She had been treated with subcutaneous (SC) terbutaline 2 mg in 24 h as well as intramuscular steroid therapy, subsequently required insulin during her pregnancy, and had a diabetic glucose tolerance test post partum. So $beta_2$ agonist therapy can unmask diabetic mellitus and cause diagnostic confusion. This report also highlights the potentiating effect of glucocorticoids in raising blood sugar and precipitating ketoacidosis in insulin-deficient individuals: steroids are often given in combination with $beta_2$ agonists in the treatment of acute asthma. Increased adrenergic drive in acute asthma can also potentiate hyperglycemia. Fetal morbidity due to disturbance of carbohydrate metabolism should not be a problem if $beta_2$ agonists are used during pregnancy.[35]

B. INSULIN

Infusion of $beta_2$ agonists causes an increase in plasma insulin in human volunteers.[36,37] This could be due to either direct stimulation of pancreatic islet cells with functional $beta_2$ receptors or a response to $beta_2$ agonist-stimulated glucose production. Insulin secretion is controlled by a number of factors including catecholamines,[38] and there is a rich adrenergic innervation of pancreatic islet tissue.[39] The $beta_2$ agonists clenbuterol and salbutamol promote insulin release from isolated human islet cells in a dose-dependent fashion,[40] indicating that a direct effect of $beta_2$ stimulation is possible. This is corroborated by the increase in C peptide, which occurred in women treated with salbutamol infusion for premature labor.[14]

The insulin response to $beta_2$ agonists occurs with both long-acting and short-acting agents,[23] is dose-dependent, reaches a maximum before plasma glucose, and differs in asthmatics and healthy volunteers. In asthmatics a significant increase in plasma insulin occurred after salbutamol injection but not after inhaled therapy.[16] Another study using salbutamol injection compared asthmatic and healthy subjects and showed no difference in response for any metabolic parameter except insulin. Asthmatic subjects had a much more marked insulin response than healthy volunteers (26.8 U/ml versus 16.4 U/ml at 5 min, $p < 0.005$).[41] Plasma insulin was the most sensitive metabolic parameter in another study of inhaled salbutamol given to asthmatics,[24] although not in diabetic patients.[31] The insulin-releasing action of $beta_2$ agonists is only relevant to acute administration because tolerance develops quickly, after 13 days oral terbutaline therapy in one study.[29] Blood glucose still rose at this time, suggesting that tolerance to the insulin response develops more rapidly.[28]

The potential clinical relevance of the insulin response to $beta_2$ receptor stimulation is twofold. First, in nondiabetics it limits the increase in blood glucose produced by $beta_2$ agonist treatment; diabetics may have a more marked hyperglycemic response. Second, cardiovascular morbidity and mortality are being increasingly linked with hyperinsulinemic states, as are hypertension, obesity, and non–insulin-dependent diabetes mellitus.[30] $Beta_2$ agonist-induced increases in plasma insulin may therefore be important. However, the swift development of tolerance may make this less of a problem.

C. LIPOLYSIS

Free fatty acids (FFAs) provide energy during exercise and stress, and lipolysis, the process of their release from adipose tissue, is stimulated by catecholamines. This action is mediated by beta adrenoceptor activation, although which subtype is involved remains undecided. Lipolysis was originally considered to be under $beta_1$ receptor control.[41-43] However, $beta_1$ blockers have less impact on lipolysis than on the heart. Furthermore, $beta_2$ agonist drugs promote lipolysis. Additional support for lipolysis being a $beta_2$-mediated process is derived from the increase in FFA induced by infusion of dilevalol, a beta blocker with $beta_2$-stimulant properties,[44] and a comparison of xamoterol, a partial $beta_1$ agonist, and terbutaline, which demonstrated a far greater lipolytic response to terbutaline.[45] Both these studies used normal volunteers. Alternatives are that human fat cell lipolysis is mediated through a mixed pool of receptors or that the receptors are different and called $beta_3$.[41] IV salbutamol produced a marked increase in plasma FFAs in normal volunteers[46] and pregnant women[14] as did nebulized salbutamol.[15] Once again, however, asthmatics behave differently; neither inhaled[26] nor IV salbutamol[16] elevated plasma FFAs. This observation was confirmed by Kallenbach et al.[41] and may be explained by the development of tolerance.[28]

The modest $beta_2$-stimulated increase in FFAs in asthmatics is unlikely to be a cause of serious morbidity. However, diabetic subjects seem more susceptible,[31] and high concentrations of FFAs have been implicated as a cause of cardiac dysfunction[47] and arrhythmias[48] under hypoxic or ischemic conditions. FFAs inhibit myocardial glucose uptake, glycolysis, and glucose oxidation.[49] FFAs and glucose can both be used as energy substrates by normally perfused myocardium, but under hypoxic conditions only glucose can be used and there is intracellular accumulation of FFAs and possibly triglycerides. All the studies documenting the toxicity of FFAs to hypoxic myocardium have been performed in animals,[49] but the results suggest a risk of myocardial depression or arrhythmias in acutely asthmatic patients who are tachycardic, hypoxic, and then administered $beta_2$ agonists.

The effect of $beta_2$ agonists on other lipids, for example, high density lipoprotein (HDL) and low density lipoprotein (LDL) cholesterol are disputed.[50,51] No changes in serum lipid levels occurred in asthmatic patients after IV salbutamol.[50] After 2 weeks of oral salbutamol an increase in HDL cholesterol was noted,[50] although in another study lower doses had no effect.[51] Thus, the lipid responses to $beta_2$ agonists may be favorable.

D. POTASSIUM

Hypokalemia is a potentially serious unwanted effect of $beta_2$ agonist therapy because it has been associated with cardiac arrhythmias. However, the contribution of hypokalemia to increased asthma mortality is difficult to establish for two reasons. First, asthma, by causing anxiety, tachycardia, tachypnea, and acid-base disturbances may also adversely affect the heart. Second, $beta_2$ agonists and other therapeutic agents used in asthma have direct actions on the heart. This subject will be considered under four headings.

1. Mechanism of Hypokalemia

The serum concentration of potassium is maintained within a narrow range because the ratio of intracellular to extracellular potassium is the principle determinant of the electrical potential across cell membranes. This, in turn, governs the behavior of cells of all types.[52] Both exercise and ingestion of food would increase serum potassium if not for several homeostatic mechanisms.[53] First, renal excretion of potassium maintains overall balance but is too slow to prevent acute increases in serum potassium. For this, extrarenal mechanisms, chiefly insulin- and catecholamine-induced cellular uptake, are vitally important. Insulin facilitates uptake of potassium into muscle, liver, and adipose tissue by stimulating Na^+/K^+-ATPase.[53] Catecholamines principally cause uptake of potassium into skeletal muscle, which is the largest single pool of body potassium and has an active Na^+/K^+-ATPase.[54] Potassium is also taken into red blood cells.[54] This is highly relevant to the action of $beta_2$ agonists on serum potassium. Finally, mineralocorticoids and glucocorticoids enhance potassium secretion from intestinal tissue in addition to increasing renal potassium excretion.[55]

Catecholamine-induced hypokalemia has been reviewed by Struthers and Reid[53] and was first described by D'Silva in 1934,[56] who showed that infusion of adrenaline into cats caused an initial transient hyperkalemia (due to an alpha adrenoceptor-mediated release from the liver) followed by hypokalemia.

Many subsequent studies using isolated animal muscle preparations[57-59] and infusing adrenaline and more specific $beta_2$ agonists into human volunteers[60-64] have shown that adrenaline stimulates muscle Na^+/K^+-ATPase through $beta_2$ adrenoceptors. Potassium uptake, for example, was blocked by ouabain and $beta_2$ receptor blockade in isolated rat skeletal muscle.[59] In human volunteers timolol, a nonselective beta adrenoceptor blocker, completely inhibited adrenaline-induced hypokalemia, whereas atenolol had a minimal effect.[65] Others[63] have demonstrated an inhibiting effect of atenolol and suggest some involvement of $beta_1$ receptors.

That the hypokalemic effect of adrenaline is in part independent of renal function or insulin has been shown in studies of animals, the kidneys and pancreas of which have been removed.[66,67] Also, salbutamol infusion (0.06 μg/kg/min) administered to five diabetic patients resulted in a decrease in plasma potassium (3.7 to 3.15 m*M*) with no increase in insulin; so the $beta_2$ effect on potassium can be produced independent of changes in insulin.[68] However, recently, somatostatin infused into ten healthy volunteers inhibited terbutaline-induced hypokalemia,[69] which suggested that $beta_2$ receptor-mediated insulin secretion may have a role. Renal excretion of potassium does not increase during salbutamol infusion.[70]

As well as stimulating cellular uptake of potassium directly and causing release of insulin, $beta_2$ agonists also increase ventilation and cause a respiratory alkalosis,[71] which promotes cellular uptake and is another reason for hypokalemia.

2. $Beta_2$ Receptor Agonist Stimulated Hypokalemia

Because bronchial dilatation and stimulation of cell membrane Na^+/K^+-ATPase are both $beta_2$-mediated functions, it could be predicted that therapeutic doses of $beta_2$ agonists for asthma would lower serum potassium. This has been demonstrated in a number of studies and has been reviewed by Spector.[72] Tables 3 to 6 report studies of how differently administered $beta_2$ agonists affect serum potassium. These reveal that parenteral administration (IV or SC) leads to the greatest decreases in serum potassium, oral dosing less so, and the inhaled route least.

The decrease in serum potassium is dose-dependent, being negligible for normal inhaled doses, and occurs most rapidly after IV or SC administered drugs. This hypokalemic response is an acute effect of $beta_2$ agonist agents and tolerance seems to develop after 2 weeks treatment.[97] Thus, chronic therapy would protect asthmatic subjects from this effect. The age of the subject does not influence the response.

Comparison between different agents shows that fenoterol seems to cause a greater decrease in serum potassium, although whether doses used were equivalent is disputed. This greater tendency of fenoterol to cause hypokalemia has been linked to the increased mortality from asthma in New Zealand, where this drug has been used more.[92,96,98]

TABLE 3
Effect of Intravenous Beta Receptor Agonists on Potassium

Medication/dose	Max K^+(mM)	Comments	Ref.
Salbutamol 10 μg/min for 1 h	−0.89	7 healthy volunteers	73
Salbutamol 4 μg/kg for 10 min	−0.45		25
Salbutamol 4 μg/kg	−0.04 (10 min)	10 asthmatics	16
Salbutamol 14.5 μg/min 10 min	−1.23 (4 h)	8 pregnant women (labor)	70
Salbutamol 300 μg/min bolus 10 μg/min infusion for 30 min	−0.4 (5–10 min) −1.1 (20–30 min)	8 asthmatics	74
Salbutamol	−0.9	4 volunteers	75
Salbutamol 0.1 mg/kg/min 0.4 mg/kg/min 0.7 mg/kg/min	 max −0.58 −1.18	4 male volunteers	23
Rimiterol 0.11 mg/kg/min 0.22 mg/kg/min 0.44 mg/kg/min	 −0.75 −1.0 −1.42		
Terbutaline 9.2 μg/min	−1.0	6 women (preterm labor)	76
Terbutaline 250 μg for 5 min	−0.6	11 healthy men	29
Terbutaline 0.5 mg	−0.85	5 pregnant women (preterm labor)	77
Salbutamol 300 μg (60 min) 600 μg (60 min)	 −0.6 (60 min) −1.0 (60 min)	7 healthy volunteers	78
Terbutaline 0.5 mg for 1 h	−0.9	8 healthy volunteers	18
Salbutamol 250 mg slow intravenous	−0.55 (30 min)	5 asthmatics	79
Salbutamol 25 μg	−0.1 (−0.1)	11 nonasthmatics	41
Salbutamol 100 μg	−0.45 (−0.55)	11 asthmatics	

TABLE 4
Effect of Subcutaneous Beta Receptor Agonists on Potassium

Medication/dose	Max K^+(m*M*)	Comments	Ref.
Terbutaline 0.5 mg	−0.81 (60 min)	29 pregnant women (preterm labor)	77
Terbutaline 0.25 mg	−0.6 (max 30 min)	7 asthmatics	80
Salbutamol 500 μg	−0.81 (max 60 min)	8 asthmatics	79
Terbutaline 0.5 mg	−0.81 (60 min)	29 pregnant women (preterm labor)	60
Terbutaline 0.25 mg 2nd dose after 30 min	−0.5 (60 min) −1.0 (90 min)	6 asthmatics (K^+ matched FEV_1 in dose-response)	81
Terbutaline 0.25 mg	−0.60 (30 min)	10 healthy subjects	69

TABLE 5
Effect of Oral Beta Receptor Agonists on Potassium

Medication	Max K^+(m*M*)	Comments	Ref.
Salbutamol 6–16 mg/day	No effect 1 h after dose on day 5	16 subjects (mainly bronchitics)	82
Salbutamol 4 mg	−0.2 at 120 min	10 healthy volunteers	83
Salbutamol 8 mg every 6 h	−0.7 24 h (5/6 patients)	6 patients	84
Salbutamol 4 mg	−0.7 no change	2 healthy volunteers	85
Salbutamol 80 mg (overdose)	Serum K^+ (no baseline) 2.3	1	86
Terbutaline 5 mg 3 times a day	Tolerance	11 healthy men	29
Day 1	−0.7		
Day 13	No change		
Pirbuterol		23 patients in heart failure	30
10 mg	−0.26		
20 mg	−0.41		
10 mg	−0.58		
20 mg 3 times a day (3/12 patients)	No change		

The concept of the selectivity of a $beta_2$ agonist is often cited as a marker of its safety, a drug more "selective" for bronchial $beta_2$ receptors being preferable. A recent study in our unit[226] of seven asthmatic subjects showed a significant correlation between plasma potassium changes and changes in peak expiratory flow rate (PEFR) during infusion of terbutaline (10 μg/kg/min), thus making it unlikely that bronchodilator and hypokalemic actions of $beta_2$ agonists could be separated (Figure 1). Also notable from the tables is how many of the studies were performed on healthy volunteers who may behave differently from asthmatic subjects in their potassium responses to $beta_2$ agonists.

3. Exacerbating Factors

The $beta_2$ agonist-induced decrease in serum potassium can be influenced by other factors. Asthmatics and those with chronic airflow limitation are often treated with other drugs that may also affect serum potassium or the response to hypokalemia. The most important of these are corticosteroids, theophyllines, diuretics, and digoxin.

The effect of oral theophylline on serum potassium during IV $beta_2$ agonist infusion in healthy volunteers is well documented.[99,100] In the first study, the decrease in potassium during terbutaline infusion changed from 0.73 m*M* to 0.93 m*M* with the addition of theophylline ($p < 0.05$). In the second study, the addition of oral slow release theophylline to a salbutamol infusion (8 μg/kg/h) in healthy volunteers increased the decrease in plasma K^+ from 1 m*M* to 1.3 m*M* and resulted in significant hypokalemia (K^+ 2.6 m*M*).[100] Theophyllines also increase adrenaline-induced hypokalemia.[101]

Many patients using $beta_2$ agonists for chronic airflow obstruction may be taking diuretics for cor pulmonale or hypertension. These may cause hypokalemia[102] and when combined with $beta_2$ agonists cause greater hypokalemia and predispose patients to cardiac arrhythmias.[103] Prior treatment with 7 days bendrofluazide 5 mg increased adrenaline-induced hypokalemia in six healthy volunteers (K^+ 2.73 m*M* versus 3.08 m*M*).[104] In 12 healthy volunteers combined treatment with bendrofluazide and inhaled salbutamol led to a lower plasma potassium (2.91 m*M*) than with salbutamol alone (3.38 m*M*) and additional therapy with oral potassium supplements, magnesium, or triamterene did not prevent this,[105] although in another study spironolactone 100 mg did.[106] These potassium changes were all associated with electrocardiographic (ECG) changes (increased QTc, T wave flattening), but no arrhythmias were demonstrated. These studies were performed on healthy volunteers, and once again care must be exercised in applying the results to asthmatics. However, greater vigilance is certainly required when patients are on therapy with $beta_2$ agonists and thiazide diuretics.

Potassium and digoxin compete for the same binding site on Na^+/K^+-ATPase in cell membranes so any drug, such as $beta_2$ agonists, causing a

TABLE 6
Effect of Inhaled Beta Receptor Agonists on Potassium

Medication	Max K^+ (m*M*)	Comments	Ref.
Salbutamol 200 μg × 4 in 1 h	Prevented rise in K^+	15 patients (familial hyperkalemic paralysis)	87
Salbutamol 200 μg	No change	Nonasthmatics	16
Nebulized salbutamol		Normal subjects	15
5 mg	−0.36		
Fenoterol		16 healthy volunteers	88
1200 μg	−0.5 (90 min)		
1800 μg	−0.5 (90 min)		
2400 μg	−0.9		
Ten doses salbutamol to 1 mg		8 asthmatics	24
Without mouth rinsing	−0.2		
With mouth rinsing	−0.2		
Fenoterol		6 healthy volunteers (more effect heart rate also)	89
1200 μg	−0.8		
1800 μg	−1.0		
2400 μg	−1.2		
Salbutamol			
1200 μg	−0.4		
1800 μg	−0.55		
2400 μg	−0.7		
Salbutamol		14 asthmatics	90
100 μg	+0.07		
200 μg	+0.05		
500 μg	−0.05		
1000 μg	−0.13		
2000 μg	−0.23		
4000 μg	−0.36		
Fenoterol		8 healthy volunteers	91
5 mg	−0.78		
Salbutamol			
5 mg	−0.33		
Terbutaline			
5 mg	−0.7		
Fenoterol 1800 μg	−0.7	6 asthmatics (took 7 h to return to predose levels)	92
Salbutamol		7 healthy volunteers	17
100 μg			
200 μg			
MDI	−0.5		
Spacer	−0.6		
Salbutamol		8 healthy volunteers	93
400 μg	0		
600 μg	−0.3		
800 μg	−0.4		

TABLE 6 (continued)
Effect of Inhaled Beta Receptor Agonists on Potassium

Medication	Max K^+ (m*M*)	Comments	Ref.
Fenoterol			
400 μg	0		
600 μg	−0.45		
800 μg	−0.8		
Isoprenaline			
400 μg	0		
600 μg	+0.25		
800 μg	+0.1		
Salbutamol		20 asthmatics	94
5 mg			
Terbutaline			
5 mg			
Acute	−0.30		
Convalescent	−0.16		
Salbutamol		7 elderly volunteers (similar to young group)	95
400 μg	−0.82		
Fenoterol		10 asthmatics (effect on FEV similar for all 3)	96
400 μg	0		
1200 μg	−0.4		
360 μg	−0.8		
Salbutamol			
200 μg	+0.1		
600 μg	0		
1800 μg	−0.4		
Terbutaline			
500 μg	0		
1500 μg	−0.2		
4500 μg	−0.45		

decrease in serum potassium could theoretically precipitate digoxin toxicity,[107] although this has not been studied clinically. Other medications commonly used by asthmatic patients in conjunction with $beta_2$ agonists are corticosteroids, which can exacerbate hypokalemia by their mineralocorticoid effect. However, there is a dearth of reports describing the effects of these drugs on plasma potassium in acute asthma.

Clearly other factors can influence the impact of $beta_2$ agonist-induced hypokalemia. Patients with preexisting ischemic heart disease are at greater risk of developing serious ventricular arrhythmias when their potassium is low. Patients with preexisting hypokalemia from whatever cause will be at a greater risk during therapy, which lowers potassium further. Sports enthusiasts are also said to be at greater risk[72] possibly related to endogenous catecholamine release and adrenaline-induced hypokalemia. All these groups of people would need closer monitoring while taking $beta_2$ agonist therapy acutely. On chronic use, tolerance should reduce the size of the problem.[28,97]

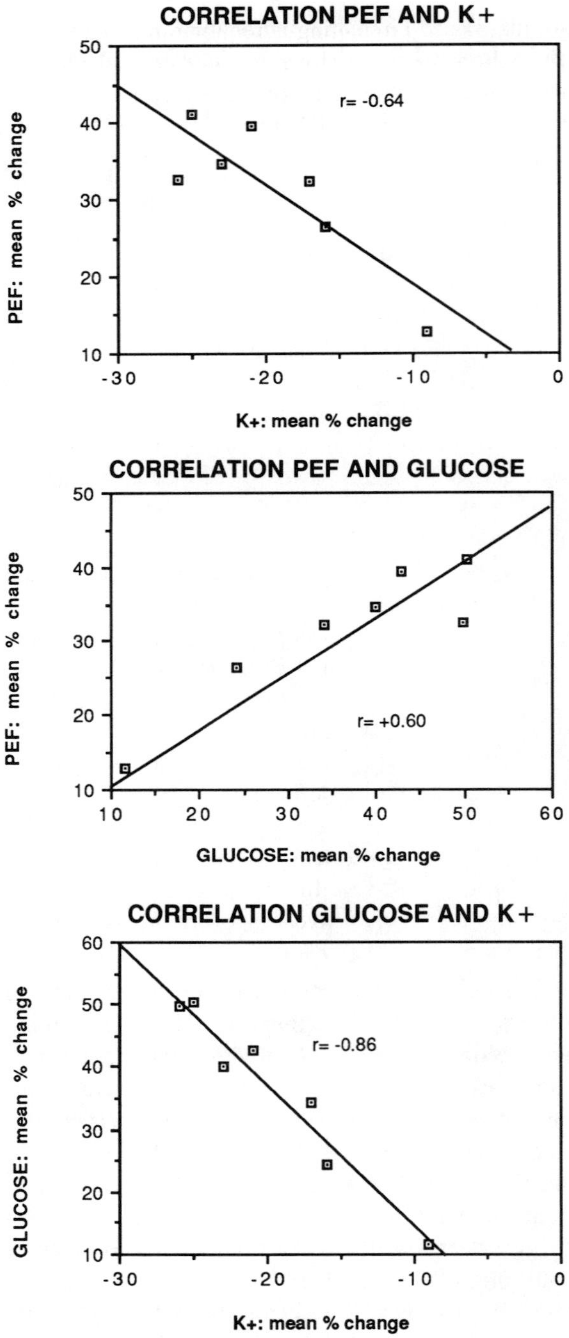

FIGURE 1. Correlations of PEFR, K^+, and glucose in seven asthmatic subjects given intravenous terbutaline.

Some claim that raised circulating adrenaline in acute severe asthma can lower serum potassium further.[88] However, infusion of adrenaline and noradrenaline into asthmatic subjects to produce physiological catecholamine concentrations only caused a decline in plasma potassium at the highest adrenaline concentration.[108] Increases in noradrenaline had no effect on potassium.

4. Clinical Relevance and Arrhythmias

The effect of a decrease in extracellular potassium concentration on the function of myocardial cells has been discussed by Hoffman et al.[109] There is an increase in the rate of their diastolic depolarization, thus increasing cardiac automaticity: the His-Purkinje cells are more sensitive to this effect than sinoatrial automatic cells so there is a shift in pacemaker site. The change in the shape of phase 4 depolarization occurs because potassium moves out across the resting membrane far less easily. Hypokalemia slows conduction velocity in the atrioventricular (AV) node in addition to increasing spontaneous ectopic activity in pacemaker cells.[110]

Certain patients with hypokalemia develop cardiac arrhythmias and some patients suffering arrhythmias have an increased risk of sudden death. However, it has not been shown that brief episodes of hypokalemia cause sudden death.[111] The link between hypokalemia and cardiac arrhythmias remains a matter of great concern in relation to $beta_2$ agonist therapy. Fisch first described a relationship between electrolyte disturbances and cardiac arrhythmias in 1933.[112] Subsequently, great concern developed about the hazards of hypokalemia associated with diuretic therapy.[103] Serum potassium decreases in proportion to the dose of diuretic and correlates with the number of ventricular premature beats.[103] Hypokalemia is particularly dangerous in the context of acute myocardial infarction. In one study of 1035 patients, the risk of ventricular fibrillation (VF) or tachycardias (VT) was greater if serum potassium were less than 3.5 m*M* (29% if $K^+ < 3.5$, 17% if $K^+ > 3.5$).[113] In another study of 151 patients with acute myocardial infarction, 37 (24.5%) had VT or VF: the risk was 67% if potassium were less than 3.1 m*M*, 40% if 3.1 to 3.8 m*M*, and 20% if there were normokalemia.[111] In Thomas' study,[114] the threshold value for potassium was higher: of 809 patients with acute myocardial infarction, 14 of 383 with potassium less than 4 m*M* had VF compared with 3 of 426 of those with potassium more than 4 m*M* (difference $p < 0.04$). Thus, it appears that the lower the serum potassium, the greater the risk of malignant arrhythmias.[115]

Arrhythmias predispose patients with impaired cardiac function or who have had a myocardial infarction to sudden death,[116,117] and treatment with beta blockers reduces this risk.[118,119] However, ventricular ectopic activity in otherwise fit young individuals has not been shown to have a bad prognosis.[120] Thus, in deciding the clinical relevance of hypokalemia induced by $beta_2$ agonists, it is necessary to establish if a person with acute severe asthma (often hypoxic, psychologically stressed, and sometimes acidotic) more closely resembles a patient with heart disease or a healthy individual. Despite all the studies demonstrating the dangers of hypokalemia and its link with $beta_2$ agonist therapy, it is difficult to directly establish that hypokalemia causes sudden death in asthma.[121,122]

E. MAGNESIUM

Magnesium is the next most abundant intracellular cation after potassium, but it is present in plasma in low concentrations,[123] which makes study of extracellular levels difficult to interpret. Magnesium acts as a co-factor to a number of enzymes and is important in activation of membrane-bound Na^+/K^+-ATPase.[123,124] Hypomagnesemia occurs in response to high catecholamine levels, for example, after myocardial infarction,[125] and during treatment with diuretics in conjunction with potassium depletion.[126] In the latter context, treatment with both magnesium and potassium is needed to restore intracellular potassium.[127] Both potassium and magnesium depletion are clinically important in the generation of ventricular arrhythmias,[128] and once again it seems that magnesium supplementation is required to prevent arrhythmias in diuretic-treated patients.[129,130]

Evidence that $beta_2$ agonists acutely affect serum magnesium was provided by Bremme et al.[124] in women receiving terbutaline infusion (20 μg/min for 30 min) for premature labor. Serum magnesium decreased significantly after 120 min and remained low. The time course for the decrease in serum potassium was much shorter (30 min). The change in magnesium was significantly inversely correlated with changes in FFAs, and previous reports of a link between magnesium and lipolysis were reviewed by Bremme et al.[124] IV salbutamol was also found to lower serum magnesium[123] in eight healthy volunteers: the decline was again slow but sustained after cessation of the infusion. Serum magnesium was not significantly affected by inhaled salbutamol, however.[17,105] The mechanism of this $beta_2$ agonist-stimulated change in serum magnesium has not been clearly elucidated. Magnesium ions do not pass easily through water-filled membrane channels due to their large hydrated size,[123] but there is evidence for membrane-binding sites of moderate affinity.[129] Thus, cellular uptake of magnesium would be one possibility with increased binding to intracellular FFAs.[130] Insulin-stimulated magnesium uptake is not likely.[123] Present evidence, however, favors $beta_2$ agonist-enhanced urinary loss of magnesium: in six healthy volunteers magnesium excretion increased during terbutaline infusion.[130] The clinical relevance of these findings is that $beta_2$ agonist-induced magnesium depletion may provoke cardiac arrhythmias and could also adversely affect asthmatic patients with coronary artery disease.[131]

F. LACTIC ACIDOSIS

Increased lactate production has been described in association with $beta_2$ agonist therapy, although the muscular exertion of premature labor or acute asthma makes it difficult to assess the role of drugs in this situation. Twenty

TABLE 7
Cardiovascular Effects of Beta$_2$ Receptor Agonists

Tachycardia related to
Nature of drug
Mode of administration
Characteristics of subject
Hemodynamic effects including
Inotropy
Systemic vasodilation
Redistribution of pulmonary blood flow
Myocardial necrosis
Myocardial ischemia
ECG changes
Arrhythmias

women treated with ritodrine infusion (0.1 to 0.35 mg/min) for premature labor[132] were found to have a mean increase of lactate from 1 to 3.5 m*M* after 6 h without change in blood *p*H. Similar findings were observed with terbutaline.[133] Lactic acidosis was suspected and confirmed in 12 patients with acute severe asthma whose *p*H was less than the value expected from their arterial p_{CO_2}. This was found to be an adverse prognostic feature; eight subsequently developed respiratory failure. Treatment with SC adrenaline has been associated with the development of lactic acidosis, although respiratory muscle overproduction of lactate[134] seemed more likely. In two case reports of lactic acidosis associated with beta$_2$ agonist therapy,[135,136] the cause was thought to be beta$_2$ stimulation of muscle glycogenolysis. Lactic acidosis has a negatively inotropic effect on the heart, but the clinical relevance of the aforementioned levels is uncertain.

III. CARDIOVASCULAR EFFECTS

The high mortality rate noted among asthmatics in the 1960s was associated with excessive use of pressurized aerosols containing the nonselective beta agonist, isoprenaline.[137] It was initially attributed to the cardiac effects, tachycardia, and arrhythmias. Despite the development of specific beta$_2$ agonists, there is still concern that their repeated use at high dosages may cause the continuing high asthma death rate.[138] The adverse cardiac effects of beta$_2$ agonists are summarized in Table 7. Before discussing these, the evidence for the existence of myocardial beta$_2$ receptors will be considered.

A. MYOCARDIAL BETA$_2$ RECEPTORS

In their classification of adrenoceptors, Lands et al.[5] differentiated beta$_1$ receptors, which showed an equal affinity for noradrenaline and adrenaline, and were found in the heart and adipose tissue, from beta$_2$ receptors, which showed greater affinity for adrenaline and were found in skeletal and smooth muscle and the liver.[139] As specific agonist and antagonist drugs were developed, and radioligand-binding studies performed, it became evident that $beta_1$ and $beta_2$ adrenoceptors coexist in human myocardium.[140] The proportion of $beta_2$ adrenoceptors in human ventricular myocardium ranges from 14% to 40% and in atrial tissue from 20% to 55%.[139,141,142] It is suggested that resting heart rate is more influenced by noradrenaline (20 $\times$ higher affinity for $beta_1$ than $beta_2$ receptors[143]) through $beta_1$ receptors. Under conditions of stress or exercise, adrenaline, which has equal affinity for $beta_1$ and $beta_2$ myocardial receptors, is released from the adrenal medulla and cardiac $beta_2$ receptors are involved in regulating heart rate[140] and contractility.[143,144] Studies of isolated human atrial and ventricular muscle have shown that stimulation of one $beta_2$ adrenoceptor leads to production of up to ten times more cyclic adenosine monophosphate (cAMP) molecules than stimulation of a $beta_1$ adrenoceptor,[143,145] indicating the greater sensitivity and perhaps functional significance of $beta_2$ receptors in the heart.

B. TACHYCARDIA

Tachycardia is the most common side effect of $beta_2$ agonist therapy, particularly when given systemically. This could arise from (1) activation of cardiac $beta_1$ receptors (suggesting the agonist is not $beta_2$-selective in cardiac muscle); (2) reflex increase in cardiac sympathetic tone from the decrease in diastolic blood pressure that occurs with peripheral vasodilation ($beta_2$ effect); (3) stimulation of cardiac presynaptic $beta_2$ receptors (leading to noradrenaline release); (4) direct stimulation of cardiac $beta_2$ receptors; (5) withdrawal of parasympathetic tone secondary to the decrease in diastolic blood pressure already mentioned;[146] and (6) central adrenergic beta receptor stimulation.[147]

Evidence that tachycardia results from direct stimulation of cardiac $beta_2$ receptors was provided by Hall et al.,[148] who infused salbutamol into the right coronary artery of subjects undergoing cardiac catheterization. This resulted in sinus tachycardia, whereas the same dose of salbutamol injected into the aortic root had no effect on heart rate. Practolol (a $beta_1$ blocker) did not prevent the action of salbutamol, but propranolol (a combined $beta_1$ and $beta_2$ blocker) did. This confirms the observations of Strauss et al.[146] who showed that the increase in heart rate induced in healthy volunteers by terbutaline infusion was not modified by atenolol (a specific $beta_1$ blocker). Further, in seven healthy volunteers salbutamol infusion produced a tachycardia, but the $beta_1$-selective agonist, prenalterol, had a predominantly inotropic effect.[149] The degree of tachycardia produced by $beta_2$ agonist treatment is clearly dependent on a number of factors, including the particular drug used, route of administration, and dose.

1. Drug

Many studies have compared the cardiovascular effects of different $beta_2$ agents to try and elucidate if any are more bronchoselective. Amory et al.[150]

used SC adrenaline and terbutaline in 23 patients with reversible airways obstruction and showed that terbutaline produced greater increases in forced vital capacity, FEV_1, other respiratory parameters, and heart rate. The drugs had comparable effects on systolic and diastolic blood pressure. Oral terbutaline has less effect on heart rate.[151] However, it seems that fenoterol is a more potent cardiac chronotropic stimulant.[98,152,153] A comparison of nebulized selective $beta_2$ agonists, salbutamol, fenoterol, and terbutaline, and saline in 12 healthy volunteers showed that fenoterol produced the most marked heart rate response.[152] However, this study was in healthy volunteers; so it is difficult to ensure that comparable bronchodilating doses were given. Fenoterol also had the greatest effect on the heart rate of 12 asthmatics in whom fenoterol, salbutamol, isoproterenol, and ipratropium bromide were compared. There was no difference between the bronchodilator effects of these drugs,[98] but fenoterol caused the greatest decrease in serum potassium, as discussed in the preceding section. Some $beta_2$ agonists, e.g., clenbuterol,[154] do not produce a tachycardia, but it is also questionable whether adequate doses of the drugs are being used for comparison. Fenoterol's greater effect may be due to better absorption.[155]

2. Mode of Administration

The mode of administration can affect the heart rate response. Both SC and nebulized $beta_2$ agonists produce tachycardia,[150,152] and oral salbutamol, used in the treatment of heart failure,[156,157] caused up to 30% increase in heart rate 2 h after dosing. $Beta_2$ agonists administered by metered dose inhaler (MDI) for asthma do not consistently raise heart rate: increasing doses of inhaled fenoterol stimulated heart rate, but salbutamol did not.[158] Equivalent bronchodilatation was achieved, suggesting that differences could not be attributed to inhalation technique. Using a pear-shaped spacer attachment reduces oropharyngeal deposition of $beta_2$ agonist drug and might therefore lessen systemic side effects including tachycardia. However, a comparison of MDI and pear-shaped spacer attachment[159] in seven healthy volunteers given four doses of salbutamol showed no difference in the degree of tachycardia induced. Mouth rinsing after inhalation of salbutamol with a standard MDI removed 24% of the total dose delivered, but the magnitude and the time course of the tachycardia induced were not affected.[24]

3. Characteristics of the Subject

Healthy subjects and asthmatics may behave differently. This could be due to differences in $beta_2$ receptor sensitivities or because a decrease in heart rate[160] in acute severe asthmatics is a response to the relief of bronchospasm.[161] The age of the patient may affect heart rate response. Kendall et al.[162] showed that IV terbutaline caused less tachycardia in a group of elderly healthy women than in young ones (28/min versus 23/min), whereas bronchial and metabolic effects were equivalent. However, in another study healthy young and elderly people showed a comparable heart rate response to increasing doses of inhaled salbutamol.[95] It may be that $beta_1$ adrenoceptor activity declines with age but $beta_2$ adrenoceptor activity remains intact.[95] Finally, other drugs, for instance, theophyllines,[161] can also alter the heart rate response to $beta_2$ agonist therapy.

The tachycardia induced by $beta_2$ agonists is important for asthmatic subjects who also suffer from coronary artery disease. There have been reports of nebulized salbutamol[163,164] causing angina and IV salbutamol causing myocardial infarction.[165] It is therefore recommended that lower doses of nebulized salbutamol (for example, 1 to 2.5 mg) should be used for those with coronary artery disease.

C. OTHER HEMODYNAMIC EFFECTS INCLUDING INOTROPY

The effect of $beta_2$ agonists on myocardial function must be considered as part of any discussion of the impact of these drugs on asthma mortality. Echocardiographic assessment in seven healthy volunteers after IV terbutaline showed an increase in cardiac index and left ventricular emptying, which were blunted by pretreatment with atenolol, suggesting that activation of cardiac $beta_1$ receptors contributed to this response.[147] However, a study of left ventricular tissue from patients undergoing mitral valve surgery showed that $beta_2$ receptors can mediate 50% of the maximal increase in contractile force induced by low concentration adrenaline and high concentration noradrenaline.[166]

Studies in patients have tended to focus on those with chronic airways limitation and impaired right ventricular (RV) function. In one such study, SC terbutaline was found to have a beneficial effect on cardiac performance increasing RV and left ventricular (LV) ejection fractions.[167] However, an increase in RV ejection fraction could adversely affect PaO_2 by redistributing pulmonary blood flow.[168] When intramuscular terbutaline was administered to patients after open heart surgery, a highly significant decrease in PaO_2 occurred, as well as an increase in cardiac output and $PaCO_2$. Increased pulmonary blood flow leading to preferential perfusion of nonventilated lung occurred.[169] This could be relevant to the initiation of therapy in acute asthma.

Pulmonary edema has also been associated with the use of terbutaline and isoxuprine in a 31-year-old woman in preterm labor[170] and with the use of salbutamol in a 28-year-old woman.[171] Even inhalation of $beta_2$ agonists by MDI causes significant hemodynamic effects, which may not be evident from simple measurement of heart rate and blood pressure.[172] The clinical relevance of these changes is less well documented, but severe hypotension has been described in two patients with quadriplegia treated with SC terbutaline for asthma.[173]

The inotropic effect of $beta_2$ agonists has been investigated in a number of studies using systolic time intervals (QS_2), the interval from the onset of the Q wave to the start of aortic valve closure. Comparison of inhaled salbutamol, fenoterol, and isoprenaline[93] showed a maximal effect 5 min after each dose, but the impact of fenoterol lasted longer. Fenoterol also increased systolic pressure significantly more than the other two drugs. Comparison of nebulized fenoterol with salbutamol and terbutaline[152] revealed that once again fenoterol decreased QS_2 and raised systolic pressure the most. These results suggest that fenoterol is less beta$_2$-selective, better absorbed, or marketed at a higher equivalent dose, and that this may make it more dangerous in a hypoxic patient.[153]

D. MYOCARDIAL NECROSIS AND ISCHEMIA

A direct toxic effect of beta$_2$ agonists on myocardium has been described. In addition, an indirect effect of beta$_2$ agonists on myocardium by increasing lipolysis and FFAs has been discussed in the preceding section. In the 1960s isoprenaline inhalers were thought to be contributing to increasing asthma mortality; so studies of the action of isoprenaline on cardiac muscle were performed. This beta agonist had an inotropic effect on cardiac muscle in micrograms per kilogram doses but caused myocardial necrosis in milligrams per kilogram doses. The studies of Collins et al.[174] showed that IV isoprenaline produced tachycardia in dogs breathing room air but bradycardia and depression of cardiac contractility in hypoxic dogs. As discussed in Chapter 7, this did not follow the development of arrhythmia or peripheral circulatory failure but was a direct drug effect. Histological examination in another animal study revealed nonhomogenous confluent necrosis and disseminated focal necrosis in papillary muscles and subendocardium.[175] No acute coronary occlusion was demonstrated: the cardiostimulatory effects of isoprenaline could increase myocardial oxygen consumption and cause relative ischemia of the myocardial cells. Another possible mechanism was demonstrated by Haft et al.[176] studying adrenaline-induced cardiac necrosis in dogs: platelet aggregation in capillaries. Another suggestion is that myocardial necrosis is due to flooding of myocardial cells with calcium, but in a study in rats,[177] propranolol administered in doses sufficient to reduce myocardial calcium did not prevent necrosis.

Whether such effects occur in humans remains debatable because histological proof is not often available. Kirkland et al.[178] described an 18-year-old girl treated with isoprenaline for status asthmaticus who had a fatal cardiac arrest on treatment. Multiple small areas of necrosis were found on post-mortem examination of her ventricular myocardium. It is difficult to conclude that this was purely a consequence of her medication. Her illness was prolonged and acute severe asthma of some days duration could adversely affect cardiac muscle. Myocardial necrosis and necrotizing coronary arteritis have been described in untreated asthma.[179]

Myocardial ischemia has been described in asthmatics treated with beta$_2$ agonists. A 14-year-old asthmatic boy given isoprenaline infusion[180] experienced chest pain and ECG evidence of myocardial ischemia with an associated pulse irregularity. The effect of isoprenaline on coronary artery caliber was studied in 13 people, nine of whom had angiographically proven coronary artery disease.[181] In this group, impaired myocardial oxygenation occurred, suggesting a mismatch between isoprenaline augmented coronary flow and local myocardial oxygen requirements. However, a study of IV terbutaline in patients with severe heart failure due to coronary artery disease did not show any evidence of reduced myocardial oxygen or lactate extraction at doses high enough to increase cardiac index. No angina or ECG evidence of ischemia occurred.[182] One conclusion to draw from these contrasting studies is that caution is required when using IV or high-dose oral or nebulized $beta_2$ agonist therapy in those with known coronary artery disease.

E. ELECTROCARDIOGRAPHIC CHANGES AND ARRHYTHMIAS

It has been suggested that $beta_2$ agonist-induced cardiac arrhythmias may be responsible for increasing asthma mortality.[183,184] This has already been mentioned in the section on hypokalemia because these two adverse effects of $beta_2$ agonist treatment may be linked.[112] As an introduction to this section, the impact of both acute asthma and $beta_2$ agonist treatment on the ECG will be considered.

1. ECG Changes and Acute Asthma

Hassan et al.[185] studied ECG changes in 70 patients with acute severe asthma and demonstrated inferior lead T wave abnormalities in 34%. The mean age was 29.3 years, making serious coexisting coronary artery disease unlikely. The abnormalities were related to asthma severity as measured by heart rate, decrease in peak expiratory flow rate, arterial oxygen pressure, and pulsus paradoxus. The changes took from 2 to 6 days to resolve depending on the ECG lead involved.

2. ECG Changes with $Beta_2$ Receptor Agonists

The effects of different $beta_2$ agonists, administered by various routes, on the ECGs of healthy volunteers have been described.[93,98,152,159,186] These show that fenoterol has the most marked effect. For example, increasing inhaled doses of fenoterol, isoprenaline, and salbutamol were compared in eight healthy men.[93] Fenoterol significantly prolonged the QTc interval early (15 min) after dosing, salbutamol and isoprenaline later (30 and 45 min). The magnitude of the changes induced by fenoterol was also greater (approximately 2 × salbutamol, 3 × isoprenaline). This was matched by a decrease in plasma potassium concentration, fenoterol again causing the greatest changes from baseline values. A similar study performed in stable asthmatic subjects[98] showed that only fenoterol caused a significant increase in QTc interval at 75 min after dosing; again, fenoterol produced the greatest decrease in plasma potassium. Comparison of inhaled salbutamol, fenoterol, and terbutaline in ten stable asthmatic patients[96] showed that all these agents produced a dose-dependent increase in QTc interval (QTc fenoterol 78 ms, salbutamol 35 ms, terbutaline 41 ms). The same order was demonstrated once again for the effect of these drugs on plasma potassium, suggesting that the latter has an etiological role in the ECG changes.

$Beta_2$ agonist stimulation also affects T wave height and can cause ST segment depression, as was shown in a study comparing administration of salbutamol to eight healthy subjects by an MDI and pear-shaped spacer device. There was no significant difference between the two devices and the ECG effects could once again be related to changes in plasma K^+ or maybe magnesium.[187,188] These effects are independent of mode of administration, occurring with nebulized[152] and SC routes.[186] In the latter study plasma K^+ and QTc interval were significantly correlated. Other medications, which affect plasma potassium, accentuate these ECG changes. Addition of bendrofluazide caused more T wave flattening, QTc lengthening, ST segment depression, and U waves and lower plasma potassium than salbutamol alone.[105] These changes were not attenuated by replacement therapy with potassium, magnesium, or potassium-sparing agents except higher doses of triamterene (200 mg) and spironolactone (100 mg). Again, a significant correlation between plasma K^+ and QTc responses was found. Prolongation of the QT interval is associated with ventricular tachyarrhythmias and sudden death;[189] so these ECG changes are relevant to the discussion of $beta_2$ agonists and asthma mortality.

3. Arrhythmias

$Beta_2$ agonist treatment can affect the ECG in both normal and asthmatic subjects, but the evidence that such therapy actually causes arrhythmias is much less convincing. Patients who have taken large overdoses of $beta_2$ agonists[122,190] rarely have cardiac arrhythmias; an overdose of SC terbutaline caused profound ST depression on ECG only.[191] This is true irrespective of the route by which the beta agonist is administered.[16,192,193]

The role of other therapeutic agents, especially theophyllines, in potentiating arrhythmias on $beta_2$ agonist treatment, has been examined. These drugs have been suggested as a cause for the recent increase in asthma mortality in New Zealand.[193] Four studies[194-197] demonstrated a greater incidence of ventricular and supraventricular premature beats (VPBs and SVPBs) in patients taking theophyllines; the other[198] showed that VPBs did not disappear on withdrawal of theophylline therapy. No serious arrhythmias occurred. Isoprenaline aerosol given to patients with chronic airways obstruction and known to have VPBs did not exacerbate their rhythm disturbances,[199] but addition of aminophylline 250 mg did.

The frequency of arrhythmias in untreated patients suffering from acute severe asthma (who are hypoxic and have high endogenous catecholamine secretion) is not well documented and needs to be known before attributing arrhythmias to therapy. In one study[200] sinus tachycardia predominated in 20 patients who underwent 24-h Holter monitoring during an acute asthma attack. In another study ten asthmatic patients who presented to hospital in incipient or actual respiratory arrest, the near-fatal nature of their asthma was the result of severe asphyxia rather than of cardiac arrhythmias (eight sinus tachycardia, one atrial fibrillation, one sinus bradycardia).[201]

The clinical state of the patients studied, their age, and the likelihood of coexisting ischemic heart disease all affect the potential to develop cardiac arrhythmias. Higgins et al.[202] described arrhythmias (ventricular tachycardia, atrial fibrillation, bigemini) occurring in six of 19 fairly elderly patients with chronic airflow obstruction given air-driven nebulized $beta_2$ agonists. Blood gas results were not significantly different between those who developed arrhythmias and those who did not, suggesting that hypoxia was not an important precipitant. Preexisting coronary artery disease seems to be more important. Serious or life-threatening arrhythmias occurred in 13 of 20 patients with chronic airflow limitation given nebulized salbutamol or terbutaline (air-driven), five of whom had suffered previous myocardial infarcts.[94] Ventricular ectopics (80% versus 40%), couplets, and tachycardia (194 episodes versus 3) were more common in these patients. However, there was no significant increase in serious arrhythmias during the 1-h periods immediately following nebulized therapy, nor was the hourly frequency of arrhythmias related to plasma potassium level.

Arrhythmias have been described on oral $beta_2$ agonist therapy using salbutamol and terbutaline.[203] Banner et al.[204] compared several oral agents in older patients with known VPBs on pretreatment monitoring. Terbutaline 5 mg daily caused VT in three patients and an increase in VPBs. No significant increase in ventricular ectopic activity occurred in six asthmatics studied following inhalation of fenoterol (at three times the recommended dose). This was true despite a significant decrease in plasma potassium.[92]

Thus, it is clear that cardiac arrhythmias do occur on $beta_2$ agonist therapy, but their clinical relevance is disputed. There seems to be increased risk in patients who are hypoxic, have coexisting coronary artery disease, and are also taking theophyllines. Fenoterol causes ECG changes more readily than other inhaled $beta_2$ agonists but has not been shown, as yet, to produce more arrhythmias. It is impossible on present evidence to extrapolate between ventricular arrhythmias and the trend in mortality in asthma.

IV. OTHER EFFECTS

In this last section a few acute unwanted effects of $beta_2$ agonists that cannot be classified as metabolic or cardiovascular will be considered. They are less likely to have an impact on mortality but can be the cause of considerable morbidity.

A. MUSCLE TREMOR

Skeletal muscle tremor is a common acute adverse effect of $beta_2$ agonist therapy for asthma, particularly when it is administered by the oral or nebulized route[192] and may be the dose-limiting factor.[161,192] Normal muscular activity is accompanied by tremor[205] and stimulation of $beta_2$ adrenoceptors increases the amplitude. $Beta_2$ receptor stimulation has different effects on slow and fast contracting muscle fibers.[206] It reduces tension and duration of maximal twitches in the former and increases these parameters in the latter. Slow contracting muscles are much more sensitive to $beta_2$ stimulation. Insulin has a similar effect but acts at a site beyond the $beta_2$ receptor.[207]

In addition to this postural tremor, body vibrations occur with skeletal muscles relaxed, chiefly as a result of cardiac pulsation (10% of finger tremor amplitude) but with a small contribution from respiratory movement. $Beta_2$ agonists would also be expected to increase this type of tremor by their chronotropic and inotropic effects and their stimulatory action on ventilation. Tremor response to IV $beta_2$ agonist increases with dose and is related to underlying basal tremor by a constant ratio,[208] so that patients with the greatest basal tremor develop the most vigorous response to $beta_2$ agonist treatment.

Different $beta_2$ agonists may have different affinities for various organ $beta_2$ receptors, for instance, muscle, heart, bronchi, and so cause less tremor. Thiringer et al.[205] studied skeletal muscle tremor in 15 healthy subjects and 13 asthmatics in response to three different dose infusions of isoprenaline and terbutaline. Graphs of tremor against heart rate were different and suggested that terbutaline had greater selectivity for $beta_2$ receptors on muscle. Larsson[209] described a $beta_2$ agonist, irbuterol, which was the di-isobutyric ester of terbutaline, and could only be activated by tissue-bound esterases. It seemed to have far less effect on tremor, blood pressure, and heart rate than terbutaline for equivalent bronchodilation. Thus, development of $beta_2$ agonists less selective for skeletal muscle could be possible.

Another study comparing terbutaline and orciprenaline[208] showed that terbutaline gave the greater bronchodilatation but also the larger subjective sensation of tremor. However, comparison of oral terbutaline with salbutamol in 34 male subjects with chronic obstructive pulmonary disease showed that bronchodilatation (as assessed by change in FEV_1) did not correlate with finger tremor response, and it was suggested that the two functions were mediated by different $beta_2$ receptor subtypes.[210] In addition, increase in tremor after SC terbutaline was significantly less in asthmatics than in healthy volunteers,[211] suggesting reduced sensitivity of $beta_2$ receptors in skeletal muscle of asthmatics. Tolerance to the tremor effect of $beta_2$ agonists develops swiftly, usually within the first 2 weeks of therapy,[212] without concomitant tolerance to bronchodilatory effects, or change in kinetics of the agonist.[213]

Among the various $beta_2$ agonists, oral terbutaline produced more tremor than oral salbutamol[214] and oral fenoterol[215]; so it may be that tremor could be alleviated by substituting one $beta_2$ agonist for another.[161] Oral theophyllines increase the likelihood but not the intensity of tremor on starting oral terbutaline therapy.[195,196] In clinical practice tremor is only a significant cause of morbidity on initiating $beta_2$ agonist therapy. Inhaled therapy rarely leads to troublesome tremor. It is likely to be more of a problem for patients with a prominent tremor prior to treatment. It will also affect the lives of elderly patients whose manual dexterity may already be adversely affected by joint problems or neurological disease.

B. MUSCLE SPASMS

A case report[216] in 1989 described intercostal muscle spasms in a 25-year-old asthmatic woman who was taking oral salbutamol. Her creatine phosphokinase (CPK) was raised and her symptoms and CPK settled on reduction of salbutamol dose. Another study[217] of 93 patients with chronic obstructive pulmonary disease treated with oral salbutamol or pirbuterol showed an increase in CPK in 20%. In practice this could confound the diagnosis of myocardial infarction in asthmatics who present with chest pain.

C. CENTRAL NERVOUS SYSTEM EFFECTS

Troublesome, but not severe, side effects caused by $beta_2$ agonist stimulation of the central nervous system have been described. A comparison of oral terbutaline and fenoterol in 33 asthmatics revealed that nervousness, insomnia, paresthesia, and instability occurred in 11 patients treated with terbutaline and six treated with fenoterol.[215] However, more serious acute adverse central nervous system effects of $beta_2$ agonists have been described. Two pregnant women with a past history of migraine developed focal cerebral ischemia while being treated with SC terbutaline.[218] Caution was advocated in administering $beta_2$ agonists to patients with migraine or vascular headache. Seizures were described in a 7.5-year-old girl treated with terbutaline[219] and in a 15-year-old abusing his salbutamol inhaler.[220] Psychosis has also resulted from $beta_2$ agonist therapy.[221] Formal electroencephalographic study of the neurophysiological effects of asthma therapy has only been performed for theophyllines to date.[222]

D. PARADOXICAL BRONCHOCONSTRICTION

Although $beta_2$ agonists normally cause bronchodilatation, there have been occasional reports of acute bronchoconstriction following oral, IV, or inhaled administration of these agents.[223,224] These are rare, and of the theories that have been proposed to account for this phenomenon, it has been suggested that increased inflammatory burden or induction of airway hyperreactivity are the best explanations.[225]

V. CONCLUSIONS

$Beta_2$ agonists are established treatment for asthma, both acutely and in conjunction with inhaled corticosteroids for long-term management. Many of the acute effects of these drugs described in this review are relevant to asthma morbidity and mortality. As tolerance develops quickly, the impact of these effects is greater in the context of acute severe asthma, when the doses used are also higher. Hypokalemia is an important acute unwanted effect of $beta_2$ agonist administration and its link with cardiac arrhythmias means it is also dangerous. Measurement of plasma potassium should be an essential part of the management of acute asthma. The cardiovascular effects of $beta_2$ agonists are most important for patients with preexisting coronary artery disease, and use of lower doses and adequate ECG monitoring are advisable. Hyperglycemia and stimulation of lipolysis are more a problem for diabetic patients. Because the new longer-acting $beta_2$ agonists, salmeterol and formoterol, are now being increasingly used for the treatment of asthma, there is a need to be vigilant for these unwanted effects of therapy. Further work is also needed to establish whether organ-specific $beta_2$ agonists can be developed.

REFERENCES

1. **Rawlins, M. D. and Thompson, J. W.,** Pathogenesis of adverse drug reactions, in *Textbook of Adverse Drug Reactions,* Davies, D. M., Ed., Oxford University Press, London, 1977.
2. **Dale, H. H.,** On some physiological actions of Ergot, *J. Physiol.,* 34, 163, 1906.
3. **Cannon, W. B. and Rosenblueth, A.,** *Automatic Neuroeffector Systems,* Macmillan, New York, 1937.
4. **Ahlquist, R. P.,** A study of adrenotropic receptors, *Am. J. Physiol.,* 153, 586, 1948.
5. **Lands, A. M., Arnold, A., McCauliff, J. P., Luduena, F. P., and Brown, T. G.,** Differentiation of receptor systems activated by sympathomimetic amines, *Nature,* 214, 597, 1967.
6. **Lees, G. M.,** A hitchhiker's guide to the galaxy of adrenoceptors, *Br. Med. J.,* 283, 173, 1981.
7. **Strosberg, A. E.,** Molecular and functional properties of beta adrenergic receptors, *Am. J. Cardiol.,* 59, 3F, 1987.
8. **Carlsson, E., Ablad, B., Brändström, A., and Carlsson, B.,** Differentiated blockade of the chronotropic effects of various adrenergic stimuli in the cat heart, *Life Sci.,* 11, 953, 1972.
9. **Minneman, K. P., Hedberg, A., and Mollinoff, P. B.,** Comparison of beta adrenergic receptor subtypes in mammalian tissues, *Pharmacol. Exp. Ther.,* 211, 502, 1979.
10. **Smith, S. R., Kendall, M. J., Worthington, D. J., and Holder, R.,** Can the biochemical responses to a beta 2 adrenoceptor stimulant be used to assess the selectivity of beta-adrenoceptor blockers?, *Br. J. Clin. Pharmacol.,* 16, 557, 1983.
11. **Morgan, D. J.,** Clinical pharmacokinetics of beta agonists, *Clin. Pharmacokinet.,* 18, 270, 1990.
12. **Jenne, J. W., Chick, T. W., Strickland, R. D., and Wall, F. J.,** A comparison of beta adrenergic function in asthma and chronic bronchitis, *J. Allergy Clin. Immunol.,* 60, 346, 1977.
13. **Ostman, J.,** β adrenergic blockade and diabetic mellitus: a review, *Acta Med. Scand.,* [*Suppl.*], 672, 69, 1983.
14. **Lunell, N. O., Joelsson, I., Larsson, A., and Persson, B.,** The immediate effect of a β adrenergic agonist (salbutamol) on carbohydrate and lipid metabolism during the 3rd trimester of pregnancy, *Acta Obstet. Gynaecol. Scand.,* 56, 475, 1977.
15. **Rolf Smith, S., Ryder, C., Kendall, M. J., and Holder, R.,** Cardiovascular and biochemical responses to nebulized salbutamol in normal subjects, *Br. J. Clin. Pharmacol.,* 18, 641, 1984.
16. **Neville, A., Palmer, J. B. D., Gaddie, J., May, C. S., Palmer, K. N. V., and Murchison, L. E.,** Metabolic effects of salbutamol: comparison of aerosol and intravenous administration, *Br. Med. J.,* 1, 413, 1977.

17. **Lipworth, B. J., Clark, R. A., Fraser, C. G., and McDevitt, D. G.,** The biochemical effects of high dose inhaled salbutamol in patients with asthma, *Eur. J. Clin. Pharmacol.*, 36, 357, 1989.
18. **Kendall, M. J., Dean, S., Bradley, D., Gibson, R., and Worthington, D. T.,** Cardiovascular and metabolic effects of terbutaline, *J. Clin. Hosp. Pharm.*, 7, 31, 1982.
19. **Ronn, O., Graffner, C., Johnsson, G., Jordo, L., Lundborg, P., and Wikstrand, J.,** Haemodynamic effects and pharmacokinetics of a new selective beta 1 adrenoceptor agonist, prenalterol and its interaction with metoprolol in man, *Eur. J. Clin. Pharmacol.*, 15, 9, 1979.
20. **Deacon, S. P. and Barnett, D.,** Comparison of atenolol and propranolol during insulin-induced hypoglycaemia, *Br. Med. J.*, 2, 272, 1976.
21. **Viberti, G. C., Keen, H., and Bloom, S. R.,** Beta blockade and diabetic mellitus: effect of oxprenolol and metoprolol on the metabolic and cardiovascular and hormonal response to insulin-induced hypoglycaemia in normal subjects, *Metabolism,* 29, 866, 1980.
22. **Lager, I.,** Adrenergic blockade and hypoglycaemia, *Acta Med. Scand.* [*Suppl.*], 672, 63, 1983.
23. **Phillips, P. J., Vedig, A. E., Jones, P. L., Chapman, M. G., Collins, M., Edwards, J. B., Smeaton, R., and Duncan, B.,** Metabolic and cardiovascular side effects of the beta 2 adrenoceptor agonists salbutamol and rimiterol, *Br. J. Clin. Pharmacol.*, 9, 483, 1980.
24. **Kung, M., Troley, S. W., and Phillips, B. A.,** Systemic cardiovascular and metabolic effects associated with the inhalation of an increased dose of albuterol: influence of mouth rinsing and gargling, *Chest,* 91, 382, 1987.
25. **Nogrady, S. G., Hartley, J. P. R., and Seaton, A.,** Metabolic effects of intravenous salbutamol in the course of acute severe asthma, *Thorax,* 32, 559, 1977.
26. **Bateman, S. M., Pidgeon, J., Spiro, S. G., and Johnson, A. J.,** The metabolic effects of inhaled salbutamol, *Br. J. Clin. Pharmacol.*, 5, 127, 1978.
27. **Harvey, J. E., Baldwin, C. J., Wood, P. J., Alberti, K. G., and Tattersfield, A. E.,** Airway and metabolic responsiveness to intravenous salbutamol in asthma: effect of regular inhaled salbutamol, *Clin. Sci.*, 60, 579, 1971.
28. **Wager, J., Fredholm, B., Lunell, N. O., and Persson, B.,** Development of tolerance to oral salbutamol in the 3rd trimester of pregnancy: a study of circulatory and metabolic effects, *Br. J. Clin. Pharmacol.*, 12, 489, 1981.
29. **Bengtsson, B. and Fagerstrom, P. O.,** Data pulmonary effects of terbutaline during prolonged administration, *Clin. Pharmacol. Ther.*, 31, 726, 1982.
30. **Canepa-Anson, R., Dawson, J. R., Kuan, P., Poolewilson, P. A., Sutton, G. C., Cockrill, B., and Reuben, S. R.,** Differences between peak and long term metabolic and endocrine effects of oral beta adrenoceptor agonist treatment with pirbuterol for cardiac failure, *Br. J. Clin. Pharmacol.*, 23, 173, 1987.
31. **Gundogdu, A. S., Juul, S., Brown, P. M., Sachs, L., and Sonksen, P. H.,** Comparison of hormonal and metabolic effects of salbutamol infusion in normal subjects and insulin requiring diabetics, *Lancet,* 2, 1317, 1979.
32. **Leslie, D. and Coats, P. M.,** Salbutamol induced diabetic ketoacidosis (letter), *Br. Med. J.*, 3, 768, 1977.
33. **Thomas, D. J. B., Stubbs, W. A., Gill, B., and Brown, P. B.,** Salbutamol induced diabetic ketoacidosis, *Br. Med. J.*, 3, 438, 1977.
34. **Bernstein, I. M. and Catalano, P. M.,** Ketoacidosis in pregnancy associated with the parenteral administration of terbutaline and betamethasone, *J. Reprod. Med.*, 35, 818, 1990.
35. **Ingemarsson, T., Westgren, M., Lindberg, C., Ahren, B., Lundquist, I., and Carlsson, C.,** Single injection of terbutaline in term labor: placental transfer and effects on maternal and fetal carbohydrate metabolism, *Am. J. Obstet. Gynecol.*, 139, 697, 1981.

36. **Massara, F., Fassio, V., Camanni, F., and Molinatti, G. M.,** Salbutamol induced increase in plasma insulin in man, *Horm. Metab. Res.*, 7, 94, 1975.
37. **Massi-Beneditti, M., Santeusanio, F., Filipponi, P., Nicoletti, R., et al.,** Effect of salbutamol infusion on insulin and glucagon secretion in normal man, *I.R.C.S. Med. Sci. Biochem.*, 10, 12, 1982.
38. **Porte, D.,** Beta adrenergic stimulation of insulin release in man, *Diabetes,* 16, 150, 1967.
39. **Ahren, B., Ericson, L. E., Lundquist, R., Loren, T., and Sundler, F.,** Adrenergic innervation of pancreatic islets and modulation of insulin secretion by the sympatho-adrenal system, *Cell Tissue Res.*, 216, 15, 1981.
40. **Lacey, R. J., Berron, N. S., London, N. O. M., Lake, S. P., James, R. F., Scarpello, J. H. B., and Morgan, N. G.,** Differential effects of beta adrenergic agonists on insulin secretion from pancreatic islets isolated from rat and man, *J. Mol. Endocr.*, 5, 49, 1990.
41. **Kallenbach, J. M., Panz, V. R., Jankelow, D., Joffe, B. R., and Seftel, H. C.,** Metabolic and hormonal responses to salbutamol in asthma, evidence of beta adrenergic over-activity?, *Respiration,* 57, 21, 1990.
42. **William-Olsson, T., Fellenius, E., Bjorntorp, P., and Smith, V.,** Differences in metabolic responses to beta adrenergic stimulation after propranolol or metoprolol stimulation, *Acta Med. Scand.*, 205, 201, 1979.
43. **Paterson, J. W., Lulich, K. M., and Goldie, R. G.,** A comment on beta 2 agonists and their use in asthma, *Trends Pharmacol. Sci.*, 4, 67, 1983.
44. **Kendall, M. J., Clark, N. W., Haffner, C. A., Kong, J., and Hughes, B. A.,** Investigation of the effects of beta 2 stimulation on FFAs in man, *J. Clin. Pharmacol. Exp. Ther.*, 16, 31, 1991.
45. **Haffner, C. A., Kendall, M. J., Maxwell, S., and Hughes, B.,** The lipolytic effect of β_1- and β_2-adrenoceptor activation in healthy human volunteers, *Br. J. Clin. Pharmacol.*, 35, 35, 1993.
46. **Goldberg, R., Joffe, B. R., Bersohn, I., Van As, M., Krut, L., and Seftel, M. C.,** Metabolic responses to selective adrenergic stimulation in man, *Postgrad. Med. J.*, 51, 53, 1976.
47. **Henderson, A. H., Most, A. S., Parmley, W. W., Gorlin, R., and Sonnenblick, E. H.,** Depression of myocardial contractility in rats by free fatty acids during hypoxia, *Circ. Res.*, 26, 439, 1970.
48. **Kurien, V. A. and Oliver, M. F.,** A metabolic cause for arrhythmias during acute myocardial hypoxia, *Lancet,* 1, 813, 1970.
49. **Opie, L. H.,** Metabolic response during impending myocardial infarction: I. Relevance of studies of glucose and fatty acid metabolism in animals, *Circulation,* 65, 483, 1972.
50. **Chazan, R., Droszcz, W., Bobilewicz, D., and Maruchin, J. E.,** Changes in plasma HDL levels after salbutamol, *Int. J. Clin. Pharmacol. Ther. Toxicol.*, 23, 427, 1985.
51. **Lehtonen, A., Vilkari, J., Sallinev, V. P., and Glo, J.,** Effect of beta 2 adrenergic stimulation on serum lipids, *Int. J. Clin. Pharmacol. Ther. Toxicol.*, 20, 530, 1982.
52. **Epstein, F. H. and Rosa, R. M.,** Adrenergic control of serum potassium, *N. Engl. J. Med.*, 309, 1450, 1983.
53. **Struthers, A. D. and Reid, J. L.,** The role of adrenal medullary catecholamines in potassium homeostasis, *Clin. Sci.*, 66, 377, 1984.
54. **Bodeman, H. H., Schluter, K. J., Irmer, M., Reininghaus, M., and Keul, J.,** Activation of sodium transport in human erythrocytes by beta adrenoceptor stimulation in vivo, *Eur. J. Appl. Physiol.*, 56, 375, 1987.
55. **Charron, R. C., Lemme, C. E., Wilson, D. R., Ing, T. S., and Wrong, O. M.,** The effect of adrenal steroids on stool composition as revealed by in vivo dialysis of faeces, *Clin. Sci.*, 37, 151, 1969.
56. **D'Silva, J. H.,** The action of adrenaline on serum potassium, *J. Physiol.*, 92, 393, 1934.
57. **Flatman, J. A. and Clausen, T.,** Combined effects of adrenaline and insulin on active Na^+/K^+ transport in rat soleus muscle, *Nature,* 281, 580, 1979.

58. **Hayes, E. T., Dwyer, J. M., Horowicz, P., and Swift, J. G.,** Epinephrine action on sodium fluxes in frog striated muscle, *Am. J. Physiol.*, 227, 1340, 1979.
59. **Clausen, T. and Flatman, J. A.,** Beta 2 adrenoceptors mediate the stimulating effect of adrenaline on active electrogenic Na+-K+ transport in rat soleus muscle, *Br. J. Pharmacol.*, 68, 749, 1980.
60. **Jonkers, R., Van Boxtel, C. J., and Oosterhuis, B.,** B-2-adrenoceptor mediated hypokalaemia and its abolishment by oxyprenolol, *Clin. Pharmacol. Ther.*, 42, 627, 1987.
61. **Brown, M. J., Brown, D. C., and Murphy, M. B.,** Hypokalaemia from beta 2 receptor stimulation by circulating epinephrine, *N. Engl. J. Med.*, 309, 1414, 1983.
62. **Struthers, A. D. and Reid, J. L.,** Adrenaline causes hypokalaemia in man by beta 2 adrenoceptor stimulation, *Clin. Endocrinol. (Oxf.)*, 20, 409, 1984.
63. **Reid, J. L., Whyte, R. F., and Struthers, A. D.,** Epinephrine induced hypokalaemia: their role of beta adrenoceptors, *Am. J. Cardiol.*, 57, 23F, 1986.
64. **Rosa, R. M., Silva, P., Young, J. B., Landsberg, L., Brown, R. S., Rowe, J. W., and Epstein, F. H.,** Adrenergic modulation of extrarenal potassium disposal, *N. Engl. J. Med.*, 302, 431, 1980.
65. **Struthers, A. D., Reid, J. L., Whitesmith, R., and Rodger, J. L.,** The effects of cardioselective and non-selective beta adrenoceptor blockade on the hypokalaemia and cardiovascular responses to adrenomedullary hormones in man, *Clin. Sci.*, 65, 143, 1983.
66. **Lundberg, P.,** The effect of adrenergic blockade on potassium concentrations in different conditions, *Acta Med. Scand.* [*Suppl.*], 672, 121, 1983.
67. **Tyler, K., Defronzo, R., and Bia, M.,** Adrenergic control of extrarenal potassium tolerance is moderated through a beta 2 receptor, *Kidney Int.*, 21, 159, 1982.
68. **Massara, F., Porta, M., and Martina, V.,** Letter to the editor, *Clin. Endocrinol.*, 22, 227, 1985.
69. **Schnack, C., Podolsky, A., Watzke, H., Schern Thaner, G., and Burghuber, O. C.,** Effects of somatostatin and oral potassium administration on terbutaline induced hypokalaemia, *Am. Rev. Respir. Dis.*, 139, 176, 1989.
70. **Smith, S. K. and Thompson, D.,** The effect of intravenous salbutamol on plasma and urinary potassium during premature labour, *Br. J. Obstet. Gynaecol.*, 84, 344, 1977.
71. **Kung, M. and Lexington, K. Y.,** Parenteral adrenergic bronchodilators and potassium, *Chest*, 89, 322, 1986.
72. **Spector, S. L.,** Adverse reactions associated with parenteral beta agonists: serum K+ changes, *N.E.R. Allergy Proc.*, 8, 317, 1987.
73. **Leitch, A. G., Clancy, L. J., Costello, J. F., and Flenley, D. C.,** Effect of intravenous infusion of salbutamol on ventilatory response to CO_2 and hypoxia on heart rate and plasma potassium in normal man, *Br. Med. J.*, 1, 365, 1976.
74. **Elegbeleye, O. O., Williams, K. O., and Femipearse, D.,** Comparison of the metabolic effects of salbutamol administered in a one minute bolus and a continuous infusion in patients with bronchial asthma, *Isr. J. Med. Sci.*, 14, 455, 1978.
75. **Berend, N. and Marlin, G. E.,** Characterization of beta adrenoceptor subtype mediating the metabolic actions of salbutamol, *Br. J. Clin. Pharmacol.*, 5, 207, 1978.
76. **Cotton, D. B., Strassner, H. T., Lipson, L. G., and Goldstein, D. A.,** The effects of terbutaline on acid base, serum electrolytes and glucose homeostasis during the management of preterm labour, *Am. J. Obstet. Gynecol.*, 141, 617, 1981.
77. **Smythe, A. R. and Sakakini, J.,** Maternal metabolic alterations secondary to terbutaline therapy for premature labour, *Br. J. Obstet. Gynaecol.*, 57, 566, 1981.
78. **Corea, L., Bentvoglio, M., and Verdecchia, P.,** Hypokalaemia due to salbutamol overdosage (letter), *Br. Med. J.*, 1, 500, 1981.
79. **Rohr, A. S., Spector, S. L., Rachelefsky, G. S., Katz, R. M., and Siegel, S. C.,** Efficacy of parenteral albuterol in the treatment of asthma, *Chest*, 3, 348, 1986.
80. **Kung, M., White, J. R., and Burki, N. K.,** The effect of subcutaneously administered terbutaline on serum potassium in asymptomatic asthmatic adults, *Am. Rev. Respir. Dis.*, 129, 329, 1984.

81. **Clifton, G. D., Burki, N. K., Hunt, B. A., and Patel, R. C.,** Hypokalaemic effects of successive subcutaneous doses of terbutaline in asthma, *Chest,* 94, 515, 1988.
82. **Deacon, S. P.,** Salbutamol and hypokalaemia (letter), *Lancet,* 1, 1302, 1976.
83. **Taylor, M. W., Gaddie, J., Murchison, L. E., and Palmer, K. N.,** Metabolic effects of oral salbutamol, *Br. Med. J.,* 1, 22, 1976.
84. **Hastwell, G. and Lambert, B. E.,** The effect of oral salbutamol on serum potassium and blood sugar, *Br. J. Obstet. Gynaecol.,* 85, 767, 1978.
85. **McInnes, G. T. and Davies, D. L.,** Hypokalaemia due to salbutamol over-dosage, *Br. Med. J.,* 283, 500, 1981.
86. **O'Brien, I. A., Fitzgerald-Fraser, J., Lewin, I. G., and Corrall, R. G.,** Hypokalaemia due to salbutamol over-dosage, *Br. Med. J.,* 282, 1515, 1981.
87. **Wang, P. and Clausen, T.,** Treatment of attacks in hyperkalaemic familial periodic paralysis by inhalation of salbutamol, *Lancet,* 1, 221, 1976.
88. **Haalboom, J. R., Deenstra, M., and Struyvenberg, A.,** Hypokalaemia induced by inhalation of fenoterol, *Lancet,* 1, 1125, 1985.
89. **Scheinin, M., Koulu, M., Laurikainen, E., and Allonen, H.,** Hypokalaemia and other non-bronchial effects of inhaled fenoterol and salbutamol: a placebo controlled dose-response study in healthy volunteers, *Br. J. Clin. Pharmacol.,* 24, 645, 1987.
90. **Lipworth, B. J., Clark, R. A., Dhilton, D. P., Brown, R. A., and McDevitt, D. G.,** Beta adrenoceptor responses to high doses of inhaled salbutamol in patients with bronchial asthma, *Br. J. Clin. Pharmacol.,* 26, 527, 1988.
91. **Burgess, C. D., Flatt, A., Siebers, R., Crane, J., Beasley, R., and Purdie, G.,** A comparison of the extent and duration of hypokalaemia following 3 nebulized beta 2 adrenoceptor agonists, *Eur. J. Clin. Pharmacol.,* 36, 415, 1989.
92. **Haalboom, J. R., Deenstra, M., and Stuyvenberg, A.,** Effect of fenoterol on plasma K+ and cardiac ectopic activity, *Lancet,* 1, 45, 1989.
93. **Crane, J., Burgess, C., and Beasley, R.,** Cardiovascular and hypokalaemic effects of inhaled salbutamol, fenoterol and isoprenaline, *Thorax,* 44, 136, 1989.
94. **Lim, R., Walshaw, M. J., Sallissi, S., and Hind, C. K.,** Cardiac arrhythmias during acute exacerbations of chronic airflow limitation: effect of fall in plasma K+ concentration induced by nebulized beta 2 agonist therapy, *Postgrad. Med. J.,* 65, 449, 1989.
95. **Lipworth, B. J., Tregoskic, B. F., and McDevill, D. G.,** Beta adrenoceptor responses to inhaled salbutamol in the elderly, *Br. J. Clin. Pharmacol.,* 28, 725, 1989.
96. **Wong, C. S., Pavard, I. D., Williams, J., Britton, J. R., and Tattersfield, A. E.,** Bronchodilator, cardiovascular and hypokalaemic effects of fenoterol, salbutamol and terbutaline in asthma, *Lancet,* 336, 1396, 1990.
97. **Smith, S. R. and Kendall, M. J.,** Down-grading of biochemical and cardiovascular responses to an intravenous infusion of terbutaline following chronic treatment with oral terbutaline, *Int. J. Clin. Pharmacol. Ther. Toxicol.,* 24, 1, 1986.
98. **Windom, H. H., Burgess, C. D., Siebers, R. W., Purdie, G., Pearce, N., Crane, J., and Beasley, R.,** The pulmonary and extra pulmonary effects of inhaled beta agonists in patients with asthma, *Clin. Pharmacol. Ther.,* 48, 296, 1990.
99. **Smith, S. R., Gove, R., and Kendall, M. J.,** Beta agonists and potassium (letter), *Lancet,* 1, 1394, 1985.
100. **Whyte, K. F., Reid, C., Addis, G. J., Whitesmith, R., and Reid, T. L.,** Salbutamol induced hypokalaemia: the effect of theophylline alone and in combination with adrenaline, *Br. J. Clin. Pharmacol.,* 25, 571, 1988.
101. **Whyte, K. F., Addis, G. J., Whitesmith, R., and Reid, Q.,** Methylxanthines and adrenaline induced hypokalaemia: possible contribution to tachyarrhythmias in asthmatic patients, *Clin. Sci.,* 66, 578, 1984.
102. **Morgan, D. B. and Davidson, C.,** Hypokalaemia and diuretics: an analysis of publications, *Br. Med. J.,* 1, 905, 1980.
103. **Hollifield, O. N. and Slaton, P. E.,** Thiazide diuretics, hypokalaemia and cardiac arrhythmias, *Acta Med. Scand.* [*Suppl.*], 647, 67, 1981.

104. **Struthers, A. D., Whitesmith, R., and Reid, T. L.,** Prior thiazide diuretic treatment increases adrenaline-induced hypokalaemia, *Lancet,* 1, 1358, 1983.
105. **Lipworth, B. J., McDevitt, D. G., and Struthers, A. A.,** ECG changes induced by inhaled salbutamol after treatment with bendrofluazide: effects of replacement treatment with potassium, magnesium and triamterene, *Clin. Sci.,* 78, 255, 1990.
106. **Lipworth, B. J., McDevitt, D. G., and Struthers, A. D.,** Hypokalaemia and ECG sequelae of combined beta agonist/diuretic therapy: protection by conventional doses of spironolactone but not triamterene, *Chest,* 98, 811, 1990.
107. **Lown, B.,** Digitalis and potassium, *Adv. Intern. Med.,* 8, 125, 1956.
108. **Berkin, K. E., McInnes, G. T., Thomson, N. C., and Ball, S. G.,** Beta agonists and potassium (letter), *Lancet,* 1, 1394, 1985.
109. **Hoffman, B. F. and Cranefield, P. F.,** The physiological basis of cardiac arrhythmias, *Am. J. Med.,* 37, 670, 1964.
110. **Curry, P., Fitchett, D., Stubbs, W., and Krikler, D.,** Ventricular arrhythmias and hypokalaemia, *Lancet,* 2, 231, 1976.
111. **Solomon, R. J. and Cole, A. G.,** Importance of potassium in patients with acute myocardial infarction, *Acta Med. Scand.,* 647, 87, 1981.
112. **Fisch, C.,** Relationship of electrolyte disturbances to cardiac arrhythmias, *Circulation,* 47, 408, 1933.
113. **Nordehaug, J. E.,** Malignant arrhythmias in relation to serum potassium values in patients with acute myocardial infarction, *Acta Med. Scand.,* 647, 101, 1981.
114. **Thomas, R. D.,** Ventricular fibrillation and initial plasma potassium in acute myocardial infarction, *Postgrad. Med. J.,* 59, 354, 1983.
115. **Nordehaug, J. E., Johannessen, K. A., and Von Der Zippe, G.,** Serum potassium as a risk factor of ventricular arrhythmias early in acute myocardial infarction, *Circulation,* 71, 643, 1985.
116. **Pratt, C. M. and Moye, L. A.,** The Cardiac Arrhythmia Suppression Trial: background interim results and implications, *Am. J. Cardiol.,* 65, 20B, 1990.
117. **Podrid, P. J., Fucias, J., and Candinas, R.,** Role of the sympathetic nervous system in the genesis of VF, *Circulation,* 82 (Suppl. 1), 103, 1990.
118. National Heart, Lung & Blood Institute Cooperative Trial, The beta blocker heart attack trial, *J.A.M.A.,* 246, 2073, 1981.
119. **Yusuf, S., Ramsdale, D., Peto, R., Furse, L., Bennett, D., Bray, C., and Sleight, P.,** Early IV atenolol treatment in suspected acute myocardial infarction. Preliminary report of a randomized trial, *Lancet,* 1, 273, 1980.
120. **Kennedy, H. L., Whitlock, J. A., Sprague, M. K., Kennedy, L. T., Buckingham, T. A., and Goldberg, R. J.,** Long term follow up of asymptomatic healthy subjects with frequent and complicated ventricular ectopy, *N. Engl. J. Med.,* 312, 193, 1985.
121. **Chapman, K. R. and Rebuck, A. S.,** Bronchodilators, hypokalaemia and fatal asthma, *Lancet,* 1, 162, 1989.
122. **Connell, J. M. C., Cook, G. M., and McInnes, G. T.,** Metabolic consequences of salbutamol poisoning revised by propranolol, *Br. Med. J.,* 285, 779, 1982.
123. **Whyte, K., Addis, G. J., Whitesmith, R., and Reid, J. L.,** Adrenergic control of plasma magnesium in man, *Clin. Sci.,* 72, 135, 1987.
124. **Bremme, K., Eneroth, P., Nordstrom, L., and Nilsson, B.,** Effects of infusion of the beta adrenoceptor agonist terbutaline on serum magnesium in pregnant women, *Magnesium,* 5, 85, 1986.
125. **Dykner, T.,** Serum magnesium in acute myocardial infarction, *Acta Med. Scand.,* 207, 59, 1980.
126. **Swales, J. M.,** Magnesium deficiency and diuretics (editorial), *Br. Med. J.,* 285, 1377, 1982.
127. **Dycker, T. and Wester, P. O.,** Ventricular extrasystoles and intracellular electrolytes before and after potassium and magnesium infusion in patients on diuretic treatment, *Am. Heart. J.,* 97, 12, 1979.

128. **Hollifield, J. N.,** Potassium and magnesium abnormalities: diuretics and arrhythmias in hypertension, *Am. J. Med.*, 77, 28, 1984.
129. **Flatman, P. W.,** Magnesium transport across cell membranes, *J. Membr. Biol.*, 80, 1, 1984.
130. **Bos, N. J., Postma, D. S., and Doormaal, J.,** Magnesiuric and calciuric effects of terbutaline in man, *Clin. Sci.*, 74, 595, 1988.
131. **Woods, K. L.,** Possible pharmacological actions of magnesium in acute myocardial infarction, *Br. J. Clin. Pharmacol.*, 52, 3, 1991.
132. **Richards, S. R., Chang, F. E., and Stempel, L. E.,** Hyperlactacidaemia associated with acute ritidrine infusion, *Am. J. Obstet. Gynecol.*, 146, 1, 1983.
133. **Braden, G., Von Oeyen, P., Smith, M., Gingras, D., Germain, M., and Fitzgibbons, J.,** Mechanisms of Ritodrine (R) and Terbutaline (T) induced hypokalaemia (Hk) and pulmonary oedema (PE), *Kidney Int.*, 27, 304, 1985.
134. **Appel, D., Rubenstein, R., Schrager, K., and Williams, M. H.,** Lactic acidosis in severe asthma, *Am. J. Med.*, 75, 580, 1983.
135. **Assadi, F. K.,** Therapy of acute bronchospasm: complicated by lactic acidosis and hypokalaemia, *Clin. Pediatr.*, 28, 258, 1989.
136. **Braden, G. L., Johnston, S., Germain, M., Fitzgibbons, J. P., and Dawson, J. A.,** Lactic acidosis associated with therapy of acute bronchospasm, *N. Engl. J. Med.*, 313, 890, 1985.
137. **Speizer, F. E., Doll, R., Heat, P., and Strange, L. B.,** Investigation into the use of drugs preceding death from asthma, *Br. Med. J.*, 1, 339, 1968.
138. **Abbott, A.,** New direction in asthma: some cause for concern, *Trends Pharmacol. Sci.*, 9, 149, 1988.
139. **McDevitt, B. G.,** In vivo studies of the function of cardiac beta adrenoceptors in man, *Eur. Heart J.*, 10 (Suppl. B), 22, 1989.
140. **Brodde, O. E., Daul, A., Wellstrein, A., Palm, D., Michael, M. C., and Backerugh, J. J.,** Differentiation of beta 1 and beta 2 adrenoceptor mediated effects in humans, *Am. J. Physiol.*, 254, H119, 1988.
141. **Stiles, G. L., Taylor, S., and Lefkowitz, R. J.,** Human cardiac beta adrenergic receptors: subtype heterogeneity, *Life Sci.*, 33, 467, 1983.
142. **Buxton, B. F., Jones, C. R., Molenaar, P., and Summers, R. J.,** Characterization and autoradiographic localization of beta adrenoceptor subtypes in human cardiac tissues, *Br. J. Pharmacol.*, 92, 299, 1987.
143. **Kaumann, A. J., Hall, J. A., Murray, K. J., Walls, F. L., and Brown, M. J.,** A comparison of the effects of adrenaline and noradrenaline in human heart: the role of beta 1 and beta 2 adrenoceptors in the stimulation of adenylate cyclase and contractile force, *Eur. Heart J.*, 10 (Suppl. B), 29, 1989.
144. **Kaumann, A. J. and Lemoine, H.,** Increase of contractile force by adrenaline through beta 2 adrenoceptors in ventricular myocardium of man, *Br. J. Clin. Pharmacol.*, 90, 17P, 1987.
145. **Robberecht, P., Delhaye, M., Taton, G., Waelbrooeck, M., De Smet, J. M., De Neef, P., Leclerc, J. L., Chatelain, P., and Christophe, J.,** The human heart beta adrenoceptors: heterogeneity of the binding sites; presence of 50% beta 1 and 50% beta 2 receptors, *Mol. Pharmacol.*, 24, 169, 1983.
146. **Strauss, M. H., Reeves, R. A., Smith, D. L., and Lennen, F. H.,** The role of cardiac beta 1 receptors in the haemodynamic response to a beta 2 agonist, *Clin. Pharmacol. Ther.*, 40, 108, 1986.
147. **Parker, G. W., Lloyd, H., Hartley, G. J., Skinner, J. E., and Entman, M. L.,** Central adrenergic mechanisms may modulate ischaemic VF in pigs, *Circ. Res.*, 66, 259, 1990.
148. **Hall, J. A., Petch, M. C., and Brown, M. C.,** Intracoronary injections of salbutamol demonstrate the presence of functional beta 2 adrenoceptors in the human heart, *Circ. Res.*, 65, 546, 1989.

149. **Corsa, L., Benturoglio, M., Verdacchio, P., Motelese, M., and Sorbini, C. A.,** Non-invasive assessment of chronotropic and inotropic response to preferential beta 1 and beta 2 adrenoceptor stimulation, *Clin. Pharmacol. Ther.*, 35, 776, 1984.
150. **Amory, D. W., Burnham, S. C., and Chaney, P. W.,** Comparison of the cardiopulmonary effects of subcutaneously administered epinephrine and terbutaline in patients with reversible airways obstruction, *Chest,* 67, 279, 1975.
151. **Tashkin, D. P., Meth, R., Simmons, D. H., and Lee, Y. E.,** Double blind comparison of acute bronchial and cardiovascular effects of oral terbutaline and ephedrine, *Chest,* 65, 155, 1978.
152. **Flatt, A., Crane, J., Pirdie, G., Kwong, T., Beasley, R., and Burgess, C.,** The cardiovascular effects of beta adrenergic agonist drugs administered by nebulization, *Postgrad. Med. J.*, 66, 98, 1990.
153. **Gray, B. J., Frame, M. H., and Costello, J. H.,** A comparative double blind study of the bronchodilator effects and side effects of inhaled fenoterol and terbutaline administered in equipotent doses, *Br. J. Dis. Chest,* 76, 341, 1982.
154. **Pasotti, C., Gandolfi, P., and Urbelli, C.,** Cardiovascular responses in normal man to beta adrenergic stimulation with clenbuterol, *Curr. Ther. Res.*, 28, 235, 1980.
155. **Hall, J. A.,** Letter to the editor, *Postgrad. Med. J.*, 67, 21, 1991.
156. **Mattauer, B., Rouleau, J. L., and Burgess, J. H.,** Detrimental arrhythmogenic and sustained beneficial haemodynamic effects of oral salbutamol in patients in congestive heart failure, *Am. Heart J.*, 109, 840, 1985.
157. **Mifune, J., Matsushita, S., Iwasaki, T., Kwanoto, K., Veda, K., Kuramoto, K., Keiji, U., Kuwajima, I., Sakai, M., Moroki, N., and Murakami, M.,** Haemodynamic effects of salbutamol, an oral long acting beta stimulant in patients chronic congestive heart failure, *Am. Heart J.*, 104, 1011, 1982.
158. **Tandon, M. K.,** Cardiopulmonary effects of fenoterol and salbutamol aerosols, *Chest,* 77, 429, 1980.
159. **Lipworth, B. J., McDevitt, D. G., and Struthers, A. D.,** Systemic beta adrenoceptor responses to salbutamol given by metered dose inhaler alone and with pear-shaped spacer attachment. Comparison of ECG, K+ and haemodynamic effects, *Br. J. Clin. Pharmacol.*, 27, 837, 1989.
160. **Jenkins, S. C. and Maxham, J.,** High dose salbutamol in chronic bronchitis: comparison of 400 μg, 1 mg and 1.6 mg and 2 mg and placebo delivered by rotahaler, *Br. J. Dis. Chest,* 81, 242, 1987.
161. **Lulich, K. M., Goldie, R. G., Ryan, G., and Paterson, J. W.,** Adverse reaction to beta 2 agonist bronchodilators, *Med. Toxicol.*, 1, 286, 1986.
162. **Kendall, M. J., Woods, K. L., Wilkins, M. R., and Worthington, D. J.,** Responsiveness to beta adrenoceptor stimulation: the effects of age are cardioselective, *Br. J. Clin. Pharmacol.*, 14, 821, 1982.
163. **Neville, E., Carris, P. A., Uriah, J., Nariman, S., and Gibson, S. J.,** Nebulized salbutamol and angina, *Br. Med. J.*, 285, 796, 1982.
164. **Shorlin, C. L. and Tam, F. W.,** Salbutamol nebulizer and precipitation of critical cardiac ischaemia, *Lancet,* 2, 1258, 1990.
165. **Santo, M., Sidi, Y., and Pinkhas, Y.,** Acute myocardial infarction following IV salbutamol, *S. Afr. Med. J.*, 58, 394, 1980.
166. **Kaumann, A. J. and Lemoine, H.,** Increase of contractile force by adrenaline through beta 2 adrenoceptors in ventricular myocardium of man, *Br. J. Clin. Pharmacol.*, 90, 17P, 1987.
167. **Matthay, R. A., Langor, R., Brent, B. N., Mahler, D. A., Berger, H. J., and Boret, B. L.,** Cardiovascular effects of terbutaline in patients with COPD, pulmonary hypertension and decreased RV function, *Am. Rev. Respir. Dis.*, 123 (Suppl. 4), 16, 1981.
168. **Winter, R. J. D., Langford, J. A., and Rudd, R. M.,** Effects of oral and inhaled salbutamol and oral pirbuterol on R and LV function in chronic bronchitics, *Br. Med. J.*, 288, 824, 1984.

169. **Henriksen, L., Aggestrip, S., Stoczynski, Z., and Lauridsen, P.,** Cardiovascular and respiratory effects of terbutaline in patients after open heart surgery, *J. Cardiovasc. Surg.,* 21, 243, 1980.
170. **Guernsey, B., Villareal, Y., Snyder, M., and Gabert, H.,** Pulmonary edema associated with the use of beta mimetic agents in preterm labour, *Am. J. Hosp. Pharm.,* 38, 1942, 1981.
171. **Whitehead, M. I., Mauder, A. M., Hertogs, K., Williams, R. M., and Pettingole, K. W.,** Acute congestive cardiac failure in a hypertensive woman receiving salbutamol for premature labour, *Br. Med. J.,* 1, 1221, 1980.
172. **Chapman, K. R., Smith, D. L., Rebuck, A. S., and Leene, H. H.,** Haemodynamic effects of an inhaled beta 2 agonist, *Clin. Pharmacol. Ther.,* 35, 762, 1984.
173. **Pingleton, S. K.,** Hypotension associated with terbutaline therapy in acute quadriplegia, *Am. Rev. Respir. Dis.,* 126, 723, 1982.
174. **Collins, J. M., McDevitt, J. C., Shauke, R. G., and Swanton, J. G.,** The cardiotoxicity of isoprenaline during hypoxia, *Br. J. Pharmacol.,* 36, 35, 1969.
175. **Kahn, D. S., Rona, G., and Chappel, C. T.,** Isoproterenol induced cardiac necrosis, *Ann. N.Y. Acad. Sci.,* 156, 285, 1969.
176. **Halt, J. Z., Gershengam, K., Kranz, P., Albert, F., Oestreicher, R., and Fani, K.,** The role of platelet aggregation in catecholamine induced cardiac necrosis: electron microscopic and drug studies, *Am. J. Cardiol.,* 29, 268, 1972.
177. **Bloom, S. and Davie, D. L.,** Calcium as mediator of isoproterenol induced myocardial necrosis, *Am. J. Pathol.,* 69, 459, 1972.
178. **Kirkland, G., Williams, J., and Lewiston, N.,** Fatal myocardial toxicity during continuous infusion of IV isoproterenol treatment of asthma, *J. Allergy Clin. Immunol.,* 63, 407, 1979.
179. **Rhatigan, R. and Deta Torre, A.,** Myocardial necrosis and bronchial asthma, *Ann. Allergy,* 28, 434, 1970.
180. **Matson, J. R., Langlin, G. M., and Stronk, R. C.,** Myocardial ischaemia complicating the use of isoproterenol in asthmatic children, *J. Pediatr.,* 92, 776, 1978.
181. **Barker, L. D., Snow, J. A., Pomposiello, G. V. R., Sharma, K., and Messer, J. V.,** Isoproterenol induced "coronary steal": metabolic observations in human coronary artery disease, *Clin. Res.,* 17, 228, 1969.
182. **Wang, R. Y., Lee, P. K., Yu, D. Y., Tse, T. F., and Chow, M. S.,** Myocardial metabolic effects of IV terbutaline in patients with severe heart failure due to coronary artery disease, *J. Clin. Pharmacol.,* 23, 362, 1983.
183. **Sears, M. R., Rera, H. H., and Fenwick, J.,** 75 deaths in asthmatics prescribed home nebulizers, *Br. Med. J.,* 294, 477, 1987.
184. **Benatar, S. R.,** Fatal asthma, *N. Engl. J. Med.,* 314, 423, 1986.
185. **Hassan, A. B., Ormerod, O., Efthimiou, J., and Benson, M. K.,** Reversible ECG T wave abnormalities in severe acute asthma, *Thorax,* 44, 879, 1989.
186. **Clifton, G. D., Hunt, B. A., Patel, R. C., and Bwki, N. K.,** Effects of sequential doses of parenteral terbutaline on plasma levels of potassium and related CP responses, *Ann. Rev. Respir. Dis.,* 141, 574, 1990.
187. **Weaver, W. F. and Birchel, H.,** Serum K+ and the electrocardiograph and hypokalaemia, *Circulation,* 21, 505, 1960.
188. **Eisenberg, M. J.,** Magnesium deficiency and cardiac arrhythmias, *N.Y. State J. Med.,* 86, 133, 1986.
189. **Williams, S. J., Winner, S. J., and Clark, T. J.,** Comparison of inhaled and IV terbutaline in acute severe asthma, *Thorax,* 36, 629, 1981.
190. **Mamson, G. W. and Forebrother, M. J. B.,** Overdose of salbutamol, *Lancet,* 2, 681, 1973.
191. **Lawyer, C. and Pond, A.,** Problems with terbutaline, *N. Engl. J. Med.,* 296, 821, 1977.

192. **Larsson, S. and Svedmyr, N.,** Bronchodilating effect and side effects of beta 2 adrenoceptor stimulants by different modes of administration (tablets, metered aerosol, and combinations thereof), *Am. Rev. Respir. Dis.*, 116, 861, 1977.
193. **Wilson, J. D., Sutherland, D. C., and Thomas, A. L.,** Has the change to beta agonists combined with oral theophylline increased cases of fatal asthma?, *Lancet,* 1, 1235, 1981.
194. **Williams, S. J., Parrish, R. W., and Seaton, A.,** Comparison of IV aminophylline and salbutamol in severe asthma, *Br. Med. J.*, 4, 685, 1975.
195. **Billing, B., Dahlquist, R., Farle, M., Horhblad, Y., and Ripe, E.,** Separate and combined use of terbutaline and theophylline in asthmatics, *Eur. J. Respir. Dis.*, 63, 399, 1982.
196. **Laursen, L. C., Taudorf, E., Gnosspelus, Y., Gymose, E., and Weeke, B.,** Long term oral Rx of asthma with terbutaline and theophylline, alone and combined, *Eur. J. Respir. Dis.*, 66, 82, 1985.
197. **Laaban, J. P., Jung, B., Chauvet, J. P., Psychoyos, I., Proteau, J., and Rochemoure, J.,** Cardiac arrhythmias during the combined use of IV aminophylline and terbutaline in status asthmaticus, *Chest,* 94, 496, 1988.
198. **Kelly, H. W., Menendez, R., and Voyles, W.,** Lack of significant arrhythmogenicity from chronic theophylline and beta 2 adrenergic combination therapy in asthmatic subjects, *Ann. Allergy,* 54, 405, 1985.
199. **Shim, C. S., Scher, S. M., and Williams, M. H.,** Effect of bronchodilator agents on arrhythmia, *N.Y. State Med. J.*, 76, 1973, 1976.
200. **Grossman, J.,** The occurrence of arrhythmias in hospitalized asthmatic patients, *J. Allergy Clin. Invest.*, 57, 310, 1976.
201. **Molfino, N. A., Nannini, L. J., Martelli, A. N., and Slutsky, A. S.,** Respiratory arrest in near fatal asthma, *N. Engl. J. Med.*, 324, 285, 1991.
202. **Higgins, R. M., Cookson, W. O., Lane, D. J., John, S. M., McCortny, G. L., and McCarthy, S. T.,** Cardiac arrhythmias caused by nebulized beta agonist therapy (letter), *Lancet,* 2, 863, 1987.
203. **Al-Hillawi, A. H., Hayward, R., and Johnson, N. M.,** Incidence of cardiac arrhythmias in patients taking SR salbutamol and SR terbutaline for asthma, *Br. Med. J.*, 288, 367, 1984.
204. **Banner, A. S., Sundirajan, E. V., Agarwal, M. K., and Addington, W. W.,** Arrhythmogenic effects of orally administered bronchodilators, *Arch. Intern. Med.*, 139, 434, 1979.
205. **Thiringer, G. and Svedmyr, N.,** Evaluation of skeletal muscle tremor due to bronchodilator agents, *Scand. J. Respir. Dis.*, 56, 93, 1975.
206. **Fellenius, E., Hedberg, R., Holmberg, E., and Waldeck, B.,** Functional and metabolic effects of terbutaline and propranolol in fast and slow contracting skeletal muscle in vivo, *Acta Physiol. Scand.*, 109, 89, 1980.
207. **Holmberg, E. and Waldeck, B.,** The effect of insulin on skeletal muscle contractions and its relation to the effect produced by beta adrenoceptor stimulation, *Acta Physiol. Scand.*, 109, 225, 1979.
208. **Jenne, J. W., Ridley, D. J., Macuci, R. A., Druz, W. S., and Rook, J. L.,** Objective and subjective tremor responses to oral beta 2 agents on first exposure, *Am. Rev. Respir. Dis.*, 126, 607, 1982.
209. **Larsson, S.,** Long term treatment with beta 2 stimulants in asthma, *Acta Med. Scand.*, 608, 1, 1977.
210. **Levy, S., Malletts, S., and Levine, S.,** Comparison of the effects of 2 beta 2 agonists with respect to bronchodilator and skeletal muscle tremor responses, *Am. Rev. Respir. Dis.*, 133 (Suppl. 4), A63, 1986.
211. **Van den Berg, W., Forrens, J., Leferink, T. G., Kreukniet, J., Maes, R. A., and Bruynzeel, P. L.,** Tremor measurement in asthma. II. changes after terbutaline administration suggesting beta adrenergic blockade, *Eur. J. Respir. Dis.*, 63, 392, 1982.

212. **Snedmyr, N. L., Larsson, S. A., and Thiringer, G. K.,** Development of resistance in beta adrenergic receptors of asthmatic patients, *Chest,* 69, 479, 1976.
213. **Bengtsson, B.,** Plasma concentration and side effects of terbutaline, *Eur. J. Respir. Dis.,* 65 (Suppl. 134), 231, 1976.
214. **Wolfe, T. D., Yamate, M., Biedermann, A. A., and Chu, T. J.,** Comparison of the acute cardiopulmonary effects of oral albuterol, metaproterenol and terbutaline in asthmatics, *J.A.M.A.,* 253, 2068, 1985.
215. **Miller, W. C. and Rice, D. L.,** A comparison of oral terbutaline and fenoterol in asthma, *Ann. Allergy,* 44, 15, 1980.
216. **Lisi, D. M.,** Muscle spasms and CPK eleration following salbutamol administration, *Eur. Resp. J.,* 2, 98, 1989.
217. **Dyson, A. J. and MacKay, A. D.,** 2 oral beta adrenergic stimulant drugs, purbuterol and salbutemol in reversible airway obstruction, *Br. J. Dis. Chest,* 74, 70, 1980.
218. **Rosene, K. A., Featherstone, H. J., and Benedetti, T. J.,** Cerebral ischaemia associated with parenteral terbutaline use in pregnant migraine patients, *Am. J. Obstet. Gynecol.,* 143, 405, 1982.
219. **Friedman, R., Zinelli, B., Jardine, D., and Fireman, P.,** Seizures in a patient receiving terbutaline, *Am. J. Dis. Child,* 136, 1091, 1982.
220. **Pratt, H. F.,** Abuse of salbutamol inhalers in young people, *Clin. Allergy,* 12, 203, 1982.
221. **Widlocher, D., Lecrubier, Y., Jouvent, R., Peuch, A. J., and Simon, P.,** Antidepressant effect of salbutamol, *Lancet,* 2, 767, 1977.
222. **Schucard, D. W., Spector, S. L., Euner, R. L., Cummins, K. R., Schucard, J. L., and Friedman, A.,** Central nervous system effects of antiasthma medication: an ECG study, *Ann. Allergy,* 54, 177, 1985.
223. **Keighley, J. F.,** Iatrogenic asthma associated with adrenergic aerosols, *Ann. Intern. Med.,* 65, 985, 1966.
224. **Trautlein, J., Allegra, J., Field, J., and Gillin, M.,** Paradoxic bronchospasm after inhalation of isoproterenol, *Chest,* 70, 711, 1976.
225. **Morley, J., Sanjar, S., and Newta, C.,** Viewpoint: untoward effects of beta adrenoceptor agonists in asthma, *Eur. Respir. J.,* 3, 228, 1990.
226. **Haffner, C. A., Hughes, B., Kendall, M. J., and Holder, R.,** Pilot study to compare the bronchodilator and metabolic responses to terbutaline infusion in seven asthmatic subjects — are they correlated? *J. Clin. Pharm. Ther.,* 17, 229, 1992.

Chapter 9

THE LONG-TERM EFFECTS OF BETA RECEPTOR AGONIST THERAPY IN RELATION TO MORBIDITY AND MORTALITY

Colin S. Wong and Anne E. Tattersfield

TABLE OF CONTENTS

0-8493-6761-1/93/$0.00 + $.50

I. INTRODUCTION

The treatment of asthma has undergone remarkable changes in the last 30 to 40 years. Despite the development of more specific and effective drugs and improved delivery systems there has been a worldwide trend for asthma morbidity and mortality to increase.[1-4] Against this background there have also been epidemics of asthma deaths, initially in the 1960s in England and Wales, Australia, and New Zealand,[5,6] and again in New Zealand in the late 1970s.[6] As reviewed in Chapters 2 and 3, several explanations for the increase in mortality have been investigated. Although the ninth revision of the International Classification of Diseases in 1979, which in effect 'uncoupled' asthma and bronchitis, may have increased the number of deaths assigned to asthma to some extent, the effect was small[7] and does not explain the increase in deaths in the younger (5–35 years) age group or the trend for increasing asthma mortality rates after 1979. Diagnostic fashion and transfer have been examined but are also unlikely to account for the rising mortality rates from asthma.[2,3] Undertreatment[8-10] and patient delay in seeking medical attention[11,12] are recognized as being contributory factors in asthma deaths, but these are unlikely to have increased over the last two decades and cannot easily explain the asthma epidemics or the gradual increase in asthma mortality over this time. An increase in asthma prevalence and/or severity has also been considered and may be a factor underlying the gradual increase in mortality, but there is no evidence for a marked increase in prevalence at the time of the epidemics. Finally, the question of whether treatment could affect severity or mortality has been raised. Attention has focused on beta agonists and the possibility that they may be implicated in the epidemics of asthma deaths in particular and that they may, paradoxically, be causing a deterioration in asthma control. In this chapter the evidence that long-term use of beta agonists may be responsible for the observed increase in asthma mortality and morbidity is examined as well as the changes that occur in bronchial reactivity during and following treatment. The possible mechanisms that might account for these effects are then discussed.

To place the changes in mortality and morbidity in perspective, it is important to recognize how widely beta agonists are used and how much this use has increased in the last decade. The number of prescriptions for all preparations of $beta_2$ agonist bronchodilators in Great Britain was nearly 11 million in 1990 compared with approximately 4 million in 1980 (Report of the beta agonist working party, Committee on Safety of Medicines, 1992). By 1988 6% of all primary school children in Nottingham were taking a $beta_2$ agonist (R. Hill, personal communication).

II. BETA RECEPTOR AGONIST THERAPY AND ASTHMA MORTALITY

A relationship between sales of beta agonists and mortality from asthma has been demonstrated for the epidemics of asthma deaths in a number of epidemiological studies (Chapters 2 and 3). The increase in asthma mortality observed in several countries in the 1960s has commonly been ascribed to the overuse of sympathomimetic drugs from pressurized aerosols;[13,14] in particular, there appeared to be a temporal relationship between increased deaths and increased sales of the aerosol preparation of isoprenaline forte, which contained 400 μg per actuation instead of the standard 80 μg dose.[15] Three recent case-control studies in New Zealand demonstrated an association between the $beta_2$ agonist fenoterol and an increased risk of asthma death, with patients who died of asthma being more likely to have been prescribed fenoterol than other beta agonists, in effect salbutamol.[16-18] In the two later New Zealand studies, the association was based on the long-term treatment with fenoterol, the drug history being obtained from records from a previous discharge from hospital. What is less clear from these studies is whether fenoterol caused the deaths or whether patients at risk of death were more likely to be prescribed fenoterol. Although there is no positive evidence for the latter suggestion, fenoterol was marketed at a higher dose relative to other $beta_2$ agonists[19] and may therefore have been perceived as being more beneficial; also, as with any new drug on the market, it was likely to be tried in patients with more 'difficult' asthma. Although matching the cases and controls for severity attempts to correct for differences in susceptibility to dying, retrospective matching is of necessity rather crude and cannot exclude entirely the possibility of a difference between the two groups. These issues are discussed in Chapter 5. These studies are also not able to address the mechanism whereby drugs might cause death.

III. BETA RECEPTOR AGONIST THERAPY AND ASTHMA MORBIDITY

Paradoxical bronchoconstriction following an inhaled $beta_2$ agonist has been reported but is uncommon.[20-22] The main concern with beta agonists is the suggestion that when taken regularly they can make asthma worse. The evidence for this is reviewed.

A. STUDIES OF FEV_1 AND SYMPTOMS

Two studies from the 1960s are relevant. In a retrospective study Van Metre[23] reviewed the records of 17 patients who had died in hospital of asthma; 9 were considered to have used excessive amounts of inhaled isoprenaline, although this was not quantified. He also presented data from 30 patients with severe, refractory asthma who were using 6 to 50 times the recommended dose of inhaled isoprenaline (the "safe" daily dose was considered to be 750 μg). The dose of isoprenaline was reduced and asthma control improved in all patients; a bronchodilator response to isoprenaline was demonstrated in the ten patients studied after reducing their isoprenaline but was absent in the one patient studied while on high doses of isoprenaline. Reisman[24] made similar observations in a prospective study of 30 symptomatic asthmatic patients, 17 of whom were considered to be overusing their isoprenaline aerosol (more than one 30 mg isoprenaline aerosol in 2 weeks). When the patients were asked to discontinue their isoprenaline aerosol there was a marked improvement in asthma symptoms in 8 of the 12 patients who had previously demonstrated an increase in forced expiratory volume in 1s (FEV_1) of less than 10% in response to inhaled isoprenaline, and an increase in bronchodilator responsiveness.

Regular $beta_2$ agonist therapy has caused a reduction in FEV_1 in subjects with asthma in some short-term studies. In three studies without a placebo control there has been a decrease in FEV_1 following regular treatment with a beta agonist, a large decrease of 0.60 l after 6 weeks of treatment with oral fenoterol 10 mg daily,[25] a reduction of 0.33 l after 4 weeks of treatment with inhaled fenoterol 600 to 1600 μg daily,[26] and a reduction of 0.35 l after 4 weeks of treatment with inhaled salbutamol 500 μg four times daily.[27] In a recent study salbutamol 200 μg three times daily for 3 weeks caused a 10% decrease in FEV_1 compared with placebo 12 h after stopping treatment.[28] Finally, in a long-term study of 223 patients with asthma or chronic obstructive airways disease, the decrease in FEV_1 was greater (72 ml) after 1 year of regular bronchodilator (salbutamol 400 μg or ipratropium bromide 40 μg four times daily) than the decrease after intermittent bronchodilator use (20 ml).[29] Some care is needed in interpreting these data, however, because in general change in FEV_1 was not a primary end point of the studies in question and several studies of beta agonists have not shown a decrease in FEV_1,[30-32] although again few have been placebo-controlled. The timing of the measurement of FEV_1 after the last dose of beta agonist is also important. Despite these reservations it appears on balance that a decrease in FEV_1 can occur after regular beta agonist treatment.

A recent prospective study from New Zealand provided evidence that regular administration of high doses of the beta agonist fenoterol may increase asthma morbidity. Sears et al.[33] studied the effects of regular fenoterol versus on-demand inhaled $beta_2$ agonist therapy in 89 subjects with stable asthma in a placebo-controlled, crossover study. Subjects continued their inhaled corticosteroids and/or sodium cromoglycate but other medication was withdrawn before entry. Fenoterol 400 μg or matched placebo was administered four times daily for 24 weeks. Subjects recorded daily symptoms and peak expiratory flow rates (PEFRs), and spirometry and bronchial reactivity to methacholine was measured every 4 weeks. The investigators determined for each patient which treatment period was associated with significantly better control of asthma, using the various measures in ranked order (the need for short courses of prednisone, morning PEFR, nocturnal bronchodilator use, nocturnal symptoms, daytime symptoms, evening PEFR, and daytime bronchodilator use) if all the differences were not in the same direction. Of the 64 subjects who completed the study, 57 showed a significant difference between treatment periods; 17 experienced better asthma control during reg-

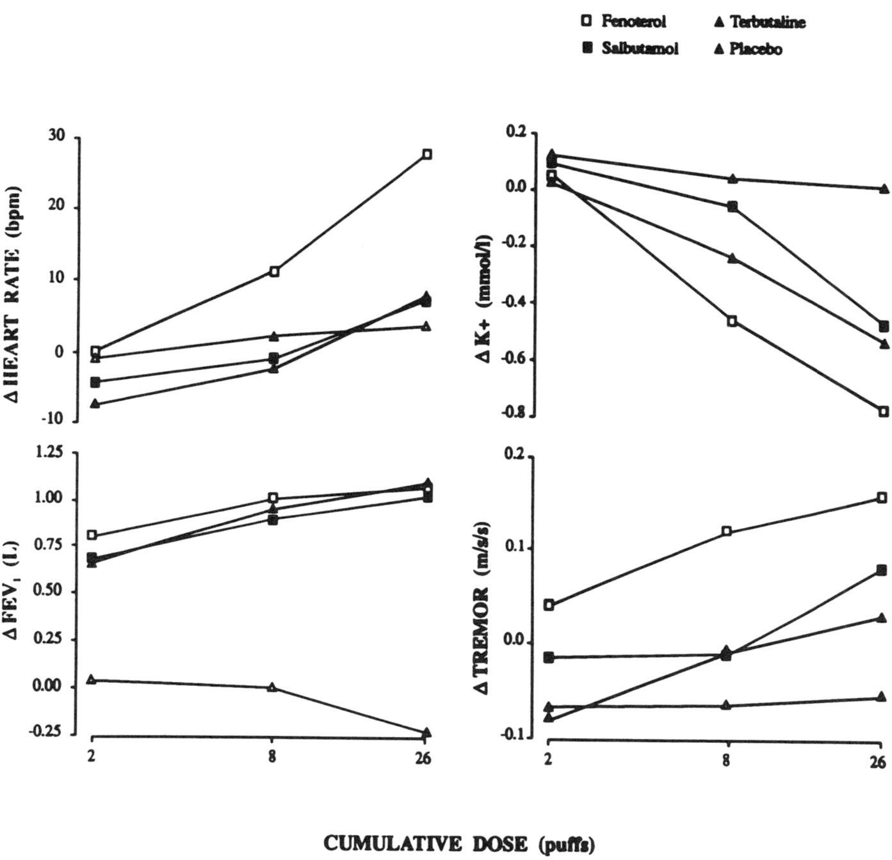

FIGURE 1. The change in FEV_1, heart rate, plasma potassium, and tremor with cumulative doses (log scale) of fenoterol (200 μg/puff), salbutamol (100 μg/puff), terbutaline (250 μg/puff), and placebo. (Adapted from Wong, C. S., Pavord, I. D., Williams, J., Britton, J. R., and Tattersfield, A. E., *Lancet,* 1, 1396, 1990. With permission.)

ular fenoterol treatment compared and 40 during intermittent bronchodilator treatment.

This study provides convincing evidence that fenoterol when given in the dose 400 μg four times daily causes some deterioration in asthma control. The magnitude of the deterioration is more difficult to determine from this study but is probably fairly small. The relevance of this finding to other beta agonists is uncertain because the dose of fenoterol used in this study was relatively high. In a dose equivalence study fenoterol caused more cardiovascular effects and greater hypokalemia (i.e., both $beta_1$ and $beta_2$ effects) than salbutamol and terbutaline, suggesting that it has been marketed at between two and four times the dose of these $beta_2$ agonists (Figure 1).[19] These findings are in keeping with several previous studies[34-36] and a review by

Svedmyr.[37] Fenoterol may also be less selective for $beta_2$ receptors,[38,39] although studies so far have not compared equipotent doses.

B. STUDIES OF BRONCHIAL REACTIVITY

When given acutely to subjects with asthma, $beta_2$ agonists provide protection against all constrictor stimuli including exercise, allergen, histamine, and methacholine; the degree of protection is related to the dose, timing, and mode of administration of the drug. In single-dose studies in asthmatic subjects, inhaled $beta_2$ agonists reduce the provocative dose of histamine or methacholine which causes a 20% decrease in FEV_1 (PD_{20}) by two to four doubling doses.[40] Small doses of $beta_2$ agonists inhibit the constrictor response to exercise[41] and the early response to antigen;[42] the late response to antigen is inhibited by high doses of salbutamol[43] and by the long-acting $beta_2$ agonist salmeterol.[44]

Following regular administration of $beta_2$ agonists there is some evidence that the protection afforded by $beta_2$ agonists against constrictor stimuli may be reduced and that after stopping treatment a rebound increase in bronchial reactivity occurs. Gibson et al.[45] found that oral salbutamol (16 mg daily for between 4 and 20 weeks) caused a reduction in the protective effect of inhaled salbutamol (200 μg) against an exercise challenge in asthmatic subjects, although the bronchodilator response was maintained. There was a similar but nonsignificant trend in subjects receiving regular inhaled salbutamol (800 μg daily). Reduced protection against histamine-induced bronchoconstriction was seen in subjects with mild asthma after 2 weeks of regular treatment with inhaled terbutaline[46] (Figure 2). A nonsignificant trend in the same direction has been seen in other studies.[47,48]

Six studies to date have shown a rebound increase in bronchial reactivity to histamine and methacholine in asthmatic subjects after treatment with regular $beta_2$ agonists[33,46,48-51] (Table 1). The increase in reactivity has occurred after fenoterol, salbutamol, and terbutaline following treatment for periods ranging from 2 to 52 weeks. The decrease in PD_{20} has ranged from 0.6 to 1.7 doubling doses of histamine or methacholine. The challenge tests were carried out at least 6 h, and in four of the studies at least 11 h, after the last dose of beta agonist. The time after cessation of treatment when the greatest change in bronchial reactivity occurs is still not clear. In the study by Vathenen et al.[46] the greatest increase in bronchial reactivity to histamine (1.5 doubling doses) was seen 21 h after cessation of treatment, the final time of measurement (Figure 3). Wahedna et al.[48] continued to measure histamine reactivity for up to 59 h after stopping regular salbutamol and found the greatest increase in bronchial reactivity (1.7 doubling doses) at this time.

It therefore appears that the regular use of $beta_2$ agonists for a period between 2 weeks and 1 year causes a rebound increase in bronchial reactivity upon cessation of treatment, and this increase continues for the following 2 to 3 days (Figure 4). An increase in bronchial responsiveness presumably

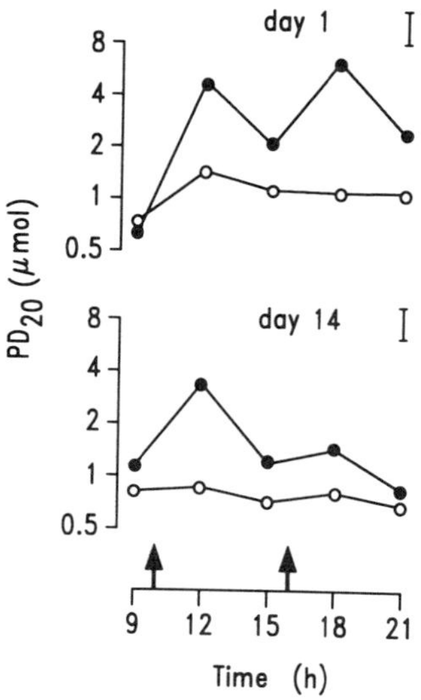

FIGURE 2. Change in PD_{20} histamine following terbutaline (●) or placebo (○) at 10 AM and 4 PM on day 1 of treatment and day 14. The increase in PD_{20} histamine following terbutaline is a measure of the protection afforded by terbutaline against histamine challenge. On day 14 terbutaline caused significantly less protection against histamine compared with the change on day 1. (From Vathenen, A. S., Knox, A. J., Higgins, B. G., Britton, J. R., and Tattersfield, A. E., *Lancet,* 1, 554, 1988. With permission.)

TABLE 1
Studies that Have Demonstrated Increased Bronchial Reactivity Following Regular Beta$_2$ Receptor Agonist Treatment

Subjects	Treatment	Time after last dose (h)	Challenge	Increase in bronchial reactivity	Ref.
7 asthma	Terbutaline 500 μg tid[b] for 26 weeks	12–16	Methacholine	0.9 DD[d] after 4 weeks	50
17 asthma	Terbutaline 500 μg qid[c] for 4 weeks	12–16	Histamine	0.6 DD after 2 weeks	49
64 asthma	Fenoterol 400 μg qid for 24 weeks	6	Methacholine	0.6 DD	33
15 asthma or COPD[a]	Salbutamol 400 μg qid for 1 year	8	Histamine	0.7 DD	51
8 asthma	Terbutaline 750 μg tid for 2 weeks	11–23	Histamine	1.5 DD at 23 h	46
11 asthma	Salbutamol 200 μg tid for 3 weeks	12–59	Histamine	1.7 DD at 59 h	48

[a] Chronic obstructive pulmonary disease.
[b] Three times a day.
[c] Four times a day.
[d] Doubling doses.

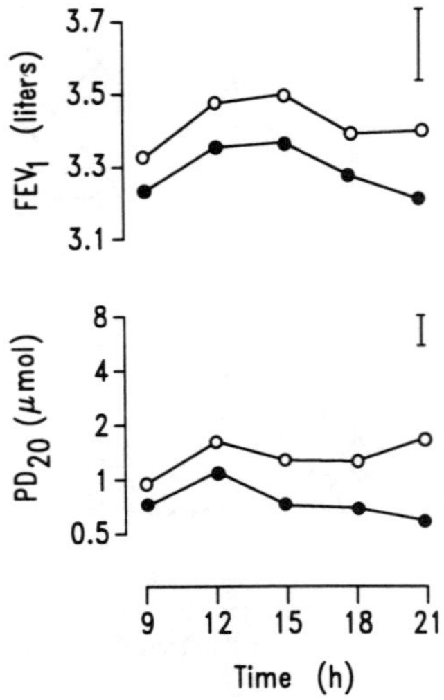

FIGURE 3. Mean values of FEV_1 and PD_{20} following cessation of treatment with terbutaline (●) and placebo (○) for the 21 h after treatment. The difference in PD_{20} (1.5 doubling doses of histamine) was statistically significant at 21 h, indicating increased reactivity following the beta agonist at this time. (From Vathenen, A. S., Knox, A. J., Higgins, B. G., Britton, J. R., and Tattersfield, A. E., *Lancet,* 1, 554, 1988. With permission.)

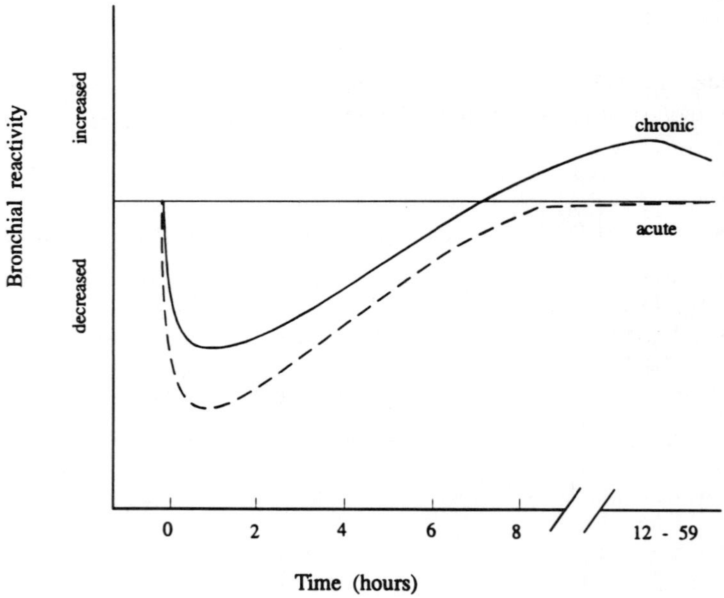

FIGURE 4. Schematic representation of the changes in bronchial reactivity following a single dose (acute) and regular doses (chronic) of inhaled $beta_2$ agonists. (Based on data from Vathenen, A. S., Knox, A. J., Higgins, B. G., Britton, J. R., and Tattersfield, A. E., *Lancet,* 1, 554, 1988. With permission.)

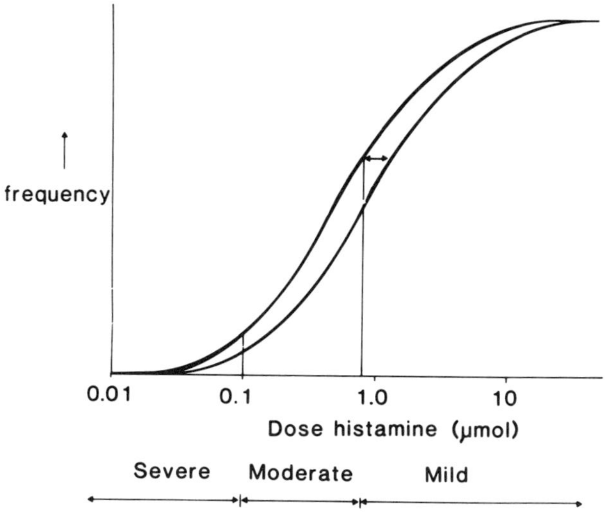

FIGURE 5. Frequency distribution showing the provocative dose of histamine which causes a 20% reduction in FEV_1 (PD_{20}). In a population of asthmatic patients a small increase in bronchial reactivity causes a large increase in the proportion with marked hyperresponsiveness. (From Mitchell, E. A., *Thorax,* 44, 81, 1989. With permission.)

means that patients would be more vulnerable to constrictor stimuli such as exercise or allergen. Although the mean changes are fairly small, any increase in bronchial responsiveness could be important in a small proportion of patients with more severe hyperresponsiveness and could conceivably cause a severe or even fatal attack of asthma on rare occasion. The effect of a small increase in airway reactivity in all patients would cause a disproportionate increase in the number of patients with marked hyperreactivity, as highlighted by Mitchell[52] (Figure 5).

Thus, there is a considerable body of evidence to suggest that the regular use of $beta_2$ agonists may cause detrimental effects in asthma. Various studies have shown a reduction in airway caliber, increase in symptoms and increase in bronchial reactivity following regular inhaled $beta_2$ agonists. How often such changes occur and their contribution to asthma morbidity overall is less certain. Further studies are needed to determine whether these adverse effects are class effects, whether they occur only with high doses of beta agonists, whether steroids protect against them and the nature of the mechanism underlying the changes.

IV. POSSIBLE MECHANISMS LINKING BETA RECEPTOR AGONIST THERAPY TO ASTHMA MORBIDITY AND MORTALITY

This section looks at the potential mechanisms by which beta agonists may increase asthma mortality and/or morbidity. Failure to take other treat-

TABLE 2
Mechanisms that May Potentially Explain the Associations with $Beta_2$ Receptor Agonists

Potential mechanism	Increase in bronchial reactivity	Deterioration in asthma	Increase in mortality
Failure to take other treatment	Yes	Yes	Yes
Dysrhythmia	No	No	Yes
Tolerance	Yes	Yes	Yes
Increased allergen load	Yes	Yes	Yes
Loss of anti-inflammatory effect of mast cells	Yes	Yes	Yes
Increased bronchial secretions	Possibly	Yes	No
Effect of bromide[a]	No	Yes	Yes
Effect of dextroisomer[b]	Yes	Yes	Yes

[a] Fenoterol only.
[b] Isoprenaline and salbutamol.

ment as a result of obtaining symptomatic relief from a $beta_2$ agonist and induction of cardiac dysrhythmias are potential causes of death in patients with asthma, although they cannot explain the decrease in FEV_1, increase in bronchial reactivity, or deterioration in asthma control discussed previously. Suggested mechanisms that could make asthma worse include beta receptor desensitization causing tolerance to beta agonists, increased deposition of allergen in the airways, loss of the anti-inflammatory effect of mast cell mediators, such as heparin, and increased bronchial secretions. More specific suggestions relate to an effect of bromide oxidants in the case of fenoterol and the role of dextroisomers in the case of isoprenaline and salbutamol in particular (Table 2). The various mechanisms are not mutually exclusive, and more than one mechanism may be contributing to the apparent increase in mortality and morbidity.

A. FAILURE TO TAKE OTHER TREATMENT

$Beta_2$ agonists provide rapid symptomatic relief from symptoms of asthma and effective prophylaxis against bronchoconstrictor stimuli, such as cold air and exercise. Regular use of a $beta_2$ agonist may therefore cause the patient to become noncompliant with other medications for asthma. Overreliance on a beta agonist can cause delay in seeking medical attention and may have contributed to some asthma deaths.[11,12] It cannot easily explain the gradual increase in mortality seen in several countries over the last two decades as the use of prophylactic treatment has increased progressively over this time. It also fails to explain why New Zealand alone should have had a more recent epidemic. Finally, it clearly does not explain the deterioration in asthma control or increase in reactivity seen with beta agonists in controlled studies.

B. DYSRHYTHMIAS

Beta agonists cause heart rate to increase due to direct stimulation of cardiac $beta_2$ receptors and the reflex baroreceptor-mediated response to peripheral vasodilatation. Tachycardia is observed with higher doses of $beta_2$-selective drugs such as salbutamol; whether $beta_2$ agonists cause more serious dysrhythmias and whether this is a cause of sudden death from asthma are more difficult to determine.

In animal studies serious cardiac dysrhythmias have been induced with high doses of both nonselective and selective beta agonists and with lower doses of beta agonists when combined with theophylline.[53,54] Hypoxia has been shown to be important in determining the cardiac response to high doses of beta agonists in animals, as outlined in Chapter 7.

Greenberg[55] reported the sudden deaths of eight asthmatic patients known to have overused their sympathomimetic inhalers, proposing that the mechanism of death was cardiac rather than respiratory. The only evidence to support this was ventricular tachycardia in the one patient in whom electrocardiographic recordings were available. Most asthma deaths occur outside hospital, and autopsy cannot determine whether or not a cardiac dysrhythmia has contributed to death. There are several anecdotal reports of cardiac dysrhythmias associated with beta agonists[56] but despite a close temporal relationship in some instances a coincidental association is always possible.

Prospective studies of oral $beta_2$ agonists in small numbers of subjects have demonstrated an increased incidence of ventricular premature beats and paroxysmal atrial tachycardia,[57] and ventricular tachycardia was seen in three of 20 patients in one study.[58] An increased incidence of cardiac dysrhythmias has also occurred with high doses of beta agonists administered by nebulizer.[59,60] The threshold for the development of cardiac dysrhythmias from $beta_2$ agonists appears to be lower in elderly patients and in those with preexisting heart disease.[58,60] Most of the dysrhythmias that have been demonstrated are clinically unimportant, but they serve to indicate that beta agonists are having an effect on the heart.

Anecdotal information and data from a small number of subjects studied for a short period are unlikely to be able to determine whether beta agonists cause fatal dysrhythmias or the extent to which they do so. If beta agonists cause fatal dysrhythmias, it must be uncommon in relation to drug usage and large prospective studies would be needed to resolve this question.

C. BETA RECEPTOR DESENSITIZATION CAUSING TOLERANCE TO BETA RECEPTOR AGONISTS

Receptor desensitization can cause tolerance, the reduction in a biological response to an agonist following continuous agonist stimulation (also referred to as tachyphylaxis, refractoriness, and resistance). Following the increase in asthma deaths in the 1960s, it was suggested that overuse of sympathomimetic aerosols may have led to the development of tolerance to the effects of these drugs and possibly to endogenous catecholamines, which may be important during an acute attack.[61] Desensitization of beta receptors on airway smooth muscle or on inflammatory cells could be responsible for a deterioration in asthma by reducing the effect of catecholamines on airway smooth muscle tone and their inhibitory effect on mediator release from inflammatory cells, such as mast cells.

Beta receptor desensitization is easily demonstrated *in vitro* and the mechanisms underlying the phenomenon have been studied in detail over the last decade. The main changes that cause loss of function in response to beta agonist stimulation include the following:

1. *Uncoupling of the beta receptor from adenylate cyclase.* The receptor may be modified by the agonist so that the agonist-receptor complex is unable to activate adenylate cyclase. Phosphorylation of the intracellular domain of the beta receptor by beta adrenergic receptor kinase and protein kinase A has been shown to be responsible. Uncoupling occurs rapidly and after short exposure to a beta agonist.
2. *Reversible internalization (sequestration) of the beta receptor.* Radioligand-binding studies have shown early and rapid (seconds to minutes) loss of beta receptors on various cells following stimulation by isoprenaline due to internalization of the receptors from the cell surface into the cytoplasm.[62] The receptors are removed transiently from the cell surface. This is probably not the major mechanism underlying rapid desensitization because desensitization can be demonstrated after sequestration has been blocked by specific reagents.[63,64]
3. *Down-regulation of the beta receptor.* Receptors are internalized and broken down by an enzyme, possibly protein kinase A, and/or cyclic adenosine monophosphate (cAMP)-independent mechanisms.[63] This occurs more slowly than sequestration and requires more prolonged exposure to the agonist. Recovery of beta receptor numbers then involves new protein synthesis.

1. Evidence for Beta Receptor Desensitization *Ex Vivo*

Studies of beta receptor desensitization in human tissue from subjects treated with a beta agonist have looked mainly at white blood cells because these are rich in beta receptors and obtained easily. All have shown a marked reduction in beta receptor numbers and function after treatment with a beta agonist and the opposite effect when treatment was discontinued. Treatment with oral terbutaline 10 mg daily for only 6 days caused an 85% reduction in receptor-binding sites on polymorphonuclear leukocytes from both asthmatic and normal subjects.[65] Another study of asthmatic patients on regular treatment with an oral beta agonist showed a reduced number of leukocyte beta receptors, which increased fourfold to control values within 7 days of cessation of terbutaline;[65] during this time the patients required additional treatment for increased symptoms of asthma. In eight healthy subjects who took oral terbutaline 15 mg daily for 2 weeks, there was a 75% reduction in lymphocyte cAMP response to isoprenaline and a 40% reduction in beta adrenoceptor numbers 12 h after the last dose of $beta_2$ agonist.[66] There was a corresponding attenuation of the plasma cAMP response to infused isoprenaline *in vivo,* and this had not returned to baseline 72 h after stopping terbutaline.

2. *In Vitro* Evidence for Beta Receptor Desensitization

Frog erythrocytes exposed to isoprenaline for 10 to 24 h show a 50% reduction in beta receptor numbers, with a reduction of receptors in the high affinity state and a reduction in adenylate cyclase activity.[67,68] Similar results have been demonstrated in erythrocytes from other animals and in other animal tissues.[69]

Data on human airways are limited. The relaxation responses to isoprenaline, adrenaline, noradrenaline, and salbutamol were studied in isolated human bronchial smooth muscle preconstricted with histamine.[70] After incubation of the tissue with isoprenaline, there was a concentration-dependent reduction in the response to all sympathomimetic agents. Isolated human airway smooth muscle incubated with isoprenaline has also shown cross-desensitization to isoetharine and terbutaline but not to aminophylline.[71] Cultured human airway smooth muscle cells show a markedly reduced cAMP response to challenge with isoprenaline following incubation with isoprenaline for 16 h, whereas the response to forskolin was maintained in keeping with uncoupling of the beta receptors from adenylate cyclase.[72]

3. Clinical Studies of Tolerance

a. Tolerance to Nonairway Effects of $Beta_2$ Receptor Agonists

Following intravenous infusions of isoprenaline for 15 to 45 min, the heart rate response to isoprenaline, terbutaline, and isoetharine was impaired.[61] Most studies in patients with asthma have looked at the effects of beta agonists given for weeks or months. Several have looked at the development of tolerance in tissues other than airways, and in general nonairway responses have developed tolerance with regular treatment. These include tremor,[36] tachycardia,[73] the increase in blood glucose, pyruvate, and cAMP responses to salbutamol,[47] and the decrease in serum potassium.[32] Some studies have shown tolerance to the metabolic and cardiovascular effects in asthmatic subjects at a time when the bronchodilator effects of the $beta_2$ agonist appeared to be maintained.[32,47]

b. Tolerance to the Bronchodilator Effects of $Beta_2$ Receptor Agonists

The important question is whether tolerance develops to the airway response to $beta_2$ agonists. The improvement in symptoms and FEV_1 seen in asthmatic patients in the two early studies from the 1960s following the reduction in use of isoprenaline aerosols[23,24] would be in keeping with the development of tolerance. This is supported by the improvement in the FEV_1 response to isoprenaline after beta agonist reduction in some patients. A large number of prospective clinical studies in the 1970s addressed the question of whether regular treatment with $beta_2$ agonists caused a reduction in the bronchodilator response to beta agonists, and the results were conflicting. A number of studies in asthmatic subjects were able to demonstrate a reduced bronchodilator response to a beta agonist following regular $beta_2$ agonist treatment whether given in oral form[74-76] or by inhalation.[77-79] Most studies, however, were unable to show any loss of bronchodilator responsiveness.[36,47,80-82] The reason for the different findings in different studies is unclear but includes small numbers of subjects, lack of a control group, and the effects of concomitant medications.[83]

The lack of development of tolerance to $beta_2$ agonists in many studies of asthmatic subjects appears to contrast with studies in healthy subjects. Following regular $beta_2$ agonist treatment healthy subjects have shown a reduction in the bronchodilator response (change in specific airways conductance) to a beta agonist challenge.[27,84-86] This was not observed in asthmatic and atopic nonasthmatic subjects studied in the same way.[27,86]

c. Loss of Protection from Beta$_2$ Receptor Agonists

More recent studies in asthmatic patients have looked at the ability of beta agonists to protect against a bronchoconstrictor stimulus after regular use. The loss of protection against histamine[46] and exercise challenge[45] following regular beta agonist treatment would be in keeping with beta receptor desensitization.

4. Summary

Regular administration of beta agonists causes rapid and marked reductions in beta receptor numbers and function in human white cells *ex vivo* and incubation with isoprenaline *in vitro* causes clear-cut desensitization to beta agonists in human airway smooth muscle. Studies of tolerance to beta agonists in humans have been less clear-cut. There is good evidence in both asthmatic and non-asthmatic subjects that tolerance occurs to non-airway responses following regular $beta_2$-agonist treatment, including heart rate and tremor. The evidence for tolerance occurring in the airways is less conclusive, but it may occur in some subjects or with high doses of beta agonists and may be reflected in loss of protection against bronchoconstrictor challenge.

The disparity between the ease with which beta receptor desensitization can be demonstrated *in vitro* and *ex vivo* and the relative difficulty in demonstrating tolerance in bronchodilator studies is marked. The increase in bronchial reactivity, decrease in FEV_1, and clinical deterioration following beta agonist treatment would fit with desensitization of beta receptors on inflammatory cells, causing increased release of pro-inflammatory mediators.

The development of tolerance to beta agonists by inflammatory cells rather than airway smooth muscle is a possible explanation for these various findings. This might occur if airway smooth muscle in asthmatic patients had a larger number of spare beta receptors than other tissues; alternatively, some feature of asthmatic airways may somehow protect smooth muscle beta receptors against desensitization.

D. INCREASED ALLERGEN LOAD

It has been suggested that regular $beta_2$ agonists may cause deterioration in asthma by allowing more allergen to be deposited in the airways.[33,87] The early bronchoconstrictor response to inhaled allergen by asthmatic subjects may act as a defense mechanism to reduce the amount of allergen inhaled and hence reduce the late bronchoconstrictor reaction[88] and subsequent increase in nonspecific bronchial reactivity.[89] This argument is not convincing, however, because the amount of allergen inhaled would be expected to relate more to minute ventilation than to FEV_1 or peak flow rate. Although $beta_2$ agonists can increase minute ventilation,[90] this effect is small in relation to the increase seen with regular exercise, for example, which is not usually associated with a late deterioration in asthma.[91] Alveolar ventilation would be expected to decrease as asthma improves.

E. LOSS OF ANTI-INFLAMMATORY EFFECT OF MAST CELLS

Page proposed that $beta_2$ agonists may increase asthma morbidity by inhibiting the release of mast cell anti-inflammatory mediators such as heparin and related proteoglycans.[92] Heparin is able to neutralize some of the cytotoxic products released by eosinophils such as major basic protein, eosinophil cationic protein, and eosinophil peroxidase *in vitro* and to limit inflammatory cell activation and recruitment. Heparin and related proteoglycans may also inhibit the fibroblast proliferation and smooth muscle hypertrophy that occur in asthmatic airways. $Beta_2$ agonists are potent inhibitors of mast cell degranulation[93] and could therefore increase inflammation by inhibiting mast cell release of anti-inflammatory mediators. This hypothesis assumes that mast cell anti-inflammatory mediators are more important than the pro-inflammatory mediators such as leukotriene C_4 and histamine. Page[92] cited the failure of many drugs with mast cell stabilizing activity to help in the management of asthma. If this hypothesis were true, nedocromil sodium and sodium cromoglycate, which are mast cell stabilizers *in vitro,* would be expected to induce inflammation in the airways.

F. INCREASED BRONCHIAL SECRETIONS

The effect of $beta_2$ agonists on human airway secretions is difficult to study. In animals beta agonists cause an increase in glandular secretion of viscous fluid with a high protein content,[94] and human bronchi stimulated with salbutamol *in vitro* show increased secretion of radiolabelled glycoproteins.[95] Mucus plugging of the airways is a characteristic pathological finding in patients dying of acute asthma.[96] $Beta_2$ agonists may be causing adverse effects in asthma by changing the volume or consistency of mucus, although there is no direct evidence.

G. DRUG-SPECIFIC MECHANISMS

1. Formulation of Fenoterol as a Bromide

Fenoterol is formulated as a bromide, and it was suggested that this might be responsible for the problems with fenoterol.[97] Eosinophils oxidize bromide in preference to chloride and bromide oxidants are capable of damaging many cells, including the myocardium in animals.[98] The amount of bromide delivered with each inhalation of fenoterol is small, however, and unlikely to alter the bromide concentration in the lung or blood sufficient to affect eosinophil oxidants appreciably.[99]

2. Effect of Dextroisomers on Beta Agonists

Work in guinea pigs has suggested that the dextro-enantiomers of salbutamol and isoprenaline, which have no bronchodilating effects, may increase bronchial reactivity.[100,101] The authors suggested that the bronchodilator response to racemic salbutamol may not last as long as the adverse effects of (+)salbutamol. Many of the effects of salbutamol in the guinea pig differ from those in humans, and there is no evidence to suggest that these effects are relevant to humans.

V. CONCLUSIONS

Epidemiological studies have linked $beta_2$ agonists to epidemic increases in asthma deaths in several countries in the 1960s and more recently in New Zealand. Although these studies cannot prove a causal association, several studies suggest that some adverse effects can occur during treatment with beta agonists or following cessation of treatment. A few studies have shown a small decrease in FEV_1 after regular treatment with inhaled $beta_2$ agonists, and bronchial reactivity has been shown to increase progressively over the 2 to 3 days after cessation of beta agonist treatment. A recent large study showed an increase in asthma morbidity after regular treatment with relatively high doses of fenoterol compared with intermittent beta agonist.

There is therefore a reasonable body of evidence to suggest that $beta_2$ agonists may increase asthma morbidity and that following cessation of treatment bronchial reactivity may increase. The clinical importance of these changes is more difficult to determine. Of the various mechanisms that have been investigated, the possibility that beta receptor desensitization might cause tolerance to beta agonists has been studied in most detail. Although beta receptor desensitization can be demonstrated easily in white cells *ex vivo* and in human smooth muscle *in vitro,* the evidence for tolerance to beta agonists in humans is more controversial. There is some evidence that protection against constrictor stimuli may be reduced after regular beta agonist treatment, and the rebound increase in bronchial reactivity that occurs after cessation of treatment could be due to desensitization of beta receptors on inflammatory cells. In general, however, bronchodilator responses to beta agonists have been maintained. The data would fit with relatively greater desensitization of beta receptors on inflammatory cells compared with airway smooth muscle. Other mechanisms have been suggested, but there are few data to support any of these at present.

REFERENCES

1. **Burney, P. G. J.,** Asthma mortality in England and Wales: evidence for a further increase, 1974–84, *Lancet,* 2, 323, 1986.
2. **Jackson, R., Sears, M. R., Beaglehole, R., and Rea, H. H.,** International trends in asthma mortality: 1970 to 1985, *Chest,* 94, 914, 1988.
3. **Sly, R. M.,** Mortality from asthma, 1979–1984, *J. Allergy Clin. Immunol.,* 82, 705, 1988.
4. **Anderson, H. R.,** Trends and district variations in the hospital care of childhood asthma: results of a regional study 1970–85, *Thorax,* 45, 431, 1990.
5. **Speizer, F. E., Doll, R., and Heaf, P.,** Observations on recent increase in mortality from asthma, *Br. Med. J.,* 1, 335, 1968.
6. **Jackson, R. T., Beaglehole, R., Rea, H. H., and Sutherland, D. C.,** Mortality from asthma: a new epidemic in New Zealand, *Br. Med. J.,* 285, 771, 1982.
7. **Stewart, C. J. and Nunn, A. J.,** Are asthma mortality rates changing?, *Br. J. Dis. Chest,* 79, 229, 1985.
8. **Ormerod, L. P. and Stableford, D. E.,** Asthma mortality in Birmingham 1975-7: 53 deaths, *Br. Med. J.,* 280, 687, 1980.
9. British Thoracic Association, Death from asthma in two regions of England, *Br. Med. J.,* 285, 1251, 1982.
10. **Rea, H. H., Scragg, R., Jackson, R., Beaglehole, R., Fenwick, J., and Sutherland, D. C.,** A case-control study of deaths from asthma, *Thorax,* 41, 833, 1986.
11. **Johnson, A. J., Nunn, A. J., Somner, A. R., Stableforth, D. E., and Stewart, C. J.,** Circumstances of death from asthma, *Br. Med. J.,* 288, 1870, 1984.
12. **Sears, M. R., Rea, H. H., Beaglehole, R., Gillies, A. J. D., Holst, P. E., O'Donnell, T. V., Rothwell, R. P. G., and Sutherland, D. C.,** Asthma mortality in New Zealand: a two year national study, *N. Z. Med. J.,* 98, 271, 1985.
13. **Stolley, P. D.,** Asthma mortality: why the United States was spared an epidemic of deaths due to asthma, *Am. Rev. Respir. Dis.,* 105, 883, 1972.
14. **Inman, W. H. W. and Adelstein, A. M.,** Rise and fall of asthma mortality in England and Wales in relation to use of pressurised aerosols, *Lancet* 2, 279, 1969.
15. **Stolley, P. D. and Schinnar, R.,** Association between asthma mortality and isoproterenol aerosols: a review, *Prev. Med.,* 7, 319, 1978.
16. **Crane, J., Pearce, N., Flatt, A., Burgess, C., Jackson, R., Kwong, T., Ball, M., and Beasley, R.,** Prescribed fenoterol and death from asthma in New Zealand, 1981–83: case-control study, *Lancet,* 1, 917, 1989.

17. **Pearce, N., Grainger, J., Atkinson, M., Crane, J., Burgess, C., Culling, C., Windom, H., and Beasley, R.,** Case-control study of prescribed fenoterol and death from asthma in New Zealand, 1977–81, *Thorax,* 45, 170, 1990.
18. **Grainger, J., Woodman, K., Pearce, N., Crane, J., Burgess, C., Keane, A., and Beasley, R.,** Prescribed fenoterol and death from asthma in New Zealand, 1981-7: a further case-control study, *Thorax,* 46, 105, 1991.
19. **Wong, C. S., Pavord, I. D., Williams, J., Britton, J. R., and Tattersfield, A. E.,** Bronchodilator, cardiovascular, and hypokalaemic effects of fenoterol, salbutamol, and terbutaline in asthma, *Lancet,* 1, 1396, 1990.
20. **Keighley, J. F.,** Iatrogenic asthma associated with adrenergic aerosols, *Ann. Intern. Med.,* 65, 985, 1966.
21. **Drexel, H., Regele, M., and Langle, U.,** Successful treatment of terbutaline-induced bronchospasm with orciprenaline sulphate, *Lancet,* 2, 446, 1982.
22. **Nicklas, R. A.,** Paradoxical bronchospasm associated with the use of inhaled beta agonists, *J. Allergy Clin. Immunol.,* 85, 959, 1990.
23. **Van Metre, T. E.,** Adverse effects of inhalation of excessive amounts of nebulised isoproterenol in status asthmaticus, *J. Allergy,* 43, 101, 1969.
24. **Reisman, R. E.,** Asthma induced by adrenergic aerosols, *J. Allergy,* 46, 162, 1970.
25. **Van Arsdel, P. P. Jr., Schaffrin, R. M., Rosenblatt, J., Sprenkle, A. C., and Altman, L. C.,** Evaluation of oral fenoterol in chronic asthmatic patients, *Chest,* 73, 997, 1978.
26. **Trembath, P. W., Greenacre, J. K., Anderson, M., Dimmock, S., Mansfield, L., Wadsworth, J., and Green, M.,** Comparison of four weeks' treatment with fenoterol and terbutaline aerosols in adult asthmatics. A double-blind crossover study, *J. Allergy Clin. Immunol.,* 63, 395, 1979.
27. **Harvey, J. E. and Tattersfield, A. E.,** Airway response to salbutamol: effect of regular salbutamol inhalations in normal, atopic, and asthmatic subjects, *Thorax,* 37, 280, 1982.
28. **Wahedna, I., Wong, C. S., Wisniewski, A. F. Z., Pavord, I. D., and Tattersfield, A. E.,** Asthma control during and after cessation of regular $beta_2$ agonist treatment, ARRD (in press).
29. **van Schayck, C. P., Dompeling, E., van Herwaarden, C. L. A., Folgering, H., Verbeek, A. L. M., van der Hoogen, H. J. M., and van Weel, C.,** Bronchodilator treatment in moderate asthma or chronic bronchitis: continuous or on demand? A randomised controlled study, *Br. Med. J.,* 303, 1426, 1991.
30. **Larsson, S., Svedmyr, N., and Thiringer, G.,** Lack of bronchial beta-adrenoceptor resistance in asthmatics during long-term treatment with terbutaline, *J. Allergy Clin. Immunol.,* 59, 93, 1977.
31. **Peel, E. T. and Gibson, G. J.,** Effects of long-term inhaled salbutamol therapy on the provocation of asthma by histamine, *Am. Rev. Respir. Dis.,* 121, 973, 1980.
32. **Lipworth, B. J., Struthers, A. D., and McDevitt, D. G.,** Tachyphylaxis to systemic but not to airway responses during prolonged therapy with high dose inhaled salbutamol in asthmatics, *Am. Rev. Respir. Dis.,* 140, 586, 1989.
33. **Sears, M. R., Taylor, D. R., Print, C. G., Lake, D. C., Li, Q., Flannery, E. M., Yates, D. M., Lucas, M. K., and Herbison, G. P.,** Regular inhaled beta-agonist treatment in bronchial asthma, *Lancet,* 1, 336, 1990.
34. **Gray, B. J., Frame, M., and Costello, J. F.,** A comparative double-blind study of the bronchodilator effects and side-effects of inhaled fenoterol and terbutaline administered in equipotent doses, *Br. J. Dis. Chest,* 76, 341, 1982.
35. **Lawford, P., Dowd, D. E., and Palmer, K. N. V.,** A comparison of the duration of action of fenoterol and salbutamol in asthma, *Curr. Med. Opin.,* 7, 349, 1981.
36. **Larsson, S. and Svedmyr, N.,** Cumulative dose-response curves for comparison of oral bronchodilating drugs: a study of salbutamol and fenoterol, *Ann. Allergy,* 39, 362, 1977.
37. **Svedmyr, N.,** Fenoterol: a $beta_2$-adrenergic agonist for use in asthma, *Pharmacotherapy,* 5, 109, 1985.

38. **Tandon, M. K.,** Cardiopulmonary effects of fenoterol and salbutamol aerosols, *Chest,* 77, 429, 1980.
39. **Burgess, C. D., Windom, H. H., Pearce, N. E., Marshall, S., Beasley, R., Siebers, R. W. L., and Crane, J.,** Lack of evidence for $beta_2$ receptor selectivity: a study of metaproterenol, fenoterol, isoproterenol and epinephrine in patients with asthma, *Am. Rev. Respir. Dis.,* 143, 444, 1991.
40. **Tattersfield, A. E.,** Effect of beta-agonists and anticholinergic drugs on bronchial reactivity, *Am. Rev. Respir. Dis.,* 136 (Suppl.) 64, 1987.
41. **Anderson, S. D., Seale, J. P., Rozea, P., Bandler, L., Theobald, G., and Lindsay, D. A.,** Inhaled and oral salbutamol in exercise induced asthma, *Am. Rev. Respir. Dis.,* 114, 493, 1976.
42. **Cockcroft, D. W. and Murdock, K. Y.,** Comparative effects of inhaled salbutamol, sodium cromoglycate and beclomethasone dipropionate on allergen-induced early asthmatic responses, late asthmatic responses and increased bronchial responsiveness to histamine, *J. Allergy Clin. Immunol.,* 79, 734, 1987.
43. **Twentyman, O. P., Finnerty, J. P., and Holgate, S. T.,** The inhibitory effect of nebulized albuterol on the early and late asthmatic reactions and increase in airway responsiveness provoked by inhaled allergen in asthma, *Am. Rev. Respir. Dis.,* 144, 782, 1991.
44. **Twentyman, O. P., Finnerty, J. P., Harris, A., Palmer, J., and Holgate, S. T.,** Protection against allergen-induced asthma by salmeterol, *Lancet,* 1, 336, 1990.
45. **Gibson, G. J., Greenacre, J. K., Konig, P., Conolly, M. E., and Pride, N. B.,** Use of exercise challenge to investigate possible tolerance to beta-adrenoceptor stimulation in asthma, *Br. J. Dis. Chest,* 72, 199, 1978.
46. **Vathenen, A. S., Knox, A. J., Higgins, B. G., Britton, J. R., and Tattersfield, A. E.,** Rebound increase in bronchial responsiveness after treatment with inhaled terbutaline, *Lancet,* 1, 554, 1988.
47. **Harvey, J. E., Baldwin, C. J., Wood, P. J., Alberti, K. G. M. M., and Tattersfield, A. E.,** Airway and metabolic responsiveness to intravenous salbutamol in asthma: effect of regular inhaled salbutamol, *Clin. Sci.,* 60, 579, 1981.
48. **Wahedna, I., Wisniewski, A., Wong, C., Pavord, I., and Tattersfield, A. E.,** Airway effects of regular broxaterol and salbutamol treatment in asthmatic subjects, *Thorax,* 46, 770P, 1991.
49. **Kraan, J., Koeter, G. H., van der Mark, T. H., Sluiter, H. J., and de Vries, K.,** Changes in bronchial reactivity induced by 4 weeks of treatment with anti asthmatic drugs in patients with allergic asthma: a comparison between budesonide and terbutaline, *J. Allergy Clin. Immunol.,* 76, 628, 1985.
50. **Kerrebijn, K. F., van Essen-Zandvliet, E. E. M., and Neijens, H. J.,** Effect of long term treatment with inhaled corticosteroids and beta agonists on the bronchial responsiveness in children with asthma, *J. Allergy Clin. Immunol.,* 79, 653, 1987.
51. **van Schayck, C. P., Graafsma, S. J., Visch, M. B., Dompeling, E., van Weel, C., and van Herwaarden, C. L. A.,** Increased bronchial responsiveness after inhaling salbutamol during 1 year is not caused by subsensitization to salbutamol, *J. Allergy Clin. Immunol.,* 86, 793, 1990.
52. **Mitchell, E. A.,** Is current treatment increasing asthma mortality and morbidity?, *Thorax,* 44, 81, 1989.
53. **Clark, D. G. and Tinston, D. J.,** Cardiac effects of isoproterenol, hypoxia, hypercapnia and fluorocarbon propellants and their use in asthma inhalers, *Ann. Allergy,* 30, 536, 1972.
54. **Joseph, X., Whitehurst, V. E., Bloom, S., and Balazs, T.,** Enhancement of cardiotoxic effects of beta-adrenergic bronchodilators by aminophylline in experimental animals, *Fund. Appl. Toxicol.,* 1, 443, 1981.
55. **Greenberg, M. J.,** Isoprenaline in myocardial failure, *Lancet,* 2, 442, 1965.

56. **Tattersfield, A. E. and Britton, J. R.,** Beta-adrenoceptor agonists, in *Asthma: Basic Mechanisms and Clinical Management,* Barnes, P. J., Rodger, I. W., and Thomson, N. C., Eds. Academic Press, London, 1988, 563.
57. **Al-Hillawi, A. H., Hayward, R., and Johnson, N. M.,** Incidence of cardiac arrhythmias in patients taking slow release salbutamol and slow release terbutaline for asthma, *Br. Med. J.,* 288, 367, 1984.
58. **Banner, A. S., Sunderrajan, E. V., Agarwal, M. K., and Addington, W. W.,** Arrhythmogenic effects of orally administered bronchodilators, *Arch. Intern. Med.,* 139, 434, 1979.
59. **Cookson, W. O. C. M., John, S., McCarthy, G., McCarthy, S., and Lane, D. J.,** Nebuliser therapy and cardiac dysrhythmias in patients with COAD, *Thorax,* 40, 704, 1985.
60. **Higgins, R. M., Cookson, W. O. C. M., Lane, D. J., John, S. M., McCarthy, G. L., and McCarthy, S. T.,** Cardiac arrhythmias caused by nebulised beta-agonist therapy, *Lancet,* 2, 863, 1987.
61. **Conolly, M. E., Davies, D. S., Dollery, C. T., and George, C. F.,** Resistance to beta-adrenoceptor stimulants (a possible explanation for the rise in asthma deaths), *Br. J. Pharmacol.,* 43, 389, 1971.
62. **Sibley, D. R. and Lefkowitz, R. J.,** Molecular mechanisms of receptor desensitisation using the beta-adrenergic receptor-coupled adenylate cyclase system as a model, *Nature,* 317, 124, 1985.
63. **Lefkowitz, R. J., Hausdorff, W. P., and Caron, M. G.,** Role of phosphorylation in desensitization of the β-adrenoceptor, *Trends Pharmacol. Sci.,* 11, 190, 1990.
64. **Hausdorf, W. P., Caron, M. G., and Lefkowitz, R. J.,** Turning off the signal: desensitisation of beta-adrenergic receptor function, *FASEB J.,* 4, 2881, 1990.
65. **Galant, S. P., Duriseti, L., Underwood, S., and Insel, P. A.,** Decreased beta-adrenergic receptors on polymorphonuclear leukocytes after adrenergic therapy, *N. Engl. J. Med.,* 299, 933, 1978.
66. **Martinsson, A., Larsson, K., and Hjemdahl, P.,** Studies *in vivo* and *in vitro* of terbutaline-induced beta-adrenoceptor desensitization in healthy subjects, *Clin. Sci.,* 72, 47, 1987.
67. **Mickey, J., Tate, R., and Lefkowitz, R. J.,** Subsensitivity of adenylate cyclase and decreased β-adrenergic receptor binding after chronic exposure to (−)isoproterenol *in vitro, J. Biol. Chem.,* 250, 5727, 1975.
68. **Samuelson, W. M. and Davies, A. O.,** Hydrocortisone-induced reversal of beta-adrenergic receptor uncoupling, *Am. Rev. Respir. Dis.,* 130, 1023, 1984.
69. **Avner, B. P. and Jenne, J. W.,** Comparison of *in vitro* isoproterenol induced desensitisation in human, dog, rat and rabbit respiratory smooth muscle, *Am. Rev. Respir. Dis.,* 115, 45, 1977.
70. **Davis, C. and Conolly, M. E.,** Tachyphylaxis to beta-adrenoceptor agonists in human bronchial smooth muscle: studies *in vitro, Br. J. Clin. Pharmacol.,* 10, 417, 1980.
71. **Avner, B. P. and Jenne, J. W.,** Desensitisation of isolated human bronchial smooth muscle to beta-receptor agonists, *J. Allergy Clin. Immunol.,* 68, 51, 1981.
72. **Hall, I. P., Daykin, K., Townsend, P., and Widdop, S.,** Control of beta adrenoceptor desensitization in cultured human airway smooth muscle cells, *Thorax,* 47, 212, 1992.
73. **Paterson, J. W., Conolly, M. E., Davies, D. S., and Dollery, C. T.,** Isoprenaline resistance and the use of pressurised aerosols in asthma, *Lancet,* 2, 426, 1968.
74. **Nelson, H. S., Raine, D. Jr., Doner, H. C., and Posey, W. C.,** Subsensitivity to bronchodilator action of albuterol produced by chronic administration, *Am. Rev. Respir. Dis.,* 116, 871, 1977.
75. **Jenne, J. W., Chick, T. W., Strickland, R. D., and Wall, F. J.,** Subsensitivity of beta responses during therapy with a long-acting beta-2 preparation, *J. Allergy Clin. Immunol.,* 59, 383, 1977.

76. **Plummer, A. L.,** The development of drug tolerance to $beta_2$ adrenergic agents, *Chest,* 73 (Suppl.), 949, 1978.
77. **Conolly, M. E., Tashkin, D., Hui, K. K. P., Littner, M. R., and Wolfe, R. N.,** Selective subsensitisation of beta adrenergic receptors in central airways of asthmatics and normal subjects during long term therapy with inhaled salbutamol, *J. Allergy Clin. Immunol.,* 70, 423, 1982.
78. **Weber, R. W., Smith, J. A., and Nelson, H. S.,** Aerosolized terbutaline in asthmatics: development of subsensitivity with long-term administration, *J. Allergy Clin. Immunol.,* 70, 417, 1982.
79. **Repsher, L. H., Anderson, J. A., Bush, R. K., Falliers, C. J., Kass, I., Kemp, J. P., Reed, C., Siegel, S., and Webb, D. R.,** Assessment of tachyphylaxis following prolonged therapy of asthma with inhaled albuterol aerosol, *Chest,* 85, 34, 1984.
80. **Sims, B. A.,** Investigation of salbutamol tolerance, *Br. J. Clin. Pharmacol.,* 1, 291, 1974.
81. **Formgren, H.,** The therapeutic value of oral long term treatment with terbutaline (Bricanyl) in asthma: a follow up study of its efficacy and side effects, *Scand. J. Respir. Dis.,* 56, 321, 1975.
82. **Angelici, E., Delfino, M., Carlone, S., Serra, P., Fineberg, N. S., and Farber, M. O.,** Tolerance to inhaled fenoterol, *Am. Rev. Respir. Dis.,* 129, 1014, 1984.
83. **Tattersfield, A. E.,** Tolerance to beta agonists, Bull. Eur. Physiopathol. Respir. (Clin. Respir. Physiol.), 21, 1, 1985.
84. **Holgate, S. T., Baldwin, C. J., and Tattersfield, A. E.,** Beta adrenergic agonist resistance in normal human airways, *Lancet,* 2, 375, 1977.
85. **Holgate, S. T., Stubbs, W. A., Wood, P. J., McCaughey, E. S., Alberti, K. G. M. M., and Tattersfield, A. E.,** Airway and metabolic resistance to intravenous salbutamol: a study in normal man, *Clin. Sci.,* 59, 155, 1980.
86. **Tashkin, D. P., Conolly, M. E., Deutsch, R. I., Hui, K. K., Littner, M., Scarpace, P., and Abrass, I.,** Subsensitization of beta-adrenoceptors in airways and lymphocytes of healthy and asthmatic subjects, *Am. Rev. Respir. Dis.,* 125, 185, 1982.
87. **Morley, J., Sanjar, S., and Newth, C.,** Viewpoint: untoward effects of beta-adrenoceptor agonists in asthma, *Eur. Respir. J.,* 3, 228, 1990.
88. **Lai, C. K. W., Twentyman, O. P., and Holgate, S. T.,** The effect of an increase in inhaled allergen dose after rimiterol hydrobromide on the occurrence and magnitude of the late asthmatic response and the associated change in nonspecific bronchial responsiveness, *Am. Rev. Respir. Dis.,* 140, 917, 1989.
89. **Cockcroft, D. W., Ruffin, R. E., Dolovich, J., and Hargreave, F. E.,** Allergen-induced increase in non-allergic bronchial reactivity, *Clin. Allergy,* 7, 503, 1977.
90. **Rudolf, M., Turner, J., Summers, G., Ullah, M., Good, C., and Stanley, N.,** Effect of beta-adrenergic blockade and stimulation on respiration, *Thorax,* 34, 701, 1979.
91. **Cochrane, L. M. and Clark, C. J.,** Benefits and problems of a physical training programme for asthmatic patients, *Thorax,* 45, 345, 1990.
92. **Page, C. P.,** Hypothesis: one explanation of the asthma paradox: inhibition of natural anti-inflammatory mechanism by $beta_2$-agonists, *Lancet,* 1, 717, 1991.
93. **Church, M. K. and Hiroi, J.,** Inhibition of IgE-dependent histamine release from human dispersed lung mast cells by anti-allergic drugs and salbutamol, *Br. J. Pharmacol.,* 90, 421, 1987.
94. **Borson, B. and Nadel, J.,** Neurophysiologic control of airway secretions in experimental animals, *Am. Rev. Respir. Dis.,* 134, 614, 1986.
95. **Phipps, R. J., Williams, I. P., Richardson, P. S., Pell, J., Pack, R. J., and Wright, N.,** Sympathetic drugs stimulate the output of secretory glycoproteins from human bronchi *in vitro, Clin. Sci.,* 63, 23, 1982.
96. **Dunnill, M. S.,** The pathology of asthma with special reference to changes in the bronchial mucosa, *J. Clin. Pathol.,* 13, 27, 1960.

97. **Green, W. F.,** Fenoterol and its bromide, *Lancet,* 1, 1613, 1991.
98. **Slungaard, A. and Mahoney, J. R.,** Bromide-dependent toxicity of eosinophil peroxidase for endothelium and isolated working rat hearts: a model for eosinophilic endocarditis, *J. Exp. Med.,* 173, 117, 1991.
99. **Hammer, R., Jennewein, H.-M., Kutter, E., and Lopez-Vidriero, M. T.,** Fenoterol and its bromide, *Lancet,* 1, 507, 1991.
100. **Sanjar, S., Kristersson, A., Mazzoni, L., Morley, J., and Schaeublin, E.,** Increased airway reactivity in the guinea-pig follows exposure to intravenous isoprenaline, *J. Physiol.,* 425, 43, 1990.
101. **Morley, J.,** Adverse reactions to sympathomimetics in laboratory animals, in *Beta Agonists in the Treatment of Asthma,* Costello, J. F. and Mann, R. D., Eds., Parthenon Publishing, United Kingdom, 1992.

Section 6
The Future

Chapter 10

LONG-ACTING INHALED BETA$_2$ RECEPTOR AGONIST DRUGS

K. Fan Chung and Peter J. Barnes

TABLE OF CONTENTS

0-8493-6761-1/93/$0.00 + $.50

I. INTRODUCTION

Beta$_2$ receptor agonists are by far the most effective bronchodilators currently available. Selective beta$_2$ agonists, such as salbutamol and terbutaline, induce prompt symptomatic relief of wheezing and breathlessness with a duration of action of 3 to 6 h. Repeated use of beta$_2$ agonists does not appear to lead to tachyphylaxis of the bronchodilator effect in asthmatic patients.[1] Beta$_2$ agonists are also potent in inhibiting mast cell degranulation.[2] However, their effect on various manifestations of the inflammatory events in asthma has been controversial. Studies of airway microvascular leakage has provided conflicting results,[3,4] and there is evidence to suggest that beta$_2$ agonists do not inhibit activation of human eosinophils and alveolar macrophages.[5,6] The effects of short-acting beta$_2$ agonists on the late-phase reaction after allergen provocation are also controversial because it is difficult to dissociate an effect on the inflammatory response from functional antagonism.[7,8] Currently available beta$_2$ agonists may not modify the chronic inflammatory process of asthmatic airways, and concomitant treatment with an inhaled glucocorticoid is recommended, particularly if regular use of inhaled beta$_2$ agonist is needed to control symptoms.[9]

A new group of inhaled beta$_2$ receptor agonists, formoterol and salmeterol, characterized by their prolonged bronchodilator effect, has recently been developed. In clinical studies formoterol was found to have a long duration of bronchodilatation when given by inhalation compared with the oral route where the duration of action was similar to that of salbutamol.[10] Salmeterol was the result of a specific research program to design long-acting bronchodilators by molecular modification of the beta$_2$ agonist salbutamol.[11] Apart from their improved duration of action, these new drugs, salmeterol and formoterol, may possess other properties of particular relevance to asthma compared with the shorter-acting beta$_2$ agonists. Salmeterol and formoterol are now becoming available for prescription in several European countries at a time when questions have been raised about the safety of short-acting beta$_2$ agonists. It is possible that they may have a different profile of effects than the shorter-acting drugs and their place in the current management of asthma is under discussion. In this chapter the basis for the clinical pharmacology of these drugs is discussed and the safety aspects of these long-acting beta$_2$ agonists, particularly in view of the recent concerns that have been raised concerning the regular use of short-acting beta$_2$ agonists in asthma,[13] are considered.

II. BASIC PHARMACOLOGY

A. MODE OF ACTION

The chemical structure of the two new compounds, salmeterol and formoterol, are shown together with salbutamol, terbutaline, and fenoterol in

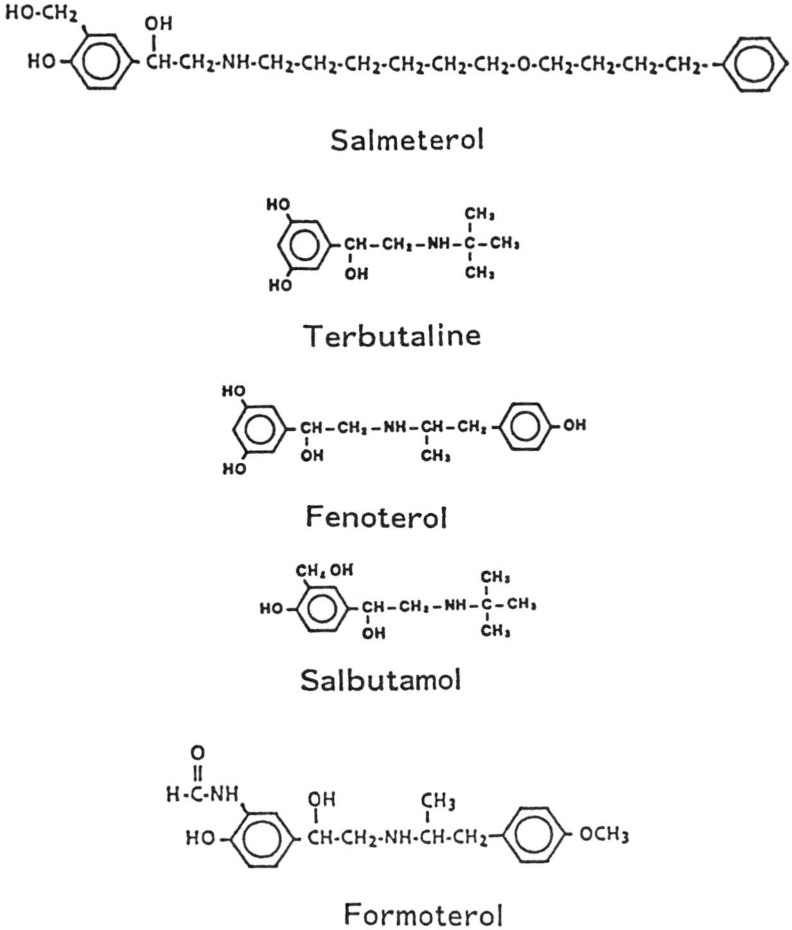

FIGURE 1. Chemical structure of beta receptor agonists.

Figure 1.[11,14,15] Both formoterol and salmeterol possess a longer side chain than salbutamol and terbutaline. However, the salmeterol side chain is considerably longer than that of formoterol, and it has been suggested that this long side chain binds to an exoreceptor near the beta receptor. The exoreceptor may help to anchor the $beta_2$ agonist to its receptor, and this may explain the prolonged duration of salmeterol.[11,16] This is an unlikely explanation because molecular analysis shows that the size of the $beta_2$ receptor is more than 500 times greater than the salmeterol molecule. It is likely that the $beta_2$ agonists bind in a cleft within the receptor and that the lipophilic tail may intersect with amino acids within the binding domain to anchor the active part of the molecule.[17] From a structural viewpoint, it seems unlikely that formoterol possesses its long duration for the same reason as salmeterol, although the lipophilic protein of the molecule may promote its retention within the binding cleft.

The long duration of bronchorelaxation for these drugs may also be related to lipophilicity. The octanol-water distribution coefficient as a measurement of lipophilicity has been found to be low for salbutamol, whereas formoterol was relatively more lipophilic and salmeterol was highly lipophilic.[18] A relatively good correlation between the lipophilicity and the *in vitro* duration of action of several beta agonists, including the long-acting agents, has been reported. However, the lipophilicity may not be the only explanation because some beta agonist drugs have a relatively high lipophilicity without having a prolonged duration of action. The prolonged duration of effect *in vitro* is unlikely to be due to effects on the airway epithelium, such as prolonged release of a relaxant factor, because there was no difference in duration of relaxant effect in guinea pig tracheal rings with or without epithelium.[19] Both compounds are highly selective for $beta_2$ receptors.[15,20] Formoterol is about 200 times more potent in inducing relaxation of the precontracted guinea pig tracheal smooth muscle than in increasing the atrial rate in isolated guinea pig atria. By comparison, salbutamol was in the same study 17 times more potent on the trachea than on the atria.[15] Formoterol and salmeterol are much more potent than salbutamol in the guinea pig trachea.[18]

B. EFFECT ON AIRWAY SMOOTH MUSCLE

Salmeterol has been shown to have a relaxant effect on isolated guinea pig trachea and human bronchial tissue lasting for many hours.[20] A prolonged bronchodilator effect of formoterol has also been demonstrated *in vitro*. In one study,[19] the remaining beta-stimulating effect on isolated guinea pig trachea after washout and continuous flushing of the organ baths for 1 h for salbutamol (0.1 μM) was only 9 $\pm$ 4%, whereas for formoterol (10 n*M*) it was 78 $\pm$ 7% and for salmeterol (50 n*M*) it was 93 $\pm$ 7%. In this study, the duration of the relaxation after continuous washing was longer for salmeterol than for formoterol.[19] In other *in vitro* experimental models and with different choices of doses, the difference between salmeterol and formoterol has been more pronounced with a longer relaxant effect for salmeterol than for formoterol.[18,21,22] In a study of the effects of salmeterol, formoterol, and salbutamol on the binding of [^{125}I]iodopindolol ([^{125}I]PIN), a beta antagonist, in rat lung membranes, both salmeterol and formoterol had similar affinities (53 and 76 n*M*, respectively) compared with 2.5 μM for salbutamol. Preincubation of membranes with salmeterol prevented [^{125}I]PIN binding, but both salbutamol and formoterol were rapidly displaced by [^{125}I]PIN.[22] Similar studies are needed in human lung membrane preparations.

The effect of salmeterol can be blocked by sotalol, a hydrophilic beta antagonist but reasserts itself after washout.[11] In a recent comparison of salmeterol and formoterol in carbachol-contracted guinea pig tracheal rings, treated with supramaximal salmeterol (1 μM) and formoterol (50 n*M*) doses, sotalol (10 μM) rapidly reversed the relaxation in all rings. After washout procedures and 30 min continuous flushing of the muscle baths, the effect of salmeterol and formoterol reasserted itself to a similar level as after the first treatment. In rings treated with supramaximal salbutamol doses, there was no reassertion of the relaxation after sotalol treatment followed by washout and flushing. After a second sotalol treatment, the washout procedures and washing were repeated with a reassertion of the relaxant effect similar to that seen after the first washing period for salmeterol, and a reduced relaxant effect for formoterol.[19] These studies suggest that both compounds are bound in the smooth muscle membrane adjacent to the beta receptor, and both compounds can reactivate the receptor after beta blockade and washout of the baths. There may be quantitative differences between the two compounds with salmeterol being more firmly attached than formoterol adjacent to the $beta_2$ receptor, and it is impossible to say whether the binding in the membrane is of a similar kind.

C. ANTI-INFLAMMATORY EFFECTS

Asthma is now considered to be a chronic inflammatory disease of the airways, and whether $beta_2$ agonists have an anti-inflammatory effect is an important question yet to resolved. It is apparent that in addition to relaxation of airway smooth muscle, $beta_2$ agonists may inhibit mediator release from mast cells[2] and reduce airway plasma exudation,[4] suggesting that they may modulate acute inflammatory responses. There is less certainty about whether they have any effect on chronic inflammatory processes or on cells, such as macrophages or eosinophils, which mediate chronic inflammation. Whether long-acting $beta_2$ agonists have effects on these cellular responses is also uncertain.

The effect of the new drugs on the release of inflammatory mediators has been partly evaluated. Formoterol is 400 times more potent than salbutamol in inhibiting the release of histamine from sensitized human lung *in vitro*.[23] Similar results have been achieved in studies of histamine release from human basophils and human lung mast cells.[24] Formoterol is also effective in inhibiting allergen-induced release of leukotrienes from sensitized rat and human lungs and in that respect it is about 40 times more potent than salbutamol.[25] Formoterol is more potent than salbutamol in inhibiting the release of hydrogen peroxide and intracellular calcium mobilization from guinea pig eosinophils stimulated by leukotriene B_4.[26] Salmeterol is also 5 to 20 times more active than salbutamol in preventing the release of histamine, leukotriene C_4 and D_4, and prostaglandin D_2 from sensitized human lung fragments, and has a considerably longer duration of effect than salbutamol.[27] Salmeterol, but not salbutamol, inhibits allergen-induced eosinophil accumulation in the lungs of sensitized guinea pigs.[27] In human alveolar macrophages, salmeterol at a relatively high concentration inhibits the release of thromboxane B_2 after zymosan stimulation, but this effect is unaffected by propranolol, indicating that salmeterol may inhibit cellular activation independent of $beta_2$ receptors, perhaps via some membrane-inhibitory effect.[28] By contrast, the inhibitory effect of formoterol is prevented by beta receptor blockade.[26] These initial results may indicate that these two different long-acting $beta_2$ agonists possess different anti-inflammatory mechanisms.

Studies of allergic responses in the skin indicate potential anti-inflammatory effects of the new $beta_2$ agonists. Inhibition of early- and late-phase reactions after cutaneous injection of anti-immunoglobulin E by formoterol or terbutaline was evaluated in healthy volunteers.[30,31] Both formoterol and terbutaline have an initial inhibitory effect on the flare-and-wheal reaction with a considerably greater duration of effect for formoterol (>24 h) than for terbutaline (8 h).[29] The edematous late-phase reaction was also more intensively inhibited by formoterol than by terbutaline at doses that had the same inhibitory effect on the acute flare-and-wheal reactions.[30] The prolonged stimulation achieved by a long-acting $beta_2$ agonist may be more effective inhibiting inflammatory events in the tissue. Formoterol was also much more potent than salbutamol in inhibiting airway microvascular leakage induced by histamine in the guinea pig.[32]

In sensitized dogs both salbutamol and formoterol have a protective effect on acute airway response to ragweed antigen challenge. However, only formoterol protects against airway hyperresponsiveness to acetylcholine 5 h after allergen provocation. Formoterol also blunts the eosinophil influx measured in bronchoalveolar lavage, whereas salbutamol is ineffective. Salbutamol and formoterol both blocked histamine release, but neither influenced leukotriene production.[33]

In a study of the late-phase response in allergic asthmatic patients,[34] salbutamol has a small protective effect on the late-phase response, but formoterol had a more pronounced effect. Both formoterol and salmeterol, in addition to inhibiting the early- and late-phase response, prevented allergen-induced bronchial hyperresponsiveness (BHR).[34,35] It has been proposed that this inhibition of induced hyperresponsiveness and late-phase response is a reflection of an anti-inflammatory effect, but these studies are difficult to interpret because they may still be a reflection of continuing functional antagonism. In the study of Twentyman et al.,[36] it was argued that functional antagonism was not involved because at the time BHR was inhibited, salmeterol had no protective effect against bronchoconstriction induced by methacholine. Obviously, more direct evidence for an anti-inflammatory effect of the long-acting beta agonists rests on studies of bronchial biopsies from asthmatic patients treated with such agents.

III. CLINICAL STUDIES

A. POTENCY

Both formoterol and salmeterol are more potent as stimulating drugs than the short-acting agonists, salbutamol, terbutaline, and fenoterol in clinical studies.[36-39]

B. SELECTIVITY

The long-acting $beta_2$ agonists have a similar range of selectivity as the short-acting ones. Formoterol was studied in cumulative dose-response experiments with both oral and inhaled administration. Similar increases in heart rate were observed for the same degree of bronchodilatation when comparing salbutamol and formoterol.[10] For salmeterol single-dose clinical studies have indicated that salmeterol has the same $beta_2$ selectivity as salbutamol,[40] and no cumulative studies have been performed.

C. ONSET OF ACTION

The increase in specific airway conductance at 1 min after inhalation of formoterol (12, 24, and 48 μg) is more pronounced than after 0.2 mg salbutamol.[41] Similar results have been reported in comparison with terbutaline and salbutamol.[42,43] Salmeterol has a slower onset of action.[37,44] Proper evaluation of its bronchodilator effect during the first minutes of inhalation has not been performed. Salmeterol was slower than salbutamol in protecting against methacholine-induced bronchoconstriction,[44] in accordance with similar results from *in vitro* studies.[18] In clinical practice, the slower response to salmeterol is unlikely to be important if these long-acting bronchodilators are to be used as regular maintenance therapy, rather than for rapid symptom relief for which the currently available short-acting $beta_2$ agonists are more suitable.

D. DURATION OF BRONCHODILATION

Formoterol and salmeterol have a bronchodilator effect lasting up to 12 h; with a longer duration of effect in some patients in whom it may be considerably longer. In an 8-h study, in eight asthmatic patients, inhaled formoterol (6 μg) and inhaled salbutamol (0.1 mg) both induced rapid bronchodilatation; with salbutamol, the bronchodilator effect disappeared after 4 to 5 h, whereas 8 h after formoterol about 75% of the initial response remained.[10,45] In other studies of formoterol, a 12-h duration of effect has been shown in adults[39,46,47] and in children.[37,38,48] A prolonged bronchodilator effect has also been shown in healthy smokers and nonsmokers.[49] The duration of effect is variable from individual to individual, and some patients seem to lose the effect after 9 to 10 h.[47,50] However, the median duration to return to baseline FEV_1 was greater than 12 h for 12 and 24 μg formoterol.[46]

Salmeterol caused sustained bronchodilatation for more than 12 h.[40] Other studies have confirmed the 12 h duration for salmeterol,[51-54] but there are no direct comparative studies between the two long-acting bronchodilators.

E. DURATION OF PROTECTION AGAINST BRONCHOCONSTRICTOR CHALLENGES

A protective effect of up to 12 h against methacholine provocation in asthmatic patients has been demonstrated;[55,56] one study showed protection lasting for at least 5 h.[57] In children the provocative methacholine or histamine dose remained elevated for more than 12 h after formoterol treatment.[58,59] For salmeterol the protection against histamine-induced bronchoconstriction in healthy subjects had a duration up to 12 h, whereas salbutamol only showed a protective effect after 1 h but not after 4 h.[60] In asthmatics salmeterol also has a protective effect up to 12 h against methacholine-induced bronchoconstriction.[61] In adults and in children formoterol had a protective effect against exercise-induced bronchoconstriction, which lasted for at least 8 h.[59,62,63] Formoterol was also found to protect against hyperventilation-induced bronchoconstriction for up to 12 h.[64]

F. LONG-TERM EFFECT ON ASTHMA

In a crossover study in 20 asthmatic patients comparing formoterol (12 μg twice daily and extra doses as when needed) with salbutamol (0.2 mg twice daily plus extra doses), an improvement in peak expiratory flow rates and subjective evaluation of symptoms was noticed during formoterol treatment.[65] Additional doses of bronchodilator were less during formoterol treatment. There was a marked preference for the formoterol period of treatment for 15 of 20 patients. No evidence of tachyphylaxis to the bronchodilator response of salbutamol was observed 2 weeks after treatment with either formoterol or salbutamol. Similar overall results have been obtained in a 1-month study comparing formoterol with salbutamol.[66] In a longer 3-month study involving 301 patients distributed in parallel groups to compare the effects of formoterol (12 μg twice daily) with salbutamol (200 μg four times daily), patients on formoterol treatment had higher morning peak flow values, lesser number of acute asthma attacks, with the need for less rescue medication.[67] In a smaller parallel group study of 66 patients, no significant difference was shown for formoterol compared with terbutaline, but there was a trend for decreased use of rescue medication in the formoterol group.[68]

In a 2-week crossover study in 12 patients comparing salmeterol (50 μg twice daily) with salbutamol (200 μg four times per day), ten patients preferred salmeterol and two could not make a choice.[69] Peak flow measurements improved and the use of rescue medication decreased during salmeterol treatment. There was no evidence of tachyphylaxis. Sleep quality and breathlessness improved. In a multicenter study involving 692 patients randomized to three different dose levels of salmeterol, a dose-dependent improvement of peak flow, a reduction in the number of nocturnal awakenings, and in the use of additional bronchodilator were observed.[70] Both salmeterol and formoterol have a protective effect on nocturnal wheeze.[71-74] In one study with formoterol, this protective effect was maintained for up to 1 year.[72] However, in one study, no difference between formoterol and salbutamol was found concerning control of nocturnal symptoms.[75]

Several studies have examined the effects of formoterol over a period of 1 year. Sustained clinical benefit was observed over that period,[72,76-78] with maintenance of high peak flow values and with lack of evidence of tachyphylaxis to salbutamol-induced bronchodilatation. In two studies in children, the ability of formoterol to protect against induced bronchoconstriction was preserved after 3 or 12 months of treatment.[58,59] No rebound BHR was observed on discontinuation of treatment. There also does not appear to be a worsening of BHR during salmeterol treatment or a rebound in BHR on stopping treatment.[79]

IV. SAFETY ASPECTS

A. SIDE EFFECTS

Several studies have investigated the side effect profile of long-acting $beta_2$ agonists. Their effects on $beta_2$ receptor-mediated responses, such as tremor, plasma potassium, and lipid profile, are similar to short-acting $beta_2$ agonists at similar bronchodilator doses. Formoterol (24 μg) was found to cause similar cardiovascular effects (increase in heart rate and prolongation of the QTc interval) and decrease in plasma potassium in healthy volunteers as salbutamol (400 μg).[80] Tachyphylaxis to the bronchodilator effect has not been observed when either salmeterol or formoterol has been given over prolonged periods in the usual therapeutic doses.[65,66,78] This is perhaps surprising given the prolonged activation of the $beta_2$ receptors in airways but presumably reflects the change in $beta_2$ receptor reserves in airway smooth muscle and the high rate of $beta_2$ receptor gene transcription in these cells.[81] It is also possible that the concomitant use of inhaled steroids in patients included in these studies could have prevented the development of tachyphylaxis.

B. LONG-TERM EFFECTS ON LUNG FUNCTION

Despite the concern that the regular use of short-acting $beta_2$ agonists, such as fenoterol and salbutamol, may result in an increase in BHR and a decrease in lung function,[13,82] there is no evidence yet available demonstrating that formoterol and salmeterol have similar effects. However, it will be necessary to design studies that specifically study these effects following long-term usage. In clinical studies set up during the development of salmeterol by Glaxo Group Research Limited, no loss of asthma control could be detected in salmeterol-treated asthmatics, as demonstrated by the constant rate of asthma exacerbations observed throughout the observation period of 1 year.[83,84] The percentage of patients who had an exacerbation when taking inhaled corticosteroids was similar to those not taking corticosteroids.[84] Hopefully, these data will be published in full.

Of greater potential concern is the likelihood that long-acting inhaled $beta_2$ agonists will be used alone for symptom control. If they do not control the underlying chronic inflammation of asthma, a worsening of the condition may eventually ''break through'', resulting in severe and perhaps fatal asthma attacks. It would be prudent to prescribe these drugs only in combination with regular inhaled steroids, which may be necessary to control the underlying inflammation. Although several cases of asthma deaths have been reported in patients taking salmeterol in the United Kingdom, it is not possible to conclude that this is causally related because it is likely that when a new drug is introduced for treatment of asthma, the patients with more severe disease and with higher risk of dying of asthma will be prescribed the new therapy.

V. PLACE OF LONG-ACTING BETA$_2$ RECEPTOR AGONIST DRUGS IN THE MANAGEMENT OF ASTHMA

A. LONG- AND SHORT-ACTING BETA$_2$ RECEPTOR AGONISTS

The new beta$_2$ agonists may be used to replace currently available short-acting beta$_2$ agonists. Crossover studies in stable asthmatic patients have shown a strong preference for the new long-acting drugs compared with salbutamol.[65,66,69] Patients experiencing nocturnal asthma have also shown a preference for the long-acting drugs.[71-74] Patients needing daily regular intake of short-acting beta$_2$ agonists with or without nocturnal symptoms should be treated with the new long-acting drugs.

Long-acting beta$_2$ agonists will be prescribed on a twice daily schedule, which raises the question of how to relieve breakthrough symptoms when these occur. It would seem cautious at this stage to educate the patient to seek medical advice when this happens to increase anti-inflammatory therapy with corticosteroids. It is not clear how frequently long-acting beta$_2$ agonists can be safely used in the face of worsening asthma. Whether a conventional beta$_2$ agonist for rescue medication would be more appropriate is not known with this approach. Patients need to be taught when to use both short- and long-acting beta$_2$ agonists.

Several studies have shown that the need for rescue medication decreases with the use of the long-acting beta$_2$ agonists. However, the patients must be informed that they may occasionally have to take rescue medication. It would be an advantage to use the long-acting bronchodilator also as a rescue medication.

Some issues must be clarified before this can be recommended. First, is the onset of action for the new drugs similar to that of short-acting beta$_2$ agonists? Recent studies with formoterol indicate a similar onset of action as salbutamol; therefore, formoterol may relieve symptoms rapidly. Second, is the therapeutic range the same for the new drugs as for the old drugs? The side effects for beta$_2$ receptor-mediated effects are skeletal muscle tremor and palpitations, which have been shown for salmeterol and formoterol for doses exceeding recommended therapeutic doses. It seems unlikely that an acute high dose could have any serious side effect compared with the short-acting drugs, such as terbutaline and salbutamol, which can be given in high doses acutely.[85]

B. LONG-ACTING BETA$_2$ RECEPTOR AGONISTS AND INHALED CORTICOSTEROIDS

The need for combining anti-inflammatory treatment when treating with a long-acting beta$_2$ agonist is an important issue. Symptomatic relief from a potent bronchodilator could "mask" the underlying inflammation, thereby decreasing the compliance both from the doctor and the patient to anti-inflammatory therapy. However, long-acting beta$_2$ agonists may have some useful anti-inflammatory effect. Further studies are needed to evaluate the long-term effect of these drugs on BHR and also on bronchial biopsies and inflammatory markers measured in bronchoalveolar lavage fluid.

At present, there is no evidence that the long-acting beta agonists have any corticosteroid-sparing effect, and the introduction of inhaled corticosteroid therapy in patients who regularly use short-acting beta$_2$ agonists is necessary, as indicated in recent national guidelines.[9,86] Therefore, we believe that only patients already stabilized on inhaled corticosteroid therapy and who are still symptomatic should be commenced on long-acting beta$_2$ agonists.

Whether long-acting beta$_2$ agonists should be given in fixed combinations with corticosteroids is another issue. This combination could improve patient compliance because both drugs are usually administered twice daily. The choice of doses will be limited particularly in many asthma patients who need higher doses of inhaled corticosteroids. Fixed combinations also make it difficult to use the same inhalation device for both maintenance and rescue use.

C. LONG-ACTING BETA$_2$ AGONISTS AND ACUTE SEVERE ASTHMA

This area remains to be evaluated. High doses of the long-acting beta$_2$ agonists could perhaps give a better prolonged stabilization of the acutely ill severe asthmatic. However, salmeterol in comparison with formoterol has a relatively slow onset of bronchodilator effect to be useful in this situation. Studies of the effects of these new beta$_2$ agonists on serum potassium and oxygen saturation are also necessary in the treatment of acute severe asthma if these drugs are to be administered at high doses via nebulizers.

VI. CONCLUSIONS

The introduction of long-acting beta$_2$ agonists represents a significant milestone in asthma management and how this will modify our practice will be revealed with time. More information is necessary, particularly with regard to any beneficial anti-inflammatory effect and to their use in more severe asthma. It is interesting that the two long-acting beta$_2$ agonists, salmeterol and formoterol, which may become available in several European countries soon, may have different mechanisms of action underlying their prolonged duration of bronchodilator effect.

In clinical studies long-acting $beta_2$ agonists are strongly preferred by the patients compared with the short-acting drugs. They may be particularly useful in controlling symptoms of nocturnal asthma and will most likely replace the use of slow-release theophylline or oral $beta_2$ agonists. If these drugs possess clinical beneficial anti-inflammatory effects, their importance in asthma treatment could be considerably more important than that of the short-acting $beta_2$ agonists used today.

Long-acting $beta_2$ agonists are now being marketed at a time when some doubts have been raised concerning the safety of long-term chronic therapy with $beta_2$ agonists.[13] One view is that the level of hazards with $beta_2$ agonists depends on the dose, potency, and selectivity of the compound.[87] Thus, full agonists with less selectivity for the $beta_2$ receptor and potent effects of the $beta_1$ receptor, such as fenoterol and isoprenaline forte, may have played a role in previous increases in asthma deaths. However, there is continuing controversy in this area. Nevertheless, $beta_2$ agonists continue to be the most effective and convenient bronchodilators currently available for the relief of symptoms in asthma. The introduction of the new long-acting drugs gives the opportunity to examine in detail the effect of $beta_2$ agonist on airway inflammation in asthma and on the natural evolution of the disease. This should lead to a more rational basis for the use of both short- and long-acting $beta_2$ agonists in asthma. In the meantime, it should be recommended that long-acting $beta_2$ agonists should only be prescribed in patients who are still symptomatic despite the use of inhaled corticosteroid therapy.

ACKNOWLEDGMENT

The authors thank Patricia Murphy for her utmost care in the preparation of the manuscript.

REFERENCES

1. **Svedmyr, N. and Lofdahl, C. G.,** Physiology and pharmacodynamics of beta-adrenergic agonists, in Jenne, J. W. and Murphy, S., Eds., *Drug Therapy for Asthma: Research and Clinical Practice,* Marcel Dekker, New York, 1987, 177.
2. **Butchers, P. R., Skidmore, I. F., Vardey, C. J., and Wheelden, A.,** Characterization of the receptor mediating the anti-anaphylactic effects of the beta-adrenocepter agonists in human lung tissue in-vitro, *Br. J. Pharmacol.,* 71, 663, 1980.
3. **Boschetto, P., Roberts, N. M., Rogers, D. F., and Barnes, P. J.,** Effect of anti-asthma drugs on microvascular leakage in guinea-pig airways, *Am. Rev. Respir. Dis.,* 139, 416, 1989.
4. **Persson, E. G. A., Ekman, M., and Erjefalt, I.,** Vascular anti-permeability effects of beta-agonists and theophylline in the lung, *Acta Pharmacol. Toxicol.,* 44, 216, 1979.

5. **Yukawa, T., Ukena, D., Kroegel, C., Chanez, P., Dent, G., Chung, K. F., and Barnes, P. J.,** Beta 2-adrenergic receptors on eosinophils: binding and functional studies, *Am. Rev. Respir. Dis.,* 141, 1446, 1990.
6. **Fuller, R. W., O'Malley, G., Baker, A. J., and MacDermot, J.,** Human alveolar macrophage activation: inhibition by forskolin but not beta-adrenoceptor stimulation or phosphodiesterase inhibition, *Pulm. Pharmacol.,* 1, 101, 1988.
7. **Cockcroft, D. W. and Murdoch, K. Y.,** Comparative effects of inhaled salbutamol, sodium cromoglycate, and beclomethasone dipropionate on allergen-induced early asthmatic responses, late asthmatic responses, and increased bronchial responsiveness to histamine, *J. Allergy Clin. Immunol.,* 79, 734, 1987.
8. **Twentyman, O. P., Finnerty, J. P., and Holgate, S. T.,** The inhibitory effect of nebulized albuterol on the early and late asthmatic reactions and increase in airway responsiveness provided by inhaled allergen in asthma, *Am. Rev. Respir. Dis.,* 144, 782, 1991.
9. British Thoracic Society, Guidelines for management of asthma in adults. I. Chronic persistent asthma, *Br. Med. J.,* 301, 651, 1990.
10. **Lofdahl, C. G. and Svedmyr, N.,** Formoterol fumarate, a new β-2-adrenoceptor agonist: acute studies of selectivity and duration of effect after inhaled and oral administration, *Allergy,* 44, 264, 1989.
11. **Bradshaw, J., Brittain, R. T., Coleman, R. A., Jack, D., Kennedy, I., Lunts, L. H. C., and Skidmore, I. D.,** The design of salmeterol, a long acting selective β2-adrenoceptor agonist, *Br. J. Pharmacol.,* 92, 590P, 1987.
12. **Barnes, P. J. and Chung, K. F.,** Questions about inhaled β_2-adrenoceptor agonists in asthma, *Trends Pharmacol. Sci.,* 13, 20, 1992.
13. **Sears, M. R., Taylor, D. R., Print, C. G., Lake, D. C., Li, Q., Flannery, E. M., Yates, D. M., Lucas, M. K., and Herbison, G. P.,** Regular inhaled beta-agonist treatment in bronchial asthma, *Lancet,* 33, 1391, 1990.
14. **Ida, H.,** Cardiorespiratory activities of 3-formyl-amino-4-hydroxy-α-(N-1-methyl-2-p-methoxyphenyl-aminomethyl)-benzylalcohol-hemifumarate (BD40A) and some other β-adrenoceptor stimulants in conscious guinea pigs, *Arzneimettelforsch.,* 26, 1337, 1976.
15. **Decker, N., Quennedey, M. S., Rouot, B., Schwarts, J., and Velly, J.,** Effects of N-aralkyl substitution of β-agonists on alpha and beta-adrenoceptor subtypes: pharmacological studies and binding assays, *J. Pharm. Pharmacol.,* 34, 107, 1982.
16. **Brittain, R. T., Jack, D., and Sumner, M. J.,** Further studies on the long duration of action of salmeterol, a new, selective beta-2-stimulant bronchodilator, *J. Pharm. Pharmacol.,* 40 (Suppl.), 93P, 1988.
17. **Strader, C. D., Sigal, I. S., and Dixon, R. A. F.,** Structural basis of β-adrenergic receptor function, *FASEB J.,* 3, 1825, 1989.
18. **Jeppsson, A. B., Lofdahl, C. G., Waldeck, B., and Widmark, E.,** On the predictive value of in vitro experiments in the evaluation of the effect duration of bronchodilator drugs for local administration, *Pulm. Pharmacol.,* 2, 81, 1989.
19. **Linden, A., Bergendal, A., Ullman, A., Skoogh, B. E., and Lofdahl, C. G.,** High concentrations of formoterol and salmeterol in the isolated guinea-pig trachea: reassertion of smooth muscle relaxation after beta blockade followed by wash-out, *Am. Rev. Respir. Dis.,* 143, A749, 1991.
20. **Ball, D. I., Coleman, R. A., Denyer, L. H., Nials, A. T., and Sheldnick, K. E.,** In vitro characterization of the beta-2 adrenoceptor agonist, salmeterol, *Br. J. Pharmacol.,* 88, 591P, 1987.
21. **Nials, A. T., Butchers, P. R., Coleman, R. A., Johnson, M., and Vardey, C. J.,** Salmeterol and formoterol: are both long-acting β2-adrenoceptor agonists?, *Br. J. Pharmacol.,* 99, 120P, 1990.
22. **Coleman, R. A., Johnsson, M., Nials, A. T., and Sumner, M. J.,** Salmeterol, but not formoterol, persists at β2-adrenoceptors in vitro, *Br. J. Pharmacol.,* 99, 121P, 1990.

23. **Mita, H. and Shida, T.,** Anti-allergic activity of formoterol, a new beta-adrenoceptor stimulant, and salbutamol in human leucocytes and human lung tissue, *Allergy,* 38, 547, 1983.
24. **Subramanian, N.,** Inhibition of immunological and non-immunological histamine release from human basophils and lung mast cells by formoterol, *Arzneimittelforsch.,* 36, 502, 1986.
25. **Tomioka, K., Yamada, T., and Tachikawa, S.,** Effects of formoterol (BD40A), a β adrenoceptor stimulant on isolated guinea-pig lung parenchymal strips and antigen-induced SRS-A release in rats, *Arch. Int. Pharmacodyn.,* 267, 91, 1984.
26. **Rabe, K., Dent, G., Giembycz, M., Ravenall, P. J., Barnes, P. J., and Chung, K. F.,** Effects of long acting beta adrenoceptor agonist formoterol vs albuterol on LTB4 induced Ca2+ mobilisation, H202 and TxB2 release in guinea pig eosinophils, *Am. Rev. Respir. Dis.,* 141, A29, 1990.
27. **Butchers, P., Cousins, S. A., and Varley, C. J.,** Salmeterol: a potent and long-acting inhibitor of the release of inflammatory and spasmogenic mediators from human lung, *Br. J. Pharmacol.,* 92, 754P, 1987.
28. **Sanjar, S., McCabe, P. J., and Reynolds, L. G.,** Salmeterol, a long-acting β_2-agonist inhibits antigen-induced bronchial eosinophil accumulation, *Am. Rev. Respir. Dis.,* 143, A755, 1991.
29. **Baker, A. J. and Fuller, R. W.,** Anti-inflammatory effect of salmeterol in human alveolar macrophages, *Am. Rev. Respir. Dis.,* 141, A394, 1990.
30. **Gronneberg, R. and Zetterstrom, O.,** Inhibition of anti-IgE induced skin response in normals by formoterol, a new β2-adrenoceptor agonist, and terbutaline, I. Dose response relation and duration of effect on the early wheal and flare response, *Allergy,* 45, 334, 1990.
31. **Gronneberg, R. and Zetterstrom, O.,** Inhibition of anti-IgE induced skin response in normals by formoterol, a new β2-adrenoceptor agonist, and terbutaline, II. Effect on the late phase reaction, *Allergy,* 45, 340, 1990.
32. **Tokuyama, K., Lotvall, J. O., Lofdahl, C. G., Barnes, P. J., and Chung, K. F.,** Inhaled histamine-induced airflow obstruction and airway microvascular leakage in guinea-pig, *Eur. J. Pharmacol.,* 193, 35, 1991.
33. **Bibi, H., Becker, A. B., Lilley, M. K., Simons, F. E. R., Simons, K. J., and Kepron, M. W.,** The effect of inhaled beta-agonists on airway responses to antigen in a canine model of asthma, *J. Allergy Clin. Immunol.,* 85, 295, 1990.
34. **Palmqvist, M., Lowhagen, O., Balder, B., Melander, B., Svedmyr, M., and Wahlander, L.,** Prevention of late asthmatic reaction by salbutamol and formoterol, *Eur. Respir. J.,* 2 (Suppl. 8), 768, 1989.
35. **Wong, B. J. O., Kamade, D. H., Ramsdale, E. H., O'Byrne, P., Denbury, J. A., Dolovich, J., and Hargreave, F. E.,** The effect of formoterol compared to beclomethasone and placebo on allergen-induced airway responses, *Thorax,* 46, 770P, 1991.
36. **Twentyman, O. P., Finnerty, J. P., Harris, A., Palmer, J., and Holgate, S. T.,** Protection against allergen-induced asthma by salmeterol, *Lancet,* 1, 1338, 1990.
37. **Ullman, A. and Svedmyr, N.,** Salmeterol, a new long-acting inhaled beta-2-agonist: comparison with salbutamol in adult asthmatic patients, *Thorax,* 43, 674, 1988.
38. **Becker, A. B. and Simons, F. E. R.,** Formoterol, a new long-acting selective β2-adrenergic receptor agonist: double blind comparison with salbutamol and placebo in children with asthma, *J. Allergy Clin. Immunol.,* 84, 891, 1989.
39. **Graff-Lonnevig, V. and Browald, L.,** 12 hours bronchodilating effect of inhaled formoterol in children with asthma, *Clin. Exp. Allergy,* 20, 429, 1990.
40. **Ullman, A. and Svedmyr, N.,** A dose-response comparison of inhaled aerosol and dry powder formulations of salmeterol in asthmatic patients, *Am. Rev. Respir. Dis.,* 137, A435, 1988.
41. **Derom, E. Y. and Pauwels, R. A.,** Time course of bronchodilating effect of inhaled formoterol, a potent and long acting sympathomimetic, *Thorax,* 47, 30, 1992.

42. **Wegener, T. and Hedenstrom, H.,** Onset of action of inhaled formoterol in asthma, *Am. Rev. Respir. Dis.*, 141, A209, 1990.
43. **Stam, J., Souren, M., and Zweers, P.,** Onset of action of formoterol, a new long acting beta-2-agonist, *Eur. Respir. J.*, 2 (Suppl. 8), 769, 1989.
44. **Beach, J. R., Young, C. L., Walters, E. H., and Hendrick, D. J.,** Reversal of methacholine-induced bronchoconstriction to compare speed of action of bronchodilators, *Am. Rev. Respir. Dis.*, 143, A428, 1991.
45. **Lofdahl, C. G. and Svedmyr, N.,** Effect duration of inhaled formoterol, a new β2-adrenoceptor agonist, compared to salbutamol in asthmatic patients, *Acta Pharmacol. Toxicol.*, 229 (Suppl. 5), A1358, 1986.
46. **Larsson, S., Lofdahl, C. G., and Arvidsson, P.,** 12 hours bronchodilating effect duration of inhaled formoterol in asthma, *Am. Rev. Respair. Dis.*, 141, A27, 1990.
47. **Maesen, F. P. V., Smeets, J. J., Gubbelmans, H. L. L., and Zweers, P. G. M. A.,** Bronchodilator effect of inhaled formoterol vs salbutamol over 12 hours, *Chest*, 97, 590, 1990.
48. **von Berg, A. and Berdel, D.,** Formoterol and salbutamol metered aerosols: comparison of a new and an established beta-2-agonist for their bronchodilating efficacy in the treatment of childhood bronchial asthma, *Pediatr. Pulm.*, 7, 89, 1989.
49. **Kronenberger, H., Kullmer, T., Schultze-Werninghaus, G., Lintl, H., Siekmeier, R., Schiller-Scotland, C., Haab, S., Mues, E., Sambale, P., Wurst, D., and Meier-Syobow, J.,** Bronchodilator effect of formoterol in healthy smokers and non-smokers, *Am. Rev. Respir. Dis.*, 141, A469, 1990.
50. **Sykes, A. P. and Ayres, J. G.,** A study of the duration of the bronchodilator effect of 12 μg and 24 μg of inhaled formoterol and 200 μg inhaled salbutamol in asthma, *Respir. Med.*, 84, 135, 1990.
51. **Sandstrom, T., Fredriksen, B., Rosenhall, L., and Sandstrom, B.,** Salmeterol: a dose response study with a long-acting beta-2-agonist, *Am. Rev. Respir. Dis.*, 139, A64, 1989.
52. **Patessio, A., Podda, A., Carone, M., Trombetta, N., and Donver, C. F.,** Protective effect and duration of action of formoterol aerosol on exercise-induced asthma, *Eur. Respir. J.*, 4, 296, 1991.
53. **Boyd, G., Anderson, K., and Carter, R.,** A 12 hour placebo controlled comparison of the bronchodilator performance of salmeterol and albuterol, *Am. Rev. Respir. Dis.*, 141, A206, 1990.
54. **Bierman, C. W., Kemp, J. P., and Cuss, F. M.,** A dose-response study of salmeterol, a long acting beta 2 agonist, *Allergology*, 12, 122, 1989.
55. **Ramsdale, E. H., Otis, J., Kline, P. A., Gontovnick, L., Hargreave, F. E., and O'Byrne, P. M.,** Prolonged protection against methacholine-induced bronchoconstriction by the inhaled β2-agonist formoterol, *Am. Rev. Respir. Dis.*, 142, 998, 1991.
56. **Boaro, D., Gullotta, C., Bardessono, F., Torchio, R., Sera, G., and Trombetta, N.,** Formoterol in the prevention of methacholine induced bronchoconstriction: a double blind, within patient study, *Eur. Respir. J.*, 2 (Suppl. 8), 777, 1989.
57. **Nix, A., Nichol, M., Robson, A., Barnes, P. J., and Chung, K. F.,** Effect of formoterol, a long-lasting β2-adrenoceptor agonist, against methacholine-induced bronchoconstriction, *Br. J. Clin. Pharmacol.*, 29, 321, 1990.
58. **Becker, A. B. and Estelle, F.,** Formoterol a new long-acting selective beta2-agonist, decreases airway responsiveness in children with asthma, *Lung*, 168 (Suppl.), 99, 1990.
59. **von Berg, A., Schmitt-Grohe, S., and Berde, D.,** Protective effect of formoterol in asthmatic children, *Am. Rev. Respir. Dis.*, 141, A208, 1990.
60. **Maconochie, J. G., Forster, J. K., Fowler, P., and Thomas, M.,** An initial comparison of salmeterol and salbutamol against histamine-induced bronchoconstriction in healthy subjects, *Br. J. Clin. Pharmacol.*, 25, 115P, 1988.
61. **Derom, E., Pauwels, R., and van der Straeten, M.,** Duration of the protective effect of salmeterol on methacholine challenge in asthmatics, *Am. Rev. Respir. Dis.*, 141, A469, 1990.

62. **Patessio, A., Podda, A., Carone, M., Trombetta, N., and Donner, C. F.,** Protective effect and duration of action of formoterol aerosol on exercise induced asthma, *Eur. Respir. J.*, 4, 296, 1991.
63. **McAlpine, L. G. and Thomson, N. C.,** Prophylaxis of exercise-induced asthma with inhaled formoterol, a long-acting β2-adrenergic agonist, *Respir. Med.*, 84, 293, 1990.
64. **Malo, J. G., Cartier, A., Trudeau, C., Ghezzo, H., and Grontovnick, L.,** Formoterol, a new inhaled beta-2 adrenergic agonist, has a larger blocking effect than albuterol on hyperventilation induced bronchoconstriction, *Am. Rev. Respir. Dis.*, 142, 1147, 1990.
65. **Arvidsson, P., Larsson, S., Lofdahl, C. G., Melander, B., Wahlander, L., and Svedmyr N.,** Formoterol, a new long-acting bronchodilator for inhalation, *Eur. Respir. J.*, 2, 325, 1989.
66. **Wallin, A., Melander, B., Rosenhall, L., Sandstrom, T., and Wahlander L.,** Formoterol, a new long acting beta2 agonist for inhalation twice daily, compared with salbutamol in the treatment of asthma, *Thorax*, 45, 259, 1990.
67. **Hekking, P., Maesen, F., Greefhorst, A., Prins, J., Tan, Y., and Zweers, P.,** Long term efficacy of formoterol compared to salbutamol, *Lung*, 168 (Suppl.), 76, 1989.
68. **Rudolf, M. and Malins, D. R.,** Trial of a new long-acting inhaled beta-2 agonist formoterol, *Am. Rev. Respir. Dis.*, 141, A210, 1990.
69. **Ullman, A., Hedner, J., and Svedmyr, N.,** Inhaled salmeterol and salbutamol in asthmatic patients: an evaluation of asthma symptoms and the possible development of tachyphylaxis, *Am. Rev. Respir. Dis.*, 142, 571, 1990.
70. **Dahl, R., Earnshaw, J. S., and Palmer, J. B. D.,** Salmeterol: a four week study of a long-acting beta-adrenoceptor agonist for the treatment of reversible airways disease, *Eur. Respir. J.*, 4, 1178, 1991.
71. **Geisler, L.,** Inhaled long-acting beta2-agonist prevents nocturnal asthma attacks and morning dips, *Am. Rev. Respir. Dis.*, 141, A208, 1990.
72. **Palmqvist, M., Lowhagen, O., Melander, B., and Svedmyr N.,** One year treatment with inhaled formoterol twice daily in patients with nocturnal asthma, *Eur. Respir. J.*, 2 (Suppl. 8), 732, 1989.
73. **Fitzpatrick, M. F., Mackay, T., Driver, H., and Douglas, N. J.,** Salmeterol in nocturnal asthma: a double-blind, placebo controlled trial of long-acting inhaled β2agonist, *Br. Med. J.*, 301, 1365, 1990.
74. **Fabel, H.,** Nocturnal asthma: comparison of inhaled long acting formoterol vs. oral terbutaline slow release, *Eur. Respir. J.*, 2 (Suppl. 8), 699, 1989.
75. **Varela, L. and Mossberg, B.,** Formoterol, a new long-acting β2-stimulating drug for inhalation, compared with salbutamol in patients with nocturnal asthma, *Eur. Respir. J.*, 2 (Suppl. 8), 867, 1989.
76. **Arvidsson, P., Larsson, S., Lofdahl, C. G., Melander, B., Svedmyr, N., and Wahlander, L.,** Inhaled formoterol during one year in asthma: a comparison with salbutamol, *Eur. Respir. J.*, 4, 1168, 1991.
77. **Clauzel, A. M., Refai, N., Godard, P., Bony, C., Vergnaud, A., and Michel, F. B.,** Efficacity and tolerance of formoterol long-term treatment (12 months) in severe asthmatic patients, *Am. Rev. Respir. Dis.*, 141, A206, 1990.
78. **Rosenhall, L., Sandstrom, T., and Wallin, A.,** Formoterol, a long-acting inhaled β2-agonist, twice daily for 1 year in asthmatic patients, *Am. Rev. Respir. Dis.*, 141, A210, 1990.
79. **Beach, J. R., Young, C. L., Harkaurat, R., Neill, P., Walter, E. H., and Hendrick, D. J.,** Measurement of airway responsiveness during regular treatment with salmeterol and salbutamol, *Eur. Respir. J.*, 4 (Suppl. 14), 199, 1991.
80. **Bremner, P. R., Woodman, K., Burgess, C. D., Crane, J., Pearce, N., and Beasley, R.,** Inhaled formoterol: a comparison of the cardiovascular and metabolic effects with salbutamol and fenoterol, *Thorax*, 47, 882P, 1992.

81. **Hamid, Q. A., Mak, J. C. W., Sheppard, M. N., Corrin, B. C., Venter, J. C., and Barnes, P. J.,** Localisation of β_2-adrenoceptor messenger RNA in human and rat lung using in situ hybridisation: correlation with receptor autoradiography, *Eur. J. Pharmacol.*, (Mol. Pharmacol.) 20, 133, 1991.
82. **Van Schayk, C. P., Graufsorm, S. J., Visch, M. B., Dompeling, E., van Wed, C., and Herwaarden, C. L. A.,** Increased bronchial hyperresponsiveness after inhaling salbutamol during 1 year is not caused by subsensitisation to salbutamol, *J. Allergy Clin. Immunol.*, 86, 786, 1990.
83. **Jenkins, M. M., Hilton, C. J., De Kock, J. C., and Palmer, J. B. D.,** Exacerbations of asthma in patients on salmeterol (letter), *Lancet,* 337, 913, 1991.
84. **Shepherd, G. L., Jenkins, W. J., and Alexander, J.,** Asthma exacerbations in patients taking regular salmeterol, or salbutamol for symptoms (letter), *Lancet,* 337, 1424, 1991.
85. **Wong, C. S., Pavord, I. D., Williams, J., Britton, J. R., and Tattersfield, A. E.,** Bronchodilator, cardiovascular and hypokalaemic effects of fenoterol, salbutamol, and terbutaline in asthma, *Lancet,* 1, 1396, 1991.
86. **Hargreave, F. E., Dolovich, J., and Newhouse, M. J.,** The assessment and treatment of asthma: a conference report, *J. Allergy Clin. Immunol.*, 85, 1098, 1990.
87. **Pearce, N., Crane, J., Burgess, C., Jackson, R., and Beasley, R.,** Beta agonists and asthma mortality: deja vu, *Clin. Exp. Allergy,* 21, 401, 1991.

Chapter 11

ASTHMA MORTALITY AND BETA RECEPTOR AGONISTS: A PERSPECTIVE

Julian Crane

TABLE OF CONTENTS

0-8493-6761-1/93/$0.00 + $.50

I. INTRODUCTION

External control over the biochemical and physiological events that proceed from stimulation or inhibition of the beta adrenoceptor have had a profound effect on therapeutics and on the lives of many patients with a variety of disorders. Nowhere has this effect been more frequently and immediately demonstrated than in the reversal of bronchoconstriction by beta agonists from metered dose inhalers (MDIs). In severe and deteriorating asthma, however, inhaled beta agonists have both a reduced therapeutic effect and duration of action, often leading patients to increase the frequency of administration. Given this common serious clinical situation, it is perhaps a testament to their safety that problems have not been more frequently reported. However, individual sudden and unexpected deaths were reported soon after the introduction of beta agonists in MDIs.[1] These deaths were thought to have occurred in patients with severe attacks of asthma who had used their inhalers excessively.[2] This was followed by evidence of increased asthma mortality from several countries in the mid 1960s, leading investigators to examine the association between inhaled bronchodilator therapy and asthma deaths.[3,4] In the late 1970s a sudden increase in asthma mortality in New Zealand again prompted speculation and debate concerning this association.[5]

II. A POLARIZED DEBATE

The association between beta agonists and asthma mortality represents a fascinating chapter in the history of modern therapeutics, with a relative paucity of definitive data and a consequent tendency for opinion rather than evidence to dominate and polarize the debate. For the clinician in the office or at the bedside of patients with severe asthma, the administration of large doses of beta agonists is frequently associated with a positive and often immediate benefit with little clinical evidence of serious untoward effects. Death from asthma is an uncommon event, and even practitioners with a special interest in asthma are unlikely to observe patterns or clear associations with particular treatments or management practices. It is therefore not surprising that clinicians were skeptical about the possible role of beta agonists in asthma mortality.[6] For the epidemiologist reviewing the broader picture, the time trend data linking isoprenaline forte and asthma mortality suggested a possible causal association.[7] This debate essentially (but not entirely) between epidemiologists and clinicians, on the one hand, saw the association as a major therapeutic disaster[8] and, on the other hand, as largely unproven, speculative, or simply incorrect.[6,9]

This first epidemic ended as abruptly as it had begun, and in the subsequent decade no new evidence was available, but further speculation and review of the studies that had been carried out led to a process of "reinterpretation", and a rejection of a direct causal association.[10] The recognition of a second sudden epidemic of asthma deaths in New Zealand and the more gradual increase in asthma mortality noted in some countries again focused attention on beta agonists in a causal role to explain the sudden increase in asthma mortality.

The chapters comprising this book have brought together in a single volume much of the evidence on which these arguments are based. The relevant pharmacology of beta agonists and the epidemiological evidence for changes in asthma mortality have been reviewed with their appropriate methods. The aim of this concluding chapter is to outline the recent New Zealand experience and to summarize and try to place in perspective the international trends in asthma mortality and the possible relationship of these trends to the use of beta agonists.

III. THE EPIDEMIOLOGY OF ASTHMA MORTALITY IN PERSPECTIVE

It is now possible to view trends in asthma mortality with some perspective and discern reasonably clearly two distinct patterns in the elevations of this mortality since the early 1960s. There have been well documented epidemics, in six countries in the mid 1960s[11] and in New Zealand alone in the mid 1970s.[12] In contrast, there have been more gradual increases in asthma mortality reported from several countries over the last 20 years, including Canada, the United Kingdom, France, Denmark, and Germany.[13]

A. THE EPIDEMICS

For the two epidemics it is difficult to escape from the conclusion that they resulted from the introduction and widespread use of two beta agonists, isoprenaline and fenoterol. Both drugs are effective bronchodilators that were marketed in high-dose formulations, had greater cardiovascular effects than other commonly used beta agonists when used in higher than recommended doses, and showed increasing sales that paralleled increases in asthma mortality.[14] Similar associations have not been reported following the introduction and rising sales of any other bronchodilator.

B. THE INTERNATIONAL EPIDEMIC IN THE 1960s

In the 1960s the epidemic occurred in six of the eight countries that licensed the high-dose preparation of isoprenaline. Both the increase and decrease in mortality paralleled the increase and decrease of sales of the medication. In two countries where an epidemic increase was not seen, the forte preparation was introduced late and sales volumes were low. No epidemic occurred in countries where this formulation was not approved.[11] This time trend association has been deemed circumstantial (as all epidemiology must be to a greater or lesser extent) rather than evidential but at the time was considered more than sufficient to dictate urgent changes to public health policy on the availability of isoprenaline. These changes resulted in (or were coincident with) the rapid extinction of the epidemic and thereby precluded more formal epidemiological study. Had this been possible, the association between isoprenaline and asthma mortality might have been more firmly established. The steady erosion or reinterpretation of the evidence for such an association would have been less pronounced and the second epidemic confined to New Zealand might conceivably have been avoided. One consensus that did arise from both sides of this debate was that the definitive epidemiological method for examining this association would have been a case-control study allowing individual exposure to be linked to outcome.[15]

C. THE SECOND NEW ZEALAND EPIDEMIC: 1976–1989

1. First Reports

A second epidemic increase in asthma deaths began in 1976. Between 1977 and 1981, the increase in asthma mortality went largely unnoticed in New Zealand; in particular, there were no case reports of sudden deaths associated with any particular treatment as had happened in the 1960s. It was not until 1981 that Wilson et al.[5] reported a cluster of asthma deaths in Auckland and tentatively suggested that this might be a result of the increasing use of a combination of inhaled beta agonists and slow-release theophyllines. The authors thought that this combination of treatment was more common in New Zealand than in many other countries.[5] In the following year the association with bronchodilators was again raised by Grant[16] who visited New Zealand at the request of the New Zealand Asthma Foundation. Grant suggested that the increase in mortality might be associated with the widespread use in New Zealand of beta agonists delivered by home nebulizers.[16] That same year an increase in asthma mortality throughout New Zealand was confirmed from examination of national mortality statistics[17] and generated considerable debate.

2. Increasing Sales of Asthma Treatments

In 1984 Keating et al.[18] published an article examining international trends in the sales of asthma medications. This study demonstrated a dramatic increase in total beta agonist sales (and all asthma medications) in New Zealand between 1979 and 1980, 3 years after the beginning of the epidemic[18] (Figure 1) This finding probably more than any other single factor led observers away from study of a direct effect of asthma treatment on the increase in mortality. The timing of the increase in sales of all asthma preparations noted in Keating's article suggested that the increased prescribing might be an appropriate response to some change in the natural history of asthma in New Zealand. This combined with the ''rethinking'' that had taken place since the isoprenaline debate in the 1960s provided a strong incentive to focus on nontreatment-related causes for the sudden increase. In retrospect, the reason for the sudden increase in prescriptions of beta agonists in 1980 was due to a change in the

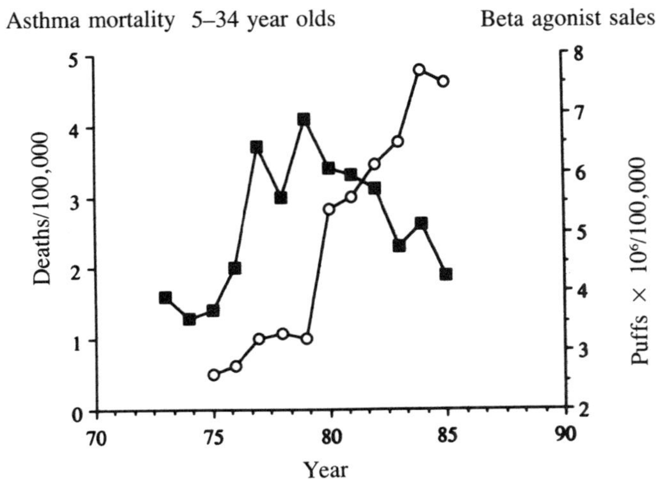

FIGURE 1. Trends in asthma mortality (■) (5–34 year olds) and total beta agonist sales (○) (puffs × 10^6/100,000) in New Zealand 1972–1985. (Adapted from Keating, G. Mitchell, E. A., Jackson, R. T., and Rea, H. H., *Br. Med. J.*, 289, 348, 1984. With permission.)

advice given to prescribers to use beta agonists regularly rather than on demand. Thus, in this second epidemic, there was no early focus on treatment as an explanation and no clear-cut time trend association with changes in drug sales on which to develop a hypothesis.

3. New Zealand Asthma Task Force

In 1980 an asthma task force was established by the New Zealand Medical Research Council to examine the increase in asthma mortality. A 2-year national survey of asthma mortality was undertaken between 1981 and 1983. This was a descriptive case survey of all deaths from asthma in New Zealand. The study was able to confirm a high mortality rate and show that it was unlikely to be due to changes in coding practices or death certification.[12] The absence of a control group meant that it was not possible to examine or quantify risk factors for a fatal outcome.[10] The study results suggested several factors that were probably important in determining a fatal outcome, such as inadequate assessment of asthma severity and inadequate use of inhaled and systemic corticosteroids, but could not define to what extent these were specific risk factors for death or explain why these factors had changed to such an extent that asthma mortality could increase almost threefold in 2 years.

Despite the previous epidemic in the 1960s, associated with isoprenaline, and the suggestions of Wilson et al.[5] and Grant[16] of a relationship with bronchodilator treatment, the specific association between asthma mortality and the use of beta agonist treatment could not be addressed by a case survey. A small case-control study was undertaken in Auckland and showed that poor medical care and psychosocial problems were risk factors for a fatal outcome but did not report findings for individual asthma treatments.[19] This led to confusing and conflicting statements regarding the possible role of bronchodilators in the epidemic. Thus, in the first report from the study it was concluded that "excessive use of bronchodilator drugs did not account for the high mortality rates."[12] This statement was based on subjective reports from relatives of the deceased rather than any specific criteria or definition of overuse. In subsequent reports, however, the authors commented that, "the most likely cause for the epidemic in New Zealand is that an excessive reliance on modern bronchodilator therapy resulted in delays in implementing appropriate treatment for acute progressive attacks."[20] Although the authors emphasized the importance of early and sufficient treatment with systemic corticosteroids in severe asthma, the ambiguity regarding beta agonists led some commentators to suggest that there was also a problem with underuse of bronchodilator treatment.[21] The authors also noted that the data did not exclude the possibility of a direct toxic effect in a susceptible subgroup of patients. This direct toxic effect is now more likely explained by a particular therapy rather than a susceptible subgroup of patients.

IV. THE FOCUS ON FENOTEROL: 1989–1991

The evidence that now incriminates fenoterol in New Zealand arose in a different way from that of isoprenaline in the 1960s and may account for some differences in the evolution and resolution of the two epidemics. Between 1989 and 1991, our group published three case-control studies that examined the specific hypothesis that the use of fenoterol might be associated with an increased risk of asthma death.[22-24] The findings from these studies suggested that fenoterol carried an increased risk, particularly among those with the most severe asthma, defined by markers of chronic asthma severity. These studies are extensively reviewed in Chapter 5.

A. FENOTEROL HYPOTHESIS

The background to the development of the hypothesis on which this series of case-control studies is based is with the benefit of hindsight disturbingly obvious and arose from four observations:[10]

1. Overrepresentation of fenoterol use in patients who had died of asthma compared with national sales figures
2. Time trend data showing that fenoterol was introduced to New Zealand in 1976 at the commencement of the epidemic with a rapid increase in market share that paralleled the increase in mortality
3. The fact that fenoterol was more potent than either salbutamol or terbutaline and marketed in twice the dose per puff by MDI, effectively rendering the formulation a forte preparation

4. Greater cardiovascular effects than either salbutamol or isoprenaline when inhaled repeatedly at frequent intervals

These observations led to a specific hypothesis concerning fenoterol that could be tested using a case-control approach similar to the studies that had been suggested to examine the epidemics in the 1960s.

B. CASE-CONTROL STUDIES

Three case-control studies have been undertaken and have been extensively reviewed in earlier chapters. They examined asthma deaths in New Zealand from 1977 to 1987, using a variety of methods for identifying cases and controls. Information on prescribed drug therapy was recorded, in the second and third studies exclusively from routine hospital records. Subgroups defined by markers of chronic asthma severity were examined to explore the issue of confounding by asthma severity. Following the initial study, the second and third were undertaken to examine potential sources of bias that had been raised by critics.[25,26] The third study examined the effect of using two different control groups to explore the issue of the validity of selecting controls with more severe asthma as an appropriate group for comparison with asthmatics who had died. In addition, it allowed the association between the severity markers used and the risk of death to be examined. The subgroup analysis repeatedly showed an increased relative risk for the most severe subgroups, suggesting that the findings were not due to confounding by asthma severity and the severity markers used were shown to identify subgroups at increased risk of death.

C. EFFECTS ON ASTHMA MORTALITY

The delay of 12 years from the first increase in mortality to developing and testing this hypothesis underlines the need to for adequate postmarketing surveillance when new therapies are introduced. The delay may account for the slow and erratic decline in the epidemic of asthma mortality in New Zealand following its identification, compatible with warnings about the dangers of acute severe asthma but without the focus on any particular risk factors. By contrast, in the 1960s, warnings about the possible dangers of isoprenaline and sympathomimetics, even before the epidemic had been studied, allowed health authorities to restrict their availability and were followed by a rapid decline in asthma mortality. This pattern now appears to have been repeated in New Zealand following warnings about the potential hazards of fenoterol in severe asthma. Our first study implicating fenoterol was published in April 1989. The Department of Health in New Zealand immediately issued warnings about fenoterol and its use in patients with severe asthma. This was immediately followed by a decline in the sales of fenoterol, and a significant reduction in mortality to one half of the level of the preceding 6 years. Figures for asthma mortality for the second half of 1989 were 1.1/100,000 for the

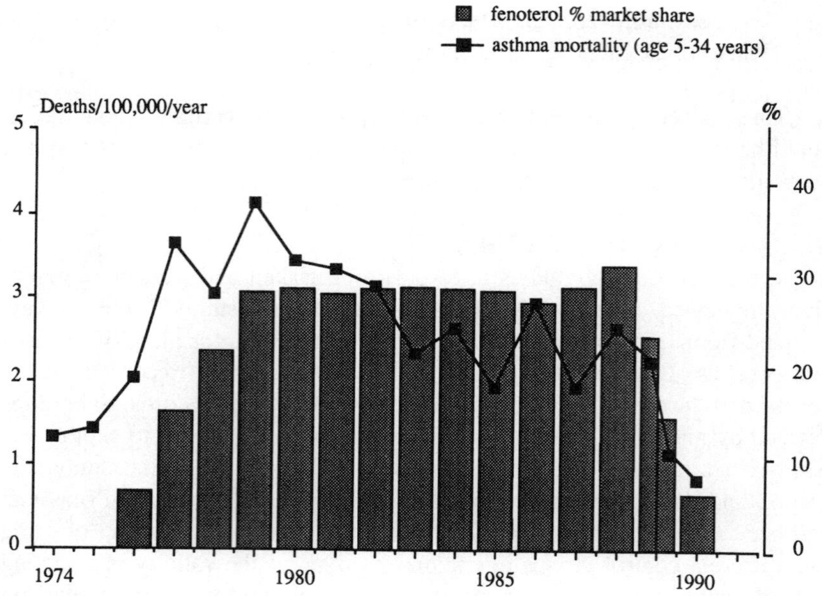

FIGURE 2. Asthma mortality (5–34 year olds) and fenoterol market share (%) in New Zealand 1974–1990. (Mortality and fenoterol market share are shown separately for the first and second six months of 1989.) (Adapted from Crane, J., et al., *Lancet,* 139, 917, 1989. With permission.)

5–34 age group, compared with 2.2/100,000 for the first half of 1989 (p = 0.04). The Department of Health then removed fenoterol from the drug tariff in 1990, which led to a further fall in the sales of fenoterol; this was associated with a further decline in mortality to 0.8/100,000 in 1990, which represented the lowest mortality rate in New Zealand in over 25 years. Figure 2 illustrates the increase and decrease of asthma mortality in relation to market share of fenoterol. This decline, however, needs to be interpreted with caution because many factors may influence improvements in asthma mortality, but they are certainly compatible with the other epidemiological findings of an increased risk of death from fenoterol.

D. SASKATCHEWAN STUDY

The epidemiological findings in New Zealand were confirmed in Canada, where a similar study found an increased risk of asthma death associated with fenoterol compared with other beta agonists.[28] The study was a nested cohort study of prescriptions for asthma medications and asthma deaths and near-deaths in a large cohort in Saskatchewan. In addition to the increased risk of death in patients using fenoterol compared with salbutamol, this study also reported a dose-response effect with an increasing risk associated with increasing prescriptions of both beta agonists. These findings suggest that the high-dose formulation of fenoterol may have been an important factor, and since the results of this study have been available, the manufacturers of fenoterol have reduced the dose in their MDI from 200 to 100 μg per puff. The authors have also suggested some increased risk for other beta agonists, based on comparisons with controls on no beta agonist therapy. Such a control group may well have had less severe asthma, and inevitably raises the concern that these findings are due to confounding by asthma severity.[29] This finding illustrates the importance of controlling for asthma severity (as was done in the New Zealand case-control studies) and the difficulties of studying a class of treatment (rather than comparisons between different agents within the same class) when almost all cases and controls are exposed. In addition, Canada has not experienced an epidemic increase in asthma mortality despite increases in beta agonist sales.

V. PATTERNS OF ASTHMA MORTALITY

Changes in asthma mortality appear to show two patterns: (1) sudden epidemic increases discretely associated both in time and place with the widespread introduction of high-dose preparations of two beta agonists, isoprenaline and fenoterol, which share a tendency for greater cardiovascular effects than other commonly used agents when used repeatedly, and (2) gradual but consistent increases in asthma mortality occurring in some countries.

A. GRADUAL INCREASES IN ASTHMA MORTALITY

While New Zealand alone experienced a sudden increase in asthma mortality in the 1970s, a more gradual increase in asthma mortality has been reported from a number of countries, including the United States, Canada, Australia, and the United Kingdom.[13] Several explanations have been proposed. These can be broadly grouped into (1) changes in diagnostic patterns and classification of cause of death, (2) changes in health care availability and utilization, (3) an increase in the prevalence and/or severity of asthma, and (4) an adverse effect of treatment.

Changes in disease classification, particularly the change from ICD version 8 to version 9 in 1979, in which "asthmatic bronchitis" was coded as asthma, would be expected to alter asthma mortality rates. However, recent studies of trends in asthma mortality in the United States have shown a steady increase in mortality from 1978, during the period of ICD version 9.[30] Changes in health care availability would also be expected to influence asthma mortality. Again, in the United States clustering of deaths in urban New York and Chicago with an excess of deaths among blacks supports the argument. However, these changes are being observed in many countries with different health care systems; furthermore, the increase in mortality is not confined to disadvantaged groups. These changes are consistent with some other effect having a greater influence on those unable to utilize health care facilities effectively. Although studies of asthma mortality over long periods of time are likely to be influenced by many factors, there is an emerging consensus that these trends cannot be wholly explained by changes in classification or health care factors and that a real and unexplained increase has indeed occurred.[13]

B. INCREASING ASTHMA MORBIDITY AND PREVALENCE

These increases in asthma mortality have arisen at the same time as substantial increases in hospital admissions, suggesting an increase in asthma severity.[31] Increasing asthma prevalence has also been observed in several recent studies from different countries.[32,33] The prevalence of hay fever appears also to have increased[34] and has prompted speculation that the frequency of atopy may be increasing.[35] However, the problems of definition and variations in the instruments used to measure prevalence over time mean that definite conclusions cannot yet be drawn. International studies of asthma prevalence in adults and children are now underway to provide a baseline from which future trends may be observed.

VI. THE ASTHMA PARADOX

Adverse effects of asthma treatment may also be involved in this more gradual increase in asthma mortality and in the increased asthma morbidity. These changes have arisen at a time of increasing sales of most antiasthma therapies, including aerosol beta agonists. It is interesting to note a particular shift in prescribing patterns in the United States with a large increase in prescriptions of beta agonist aerosols between 1977 and 1985[36] and a significant increase in asthma mortality over the same time period.[37]

These changes have recently been discussed as the asthma paradox: steadily increasing adverse mortality and morbidity statistics at a time of increasing sales of asthma treatments.[38] A tempting speculation that might explain this paradox would ascribe a variable role to different beta agonists. A sudden epidemic following the introduction and widespread use of high-dose preparations, such as isoprenaline and fenoterol, and less dramatic but more widely distributed effects from lower dose and less potent preparations, such as salbutamol and terbutaline. Alternatively, the differences between epidemic and gradual increases in mortality might relate to acute adverse effects and chronic adverse effects, respectively. There are several mechanisms by which beta agonists could directly increase the risk of death in asthma, and these have been reviewed in detail earlier in this book. They may be broadly grouped into acute and chronic adverse effects.[10]

A. ACUTE ADVERSE EFFECTS

Acute adverse effects have been detailed in previous chapters and will be summarized briefly. Essentially, acute cardiac effects resulting in increased myocardial work and hence oxygen consumption in the face of increasing systemic hypoxemia might lead to fatal cardiac arrhythmias. In addition, beta agonists could theoretically contribute to the systemic hypoxemia by pulmonary vasodilatation and the consequent worsening of ventilation-perfusion inequalities. $Beta_2$ agonist-induced hypokalemia could also theoretically increase myocardial susceptibility to arrhythmias.

B. CHRONIC ADVERSE EFFECTS

The chronic adverse effects may also be important and a variety of potentially deleterious effects have been demonstrated or postulated. Two recent studies, in particular, have shown adverse effects of beta agonists when used regularly as opposed to on demand for the treatment of asthma. Sears et al., in a study comparing the addition of regular versus on-demand fenoterol to an asthma treatment regimen, showed a significant deterioration in asthma control (using a wide range of parameters, peak flow recordings, diaries, spirometry, and measurements of bronchial hyperresponsiveness) when patients used fenoterol regularly.[39] This study suggests a possible reason for the paradox but urgently begs the question of whether the magnitude of this effect is related entirely to dose or potency or to some more specific property of fenoterol. Unfortunately, no other studies have examined overall asthma control in this way. Previous studies with terbutaline and salbutamol have found small effects on lung function[40] or small increases in bronchial hyperresponsiveness during[41] or after treatment with beta agonists.[42] They have mostly been of short duration and have rarely compared on-demand with regular therapy in a prospective way. The changes in these parameters have often been incidental findings in studies designed to answer other questions. Interestingly, the deterioration in asthma observed by Sears et al.[39] when regular fenoterol was added was not influenced by inhaled steroids to any great degree and did not appear to be predominantly due to increasing bronchial hyperresponsiveness.

The second study by van Schayk et al.[43] compared the regular versus on-demand use of two bronchodilators, salbutamol and ipratropium bromide, in parallel groups over 1 year and showed a greater deterioration in baseline forced expiratory volume in 1 s for both salbutamol and ipratropium when given regularly compared with on demand. No other parameter was significantly different for the two treatment regimens. That these effects may not relate to the beta agonists alone but to other bronchodilators suggests a more general effect associated with bronchodilatation.

A straightforward functional hypothesis would predict increasing allergen deposition in the airways both as a direct effect of prolonged bronchodilatation and an increased ability to tolerate bronchospastic stimuli. Two specific hypotheses have recently been suggested to explain the chronic adverse effects of beta agonists, although many others have been advanced. One focuses on the inhibition of mast cell degranulation by beta agonists,[38] and the other on the possible role of dextroenantiomers of beta agonists.[44]

In the mast cell hypothesis, beta agonists, by inhibiting mast cell degranulation, inhibit the release of heparin (and related proteoglycans) from the mast cell, which facilitates increased airway inflammation and its associated tissue repair. In the long term this could lead to the persistence of airway hyperresponsiveness and decreased reversibility of airway obstruction. In the enantiomer hypothesis, the dextroenantiomer of racemic mixtures might increase bronchial hyperresponsiveness, particularly in association with reduced responsivity of beta receptors.[44] There is no evidence as yet that either of these hypotheses is clinically important in humans. Further studies are clearly needed to establish whether all beta agonists share this ability to worsen asthma and to quantify the effect and tease out the underlying mechanisms.

VII. CONCLUSIONS

Adverse trends in asthma mortality and morbidity have been well documented. Although many factors may play greater or lesser roles in these changes, adverse effects associated with specific beta agonists, on the one hand, and with increasing use of all beta agonists on the other, make beta agonists the single most consistent element that might explain all of these trends. Careful evaluation and monitoring will be required following the introduction of the newer long-acting beta agonists to ensure that they are not associated with adverse trends in asthma mortality or morbidity.

How should these treatments best be used to balance the short-term improvements in symptoms with possible long-term worsening of asthma? In practice, this is probably the single most pressing question; although it cannot be clearly answered at present, two important developments in asthma management are likely to ameliorate possible adverse effects: (1) the increasing focus on anti-inflammatory therapy in the early management of asthma and in the management of increasingly mild disease and (2) the emphasis on self-management with objective assessment of asthma severity using peak flow recordings. These developments should be combined with a return to the use of short-acting beta agonists for the relief of symptomatic bronchospasm, as they were originally intended, given the present uncertainty associated with their regular use. These measures should help to reverse the adverse trends in mortality and morbidity while further studies elucidate the underlying reasons for them.

Recent years have seen the spotlight turned on beta agonists in the management of asthma with many debates, editorials, and position papers. One such editorial discussed the issues under the title, ''Beta agonists: friends or foes?''[45] This metaphor is appropriate; a good friend may be relied upon when required but equally should never be taken for granted.

REFERENCES

1. **McManis, A. G.,** Adrenaline and isoprenaline: a warning, *Med. J. Aust.*, 2, 76, 1964.
2. **Greenburg, M. J.,** Isoprenaline in myocardial failure, *Lancet,* 2, 442, 1965.
3. **Stolley, P. D.,** Asthma mortality: why the United States was spared an epidemic of deaths due to asthma, *Am. Rev. Respir. Dis.*, 105, 883, 1972.
4. **Speizer, F. E., Doll, R., and Heaf, P.,** Observations on recent increases in mortality from asthma, *Br. Med. J.*, 1, 335, 1968.
5. **Wilson, J. D., Sutherland, D. C., and Thomas, A. C.,** Has the change to beta agonists combined with oral theophylline increased cases of fatal asthma?, *Lancet,* 1, 1235, 1981.
6. **Gandevia, B.,** The changing pattern of mortality from asthma in Australia, *Med. J. Aust.*, 1, 747, 1968.
7. **Inman, W. H. W. and Adelstein, A. M.,** Rise and fall of asthma mortality in England and Wales in relation to use of pressurized aerosols, *Lancet,* 2, 279, 1969.
8. **Venning, G. R.,** Identification of adverse reactions to new drugs. I. What have been the important adverse reactions since thalidomide?, *Br. Med. J.*, 286, 199, 1983.
9. **Gandevia, B.,** Pressurised sympathomimetic aerosols and their lack of relationship to asthma mortality in Australia, *Med. J. Aust.*, 1, 273, 1973.
10. **Pearce, N. E., Crane, J., Burgess, C., Jackson, R., and Beasley, R.,** Beta agonists and asthma mortality: deja vu, *Clin. Exp. Allergy,* 21, 401, 1991.
11. **Stolley, P. D. and Schinnar, R.,** Association between asthma mortality and isoproterenol: a review, *Prev. Med.*, 7, 519, 1978.
12. **Sears, M. R., Rea, H. H., Beaglehole, R., Gillies, A. J. D., Holst, P., O'Donnell, T. V., Rothwell, R. P. G., and Sutherland, D. C.,** Asthma mortality in New Zealand: a two year national study, *N.Z. Med. J.*, 98, 271, 1985.
13. **Buist, A. S. and Vollmer, W. M.,** Reflections on the rise in asthma morbidity and mortality, *J.A.M.A.*, 264, 1719, 1990.
14. **Beasley, R., Burgess, C., Pearce, N., Crane, J., and Windom, H.,** Asthma mortality and inhaled beta agonist therapy, *Aust. N.Z. J. Med.*, 21, 753, 1991.
15. **Esdaile, J. M., Feinstein, A. R., and Horwitz, R. I.,** A reappraisal of the United Kingdom epidemic of fatal asthma, *Arch. Intern. Med.*, 147, 543, 1987.
16. **Grant, I. W. B.,** Asthma in New Zealand, *Br. Med. J.*, 286, 374, 1983.
17. **Jackson, R. T., Beaglehole, R., Rea, H. H., and Sutherland, D. C.,** Mortality from asthma: a new epidemic in New Zealand, *Br. Med. J.*, 285, 771, 1982.
18. **Keating, G., Mitchell, E. A., Jackson, R. T., and Rea, H. H.,** Trends in sales of drugs for asthma in New Zealand, Australia and the United Kingdom, *Br. Med. J.*, 289, 348, 1984.
19. **Rea, H. H., Scragg, R., Jackson, R., Beaglehole, R., Fenwick, J., and Sutherland, D. C.,** A case-control study of deaths from asthma, *Thorax,* 41, 833, 1986.
20. **Beaglehole, R., Jackson, R., Sears, M., and Rea, H.,** Asthma mortality in New Zealand: a review with some policy implications, *N.Z. Med. J.*, 100, 231, 1987.
21. **Olson, L. G.,** Acute severe asthma: what to so until the ambulance arrives, *New Ethicals,* 25, 105, 1988.
22. **Crane, J., Pearce, N., Flatt, A., Burgess, C., Jackson, R., Kwong, T., Ball, M., and Beasley, R.,** Prescribed fenoterol and death from asthma in New Zealand, 1981–83: case control study, *Lancet,* 139, 917, 1989.
23. **Pearce, N. E., Grainger, J., Atkinson, M., Crane, J., Burgess, C., Culling, C., Windom, H., and Beasley, R.,** Case-control study of prescribed fenoterol and death from asthma in New Zealand, 1977–1981, *Thorax,* 45, 170, 1990.

24. **Grainger, J., Woodman, K., Pearce, N., Crane, J., Burgess, C., Keane, A., and Beasley, R.,** Prescribed fenoterol and death from asthma in New Zealand, 1981–1987: a further case control study, *Thorax,* 46, 105, 1991.
25. **Buist, A. S., Burney, P. G. J., Feinstein, A. R., Horwitz, R. I., Lanes, S. F., Rebuck, A. S., and Spitzer, W. O.,** Fenoterol and fatal asthma, *Lancet,* 1, 1071, 1989.
26. **Poole, C., Lanes, S. F., and Walker, A. M.,** Fenoterol and fatal asthma (letter), *Lancet,* 1, 920, 1990.
27. **Crane, J., Burgess, C., Pearce, N., and Beasley, R.,** Asthma deaths in New Zealand (letter), *Br. Med. J.,* 304, 1307, 1992.
28. **Spitzer, W. O., Siussa, S., Ernst, P., Horwitz, R., Habbick, B., Cockroft, D., Boivin, J. F., McNutt, M., Buist, A. S., and Rebuck, A. S.,** The use of beta agonists and the risk of death and near-death from asthma, *N. Engl. J. Med.,* 326, 501, 1992.
29. **Gottlieb, D. J. and Celli, B. R.,** Beta agonists and death from asthma (letter), *N. Engl. J. Med.,* 327, 355, 1992.
30. **Weiss, K. B. and Wagener, D. K.,** Changing patterns of asthma mortality: identifying target populations at high risk, *J.A.M.A.,* 264, 1683, 1990.
31. **Mitchell, E. A.,** International trends in hospital admission rates for asthma, *Arch. Dis. Child.,* 60, 376, 1985.
32. **Burr, M. L., Butland, B. K., King, S., and Vaughan-Williams, E.,** Changes in asthma prevalence: two surveys 15 years apart, *Arch. Dis. Child.,* 64, 1452, 1989.
33. **Haahtela, T., Lindholm, H., Bjorksten, F., Koskenvuo, K., and Laitinen, L. A.,** Prevalence of asthma in Finnish young men, *Br. Med. J.,* 301, 266, 1990.
34. **Fleming, D. M. and Crombie, D. L.,** Prevalence of asthma and hay fever in England and Wales, *Br. Med. J.,* 294, 279, 1987.
35. **Burr, M. L.,** Is asthma increasing?, *J. Epidemiol. Community Health,* 41, 185, 1987.
36. **Bosco, L. A., Knapp, D. E., Gerstman, B., and Graham, C. F.,** Asthma drug therapy trends in the United States, 1972 to 1985, *J. Allergy Clin. Immunol.,* 80, 398, 1987.
37. **Sly, R. M.,** Increases in deaths from asthma, *Ann. Allergy,* 53, 20, 1984.
38. **Page, C. P.,** One explanation of the asthma paradox: inhibition of natural anti-inflammatory mechanisms by beta 2 agonists, *Lancet,* 1, 717, 1991.
39. **Sears, M. R., Taylor, D. R., Print, C. G., Lake, D. C., Li, Q., Flannery, E. M., Yates, D. M., Lucas, M. K., and Herbison, G. P.,** Regular inhaled beta-agonist treatment in bronchial asthma, *Lancet,* 1, 1391, 1990.
40. **Harvey, J. E. and Tattersfield, A. E.,** Airway response to salbutamol: effect of regular salbutamol inhalations in normal, atopic, and asthmatic subjects, *Thorax,* 37, 280, 1982.
41. **Kraan, J., Koëter, G. H., van der Mark, T. W., Sluiter, H. J., and de Vries, K.,** Changes in bronchial hyper-reactivity induced by four weeks of treatment with asthmatic drugs in patients with allergic asthma: a comparison between budesonide and terbutaline, *J. Allergy Clin. Immunol.,* 76, 628, 1985.
42. **Vathenen, A. S., Knox, A. J., Higgins, B. G., Britton, J. R., and Tattersfield, A. E.,** Rebound increase in bronchial responsiveness after treatment with inhaled terbutaline, *Lancet,* 1, 554, 1988.
43. **van Schayck, C. P., Dompeling, E., van Herwaarden, L. A., Folgering, H., Verbeek, A. L. M., van der Hoogen, H. J. M., and van Weel, C.,** Bronchodilator treatment in moderate asthma or chronic bronchitis: continuous or on demand?: a randomised controlled study, *Br. Med. J.,* 303, 1426, 1991.
44. **Morley, J., Sanjar, S., and Newth, C.,** Viewpoint: untoward effects of beta adrenoceptor agonists in asthma, *Eur. Respir. J.,* 3, 228, 1990.
45. **Lofdahl, C.-G. and Svedmyr, N.,** Beta agonists: friends or foes. *Eur. Respir. J.,* 4, 1161, 1991.

Index

INDEX

A

B

C

D

E

F

G

H

I

K

L

M

N

S

T

U

V

X

Z